PEARSON CUSTOM FOR
NURSING

NURS 1863
Health Promotion Family & Community
Columbus State Community College

PEARSON

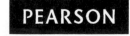

ISBN 10: 1-269-12002-6
ISBN 13: 978-1-269-12002-9

Table of Contents

The Population Context

CHAPTER OBJECTIVES

After reading this chapter, you should be able to:

1. Distinguish among neighborhoods, communities, and aggregates as populations served by community health nurses.
2. Define population health.
3. Describe changes in approaches to population health.
4. Describe the three levels at which population health care occurs.
5. Describe trends in national health objectives for 1990, 2000, and 2010.

KEY TERMS

aggregates
community
communities of identity
geopolitical community
neighborhood
population
population-based practice
population health
primary prevention
secondary prevention
tertiary prevention

MediaLink
http://www.prenhall.com/clark

Additional interactive resources for this chapter can be found on the Companion Website. Click on Chapter 2 and "Begin" to select the activities for this chapter.

Advocacy in Action

Health Care in the County Jail

Jail and prison inmates are often overlooked as populations that need health care services. In part this may be because of their invisibility, yet this population often has far greater needs for health care than the general public. Jails and prisons are intended to be places of punishment for criminal behavior, and health care services are frequently secondary to the security and retribution aspects of incarceration. What the public and policy makers often do not recognize is that providing health care services in jails and prisons is cost-effective and benefits the entire community. Several years ago, a nursing faculty member whose husband was a deputy sheriff for the southern county in which she lived started providing volunteer health services in the county jail. She took several students with her on her forays into the jail and had an uphill battle convincing the county sheriff to permit them to have access to the inmates. Gradually, they were able to win the confidence of the sheriff and the jail personnel that they were not going to create a security risk and that they could assist personnel in dealing with problems for which the staff had no training or background.

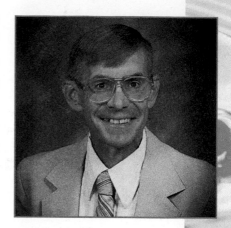

(Courtesy of Olan Mills)

After several months of volunteer work in the jail, the faculty member wrote a federal grant for a nursing clinic to be housed in the jail itself. Prior to that time, inmates with health needs that could not be addressed during the periodic visits by the volunteer faculty and students were sent to the local emergency department. The grant provided for one full-time nurse in the jail as well as for physician backup for health problems beyond the nurse's capabilities. One of the former student volunteers was hired as the nurse for the new clinic. The cost-effectiveness of the program was evaluated, and within six months of its initiation, the county's cost for health care services for inmates had decreased by 75%, primarily due to reduced emergency department visits and lost deputy time transporting inmates to the ED. With this information in hand, the sheriff was able to obtain county funding to continue the clinic after the grant period ended.

Philip Clark, RN, BSN

*T*he hallmark of community health nursing is that the primary client or recipient of care is a group of people, or population, rather than an individual or a particular family. Although nurses who engage in community health nursing practice may also provide services to individuals and families, they do so with the express purpose of improving the health of the overall population. The focus of their care is the population group, not the individuals and families who are its members. **Population-based practice** has been defined as practice that "focuses on entire populations, is grounded in community assessment, considers all health determinants, emphasizes prevention, and intervenes at multiple levels" (Keller, Strohschein, Lia-Hoagberg, & Schaffer, 2004).

DEFINING POPULATIONS AS A FOCUS FOR CARE

The population groups that form the focus for community health nursing can be many and varied. **Populations** are groups of people who may or may not interact with each other. Populations may refer to the residents of a specific geographic area, but can also include specific groups of people with some trait or attribute in common (e.g., a minority group, employees, the elderly) (Kindig & Stoddart, 2003). Three other commonly used, similar, but different terms for these smaller subgroups are *aggregate*, *neighborhood*, and *community*.

Aggregates are subpopulations within the larger population who possess some common characteristics, often related to high risk for specific health problems (Porche, 2004). School-aged children, persons with human immunodeficiency virus (HIV) infection, and the elderly are all examples of aggregates.

A **neighborhood** is a smaller, more homogeneous group than a community (Matteson, 2000) and involves an interface with others living nearby and a level of identification with those others. Neighborhoods are self-defined, and although they may be constrained by natural or man-made factors, they often do not have specifically demarcated boundaries. For example, a major highway may limit interactions between residents on either side, thus creating separate neighborhoods. Or a neighborhood may be defined by a common language or cultural heritage. Thus, non-Hispanic residents of a "Hispanic neighborhood" are not usually considered, nor do they consider themselves, part of the neighborhood.

A community may be composed of several neighborhoods (Matteson, 2000). Some authors define communities within geographic locations or settings (MacQueen et al., 2001), but the majority of writers have moved away from locale as a primary defining characteristic of communities. In addition to location, other potential defining aspects of communities include a social system or social institutions designed to carry out

 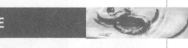

Think Advocacy

How might community health nurses in your area promote a population-health focus for local health services? What segments of the population are not currently being effectively served by existing services? How might these subpopulations be better served using a population-health approach?

specific functions; identity, commitment, or emotional connection; common norms and values; common history or interests; common symbols; social interaction; and intentional action to meet common needs. Although most of these characteristics are also true of neighborhoods, the critical distinction between neighborhoods and communities would appear to be a defined social structure containing institutions designed to accomplish designated community functions such as education, social support, and so on. For our purposes, then, a **community** is defined as a group of people who share common interests, who interact with each other, and who function collectively within a defined social structure to address common concerns. By this definition, geopolitical entities, such as the city of San Diego, a school of nursing, and a religious congregation can be considered communities. A **geopolitical community** is one characterized by geographic and jurisdictional boundaries, such as a city. All three communities (city, nursing program, and religious group), however, can be considered **communities of identity**—communities with a common identity and interests.

Community health nurses may work with any or all of these population groups—aggregates, neighborhoods, and communities—in their efforts to enhance the health status of the general public or overall population. Population health addresses the health needs of entire groups, and those health needs are affected by factors at individual, family, neighborhood, and societal levels (Northridge & Ellis, 2003).

DEFINING POPULATION HEALTH

Emphasis on the health of populations as a focus for care arose out of dissatisfaction with the limited effectiveness of individual-oriented care in improving the

CULTURAL COMPETENCE

*S*ome cultural groups traditionally think of people in the aggregate rather than as individuals. What cultural groups in your area have a community orientation? How might a community health nurse capitalize on this orientation? What aspects of traditional American culture make it more difficult to adopt aggregate thinking? What strategies by community health nurses might help people adopt a community orientation?

health of the general population (Szreter, 2003). The health of a population group goes beyond the health status of the individuals or groups who comprise it, but involves the collective health of the group (Frisch, George, Govoni, Jennings-Sanders, & McCahon, 2003). Several authors have noted the lack of a precise definition of population health (Friedman & Starfield, 2003; Kindig & Stoddart, 2003), but note that there are two basic approaches to defining population health: descriptive and analytic. Descriptive approaches focus on the health status of the population using a set of summary indicators of health (McDowell, Spasoff, & Kristjansson, 2004). In this approach, population health is viewed as the average level of health in the population and the distribution of health within the population (Friedman & Starfield, 2003). Analytic approaches define population health more broadly in terms of factors that influence health and are used to direct interventions to improving health status. Analytic approaches attempt to explain differences in the distribution of health (McDowell et al., 2004; Huttlinger, Schaller-Ayers, & Lawson, 2004).

Definitions of population health evolved from three conceptual models of health: a biomechanical model, a holistic model, and a dynamic model (McDowell et al., 2004). The biomechanical model focuses on health problems rather than on health per se and is present focused. From this perspective, a healthy population has low rates of illness and other health problems and has functioning systems equipped to deal with problems that arise. The holistic model incorporates the concept of multiple factors influencing a positive state of health (as opposed to a negative state of absence of illness). In this view, a healthy population displays aggregated indicators of individual well-being. In the dynamic model, health is viewed as a process that improves the quality of life. This last perspective has been adopted by the World Health Organization in its 1984 conception of population health.

> To be healthy, in this conception, "an individual or group must be able to identify and to realize aspirations, to satisfy needs, and to change or cope with the environment. Health is, therefore, seen as a resource for everyday life, not the object of living. Health is a positive concept, emphasizing social and personal resources as well as physical capacities." (World Health Organization, as quoted in McDowell et al., 2004, pp. 390–391)

Population health can be defined as the attainment of the greatest possible biologic, psychological, and social well-being of the population as an entity and of its individual members. Health is derived from opportunities and choices provided to the public as well as the population's response to those choices (Wilcox & Knapp, 2000). Healthy populations provide their members with the knowledge and opportunities to make choices that improve health.

In large part, the health of a population is defined and determined by the perceptions, norms, and values of its members. Despite the resulting variability in definitions of health, there are certain characteristics that healthy populations have in common. In 1999, the

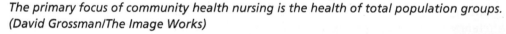

The primary focus of community health nursing is the health of total population groups. (David Grossman/The Image Works)

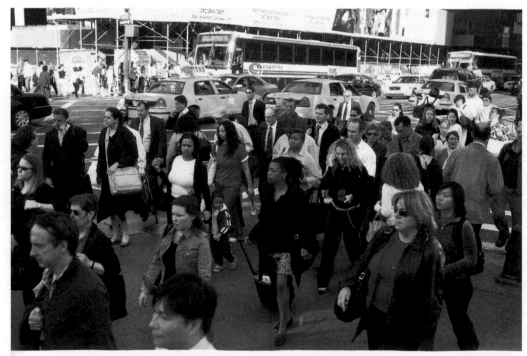

coalition for Healthier Cities and Communities, a national network of organizational partnerships dedicated to the improvement of population health, identified seven characteristics of healthy communities. Based on these characteristics, healthy communities:

- Foster dialogue among residents to develop a shared vision for the community
- Promote community leadership that fosters collaboration and partnerships
- Engage in action based on a shared vision of the community
- Embrace diversity among residents
- Assess both needs and assets
- Link residents to community resources, and
- Foster a sense of responsibility and cohesion among residents (Norris & Pittman, 2000).

Other characteristics of healthy communities include abilities to change and adapt to changing circumstances and manage conflict effectively (Duhl, 2000; Norris & Pitman, 2000).

Population health is fostered at the community level by the Healthy Cities and Healthy Communities programs. The Healthy Cities movement was initiated by the European region of the World Health Organization in 1984 (Awofeso, 2003) and was adapted as the Healthy Communities movement in the United States in the mid-1980s (Norris & Pittman, 2000). Both movements emphasize local involvement in creating conditions that support health through "a grassroots process, a way of addressing issues, making decisions, and setting policy involving the entire community" (Kesler, 2000, p. 238). They rest on the premise that healthy communities are the result of both personal choices regarding behavior and broad environmental conditions that affect health (e.g., housing, transportation, and education, as well as access to health services) (Norris & Pittman, 2000). Healthy Communities projects are based on the following eight basic principles:

- Health must be broadly defined to encompass quality-of-life issues (emotional, physical, and spiritual), not just the absence of disease.
- "Community" must also be broadly defined to encompass a variety of groups, not just populations defined by specific geographic boundaries.
- Action related to community health must arise from a shared vision derived from community values.

BUILDING OUR KNOWLEDGE BASE

*H*ow might population-focused and person/family-focused nurses collaborate in research that would improve the health of population groups? What specific research questions might be addressed? What roles might each group of nurses play in conducting the research?

EVIDENCE-BASED PRACTICE

Clark et al. (2003) described a focus-group process used to incorporate the voices of underrepresented groups in a community assessment. Review the article and answer the following questions:

1. How does this study exemplify the principles of the Healthy Communities program?
2. If you were going to conduct a community assessment of your own community, what underrepresented groups would you want to include? Would a focus-group process, as described in the article, be culturally appropriate for these groups? Why or why not?

- Actions must address the quality of life for all residents, not just a select few.
- Widespread community ownership and diverse citizen participation are required for effective community action.
- The focus of action should be on systems change in the way decisions are made and community services are delivered.
- Community health rests on the development of local assets and resources to create an environment and infrastructure that support health.
- Effectiveness is measured on the basis of specific community indicators and outcomes and promotes accountability to community residents (Healthy Community Principles, 2000; Lee, 2000).

CHANGES IN APPROACHES TO POPULATION HEALTH

Over the years, a number of approaches have been taken within public health practice to promote population health. Changes in these approaches have coincided with shifts in the mission and focus of public health practice. In the 1800s and early 1900s, the focus was on control of epidemics. Starting in the mid-1900s, the focus of practice moved to disease prevention. At present, the emphasis in public health practice is one of social justice (Drevdahl, 2002). Advocacy for social justice has always been a feature of community health nursing practice.

One author referred to these changes in the approaches to population health as the "three public health revolutions." The first revolution emphasized sanitation as a means of controlling communicable diseases. The second focused on personal behavior change to promote individual and population health. The third revolution emphasizes health as one dimension of quality of life, with a focus on "building healthy communities and healthy workplaces, strengthening the wide range of social networks for health, and increasing people's capabilities to lead healthy lives" (Kickbusch, 2003, p. 387).

Children created a mural incorporating their views of the community. (Mary Jo Clark)

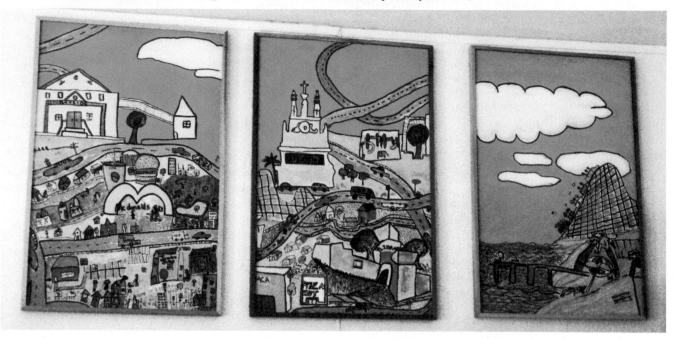

LEVELS OF POPULATION HEALTH CARE

Health care for populations takes place at three levels, often referred to as the three levels of prevention. These three levels of care are primary prevention, secondary prevention, and tertiary prevention. **Primary prevention** was defined by the originators of the term as "measures designed to promote general optimum health or . . . the specific protection of man against disease agents" (Leavell & Clark, 1965, p. 20). Primary prevention is action taken prior to the occurrence of health problems and is directed toward avoiding their occurrence (Adams et al., 2001). Primary prevention may include increasing people's resistance to illness (as in the case of immunization), decreasing or eliminating the causes of health problems, or creating an environment conducive to health rather than health problems.

Secondary prevention is the early identification and treatment of existing health problems (Adams et al., 2001) and takes place after the health problem has occurred. Emphasis is on resolving health problems and preventing serious consequences. Secondary prevention activities include screening and early diagnosis, as well as treatment for existing health problems. Screening for hypertension is an example of secondary prevention. Secondary prevention would also include the actual diagnosis and treatment of a person with hypertension. Development of health care programs to diagnose and treat hypertension in the community would be an example of secondary prevention at the population level.

Tertiary prevention is activity aimed at returning the client to the highest level of function and preventing further deterioration in health (Adams et al., 2001). Tertiary prevention also focuses on preventing recurrences of the problem. Placing a client on a maintenance diet after the loss of a desired number of pounds constitutes tertiary prevention. Legislation to promote a living wage for all workers to prevent recurrent homelessness would be an example of tertiary prevention focused on populations rather than individuals.

OBJECTIVES FOR POPULATION HEALTH

The goals and desired outcomes for population health in the United States have been operationalized in several sets of national objectives. The first set of objectives was established in 1980 in the publication *Promoting Health/Preventing Disease: Objectives for the Nation* (U.S. Department of Health and Human Services, 1980) and targeted 15 priority intervention areas in three strategic action categories: preventive health, health protection, and health promotion. The primary goal of this initiative was to reduce mortality (Friedrich, 2000). Approximately one third of the 226 objectives were met by the target date of 1990 (National Center for Health Statistics, 1992).

A subsequent set of National Health Objectives, *Healthy People 2000: National Health Promotion and Disease Prevention Objectives*, was established for the year 2000 (U.S. Department of Health and Human Services, 1990). The broad goals for this second set of objectives were to (a) increase the span of healthy life (not just longevity), (b) reduce health disparities among subpopulations, and (c) achieve access to preventive health services for all (McAlearney, 2003). The year 2000 objectives differed

GLOBAL PERSPECTIVES

*T*he chapter describes the national health objectives for population health in the United States. What other countries have adopted a similar approach to population health? What other approaches to population health have been taken in the international community? For example, see Glouberman and Millar (2003) and Coburn, Denny, Mykhalovskiy, McDonough, Robertson, and Love (2003) for a discussion of the Canadian determinants-of-health approach to population health.

ETHICAL AWARENESS

*O*ne of the major changes in the *Healthy People 2010* objectives is the shift from minimizing health disparities among various groups within the population to eliminating them altogether. What are the ethical implications of achieving this goal if it means reducing the level of service provided to groups with better health status in order to provide additional services to those with poorer health status? What models of ethical decision making would justify such an approach? What ethical arguments could be made against such reductions?

from those for 1990 in several ways. First, priority intervention areas were increased from 15 to 22 to include cancer screening, HIV infection, and preventive services. Second, the focus of the objectives was moved beyond reduction of mortality to improving the quality of life. A third difference was the special attention given to the needs of high-risk populations such as the elderly and minority groups. Fourth, the year 2000 objectives reflected concern for access to basic health services for all. Finally, responsibility for overseeing and monitoring achievement in each priority area was delegated to a specific agency of the U.S. Public Health Service (U.S. Department of Health and Human Services, 1996). A report in June of 1999 indicated that 15% of the year 2000 objectives had been met and another 44% were moving toward the established targets. Unfortunately, another 18% of objectives were moving away from the targets, and others had not been assessed due to the lack of baseline and follow-up data (Friedrich, 2000).

The most recent set of objectives was published in January 2000 in *Healthy People 2010* (U.S. Department of Health and Human Services, 2000a)◆. This most recent set of national objectives was developed with input from the Healthy People Consortium, a coalition of more than 600 national and state health agencies, organizations, and experts (Davis, Okuboye, & Ferguson, 2000). The development of the objectives was based on a systematic approach consisting of four elements: goals, objectives, determinants of health, and health status (U.S. Department of Health and Human Services, 2000b). The goals provide direction for the development of more specific objectives. The two overarching goals are to increase quality and length of healthy life and to eliminate health disparities (Smith & Bazini-Barakat, 2003). The first goal continues the emphasis of *Healthy People 2000* on improved quality of life versus reduced mortality emphasized in the objectives for 1990. The second expands the year 2000 goal of reducing disparities to eliminating them altogether (McAlearney, 2003).

The objectives specify the amount of progress expected in improving the health status of the population in the next 10 years. The 2010 objectives have been expanded to cover 28 focus areas and 467 objectives. Some of the focus areas from the year 2000 objectives have been separated and others added. Table 1 ◆

provides a summary of focus areas included in the *Healthy People 2010* document with the agencies responsible for monitoring progress toward the objectives in each area. *Healthy People 2010* incorporates a common structure for each focus area that includes:

- Identification of the lead agency responsible for monitoring progress toward achievement of objectives.
- A concise goal statement for the focus area that delineates the overall purpose of the focus area.
- An overview of context and background for the objectives related to the focus area. This overview includes related issues, trends, disparities among population subgroups, and opportunities for prevention or intervention.
- Data on progress toward meeting related objectives for 2000.
- Objectives related to the focus area. These objectives are of two types: measurable outcome objectives and developmental objectives. Measurable objectives include baseline data, the target for 2010, and potential data sources for monitoring progress toward the target. Unlike the year 2000 objectives, which set separate targets for subpopulations, a single target is set for the entire population. The targets for each objective have been set at a level that is "better than the best," resulting in improved health status for all segments of the population (U.S. Department of Health and Human Services, 2000c). Developmental objectives relate to areas for which data systems do not exist and will direct the development of data systems related to emerging health issues.
- A standard data table, including a set of population variables by which progress will be monitored. The minimum set of variables includes race and ethnicity, gender, family income, and education level. Additional categories of variables will be incorporated where relevant and include geographic location, health insurance status, disability status, and other selected populations (e.g., school grade levels) (U.S. Department of Health and Human Services, 2000a).

The third element in the systematic approach to health improvement exemplified by the document is

MediaLink Case Study: Seatbelt Safety

TABLE 1	Healthy People 2010: Focus Areas and Responsible Agencies
Focus Area	**Responsible Agencies**
Access to quality health services	Agency for Healthcare Research and Quality (AHRQ) (http://www.ahrq.gov) Health Resources and Services Administration (http://www.hrsa.gov)
Arthritis, osteoporosis, and chronic back pain	Centers for Disease Control and Prevention (http://www.cdc.gov) National Institutes of Health (http://www.nih.gov)
Cancer	Centers for Disease Control and Prevention (http://www.cdc.gov) National Institutes of Health (http://www.nih.gov)
Chronic kidney disease	National Institutes of Health (http://www.nih.gov)
Diabetes	Centers for Disease Control and Prevention (http://www.cdc.gov) National Institutes of Health (http://www.nih.gov)
Disability and secondary conditions	Centers for Disease Control and Prevention (http://www.cdc.gov) National Institute on Disability and Rehabilitation Research (http://www.ed.gov/about/offices/list/osers/nidr/index.html?src=mr) U.S. Department of Education (http://www.ed.gov)
Educational and community-based programs	Centers for Disease Control and Prevention (http://www.cdc.gov) Health Resources and Services Administration (http://www.hrsa.gov)
Environmental health	Agency for Toxic Substances and Disease Registry (http://www.atsdr.gov/atsdrhome.html) Centers for Disease Control and Prevention (http://www.cdc.gov) National Institutes of Health (http://www.nih.gov)
Family planning	Office of Population Affairs (http://opa.osophs.dhhs.gov)
Food safety	Food and Drug Administration (http://www.fda.gov) Food Safety and Inspection Service (http://fsis.usda.gov) U.S. Department of Agriculture (http://usda.gov)
Health communication	Office of Disease Prevention and Health Promotion (http://odphp.osophs.dhhs.gov)
Heart disease and stroke	Centers for Disease Control and Prevention (http://www.cdc.gov) National Institutes of Health (http://www.nih.gov)
HIV	Centers for Disease Control and Prevention (http://www.cdc.gov) Health Resources and Services Administration (http://www.hrsa.gov)
Immunization and infectious diseases	Centers for Disease Control and Prevention (http://www.cdc.gov)
Injury and violence prevention	Centers for Disease Control and Prevention (http://www.cdc.gov)
Maternal, infant, and child health	Centers for Disease Control and Prevention (http://www.cdc.gov) Health Resources and Services Administration (http://www.hrsa.gov)
Medical product safety	Food and Drug Administration (http://www.fda.gov)
Mental health and mental disorders	National Institutes of Health (http://www.nih.gov) Substance Abuse and Mental Health Services Administration (http://www.samhsa.gov)
Nutrition and overweight	Food and Drug Administration (http://www.fda.gov) National Institutes of Health (http://www.nih.gov)

Continued on next page

TABLE 1	Healthy People 2010: Focus Areas and Responsible Agencies *(continued)*
Focus Area	**Responsible Agencies**
Nutrition and overweight	Food and Drug Administration (http://www.fda.gov) National Institutes of Health (http://www.nih.gov)
Occupational safety and health	Centers for Disease Control and Prevention (http://www.cdc.gov)
Oral health	Centers for Disease Control and Prevention (http://www.cdc.gov) Health Resources and Services Administration (http://www.hrsa.gov) National Institutes of Health (http://www.nih.gov)
Physical fitness and activity	Centers for Disease Control and Prevention (http://www.cdc.gov) President's Council on Physical Fitness and Sports (http://www.fitness.gov)
Public health infrastructure	Centers for Disease Control and Prevention (http://www.cdc.gov) Health Resources and Services Administration (http://www.hrsa.gov)
Respiratory diseases	Centers for Disease Control and Prevention (http://www.cdc.gov) National Institutes of Health (http://www.nih.gov)
Sexually transmitted diseases	Centers for Disease Control and Prevention (http://www.cdc.gov)
Substance abuse	National Institutes of Health (http://www.nih.gov) Substance Abuse and Mental Health Services Administration (http://www.samhsa.gov)
Tobacco use	Centers for Disease Control and Prevention (http://www.cdc.gov)
Vision and hearing	National Institutes of Health (http://www.nih.gov)

Data from: U.S. Department of Health and Human Services. (2000). Healthy people 2010 (Conference edition, in two volumes). Washington, DC: Author. (Note: The Web address for Healthy People 2010 is http://www.health.gov/healthypeople.)

related to the determinants of health. These determinants are the "combined effects of individual and community physical and social environments and the policies and interventions used to promote health, prevent disease, and ensure access to quality health care" (U.S. Department of Health and Human Services, 2000b, p. 7).

Health status of the overall population, the fourth element of the approach, is the expected outcome and measure of success of the approach. Health status is reflected in the extent to which each of the 467 objectives is met, but is also reflected at a more general level in 10 leading health indicators (Sakamoto & Avila, 2004). These indicators are presented in Table 2◆ and are designed to reflect the major public health issues in the nation. A small set of two to three objectives is identified for each health indicator and will be used to track and report trends in the indicator. Information related to health indicators includes health impacts, trends, populations particularly affected, and related issues (U.S. Department of Health and Human Services, 2000a).

Figure 1 depicts the interrelationships among the four elements of the systematic approach taken to improving the health of the nation. Table 3◆ presents an overview of trends in the national objectives for

TABLE 2	Leading Health Indicators
Physical activity	
Overweight and obesity	
Tobacco use	
Substance abuse	
Responsible sexual behavior	
Mental health	
Injury and violence	
Environmental quality	
Immunization	
Access to care	

population health from 1990 to 2010. Information on the current status of specific *Healthy People* objectives is available from the *Healthy People* Web site at http://wonder.cdc.gov/data2010.

As we have seen in this chapter, the community or population group is the primary focus of care in community health nursing. Care is provided to individuals and families with an eye toward improving the health of the total population. National health objectives guide the provision of care and serve as a means of evaluating the effectiveness of population health care.

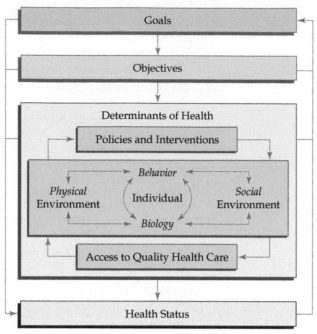

FIGURE 1 A Systematic Approach to Health Improvement
Data from: U.S. Department of Health and Human Services.
(2000). *Healthy people 2010: Understanding and improving
health* (2nd ed.). Washington, DC: Author.

TABLE 3	Trends in National Health Objectives: 1990, 2000, and 2010

Overall Goal

1990: Reduce mortality

2000: Increase the span of healthy life
Reduce disparities in health status among
    subpopulations
Achieve access to preventive health services for all

2010: Increase quality and years of healthy life
Eliminate disparities in health status among
    subpopulations

Objective Categories

1990: Preventive health objectives
Health protection objectives
Health promotion objectives

2000: Health status objectives
Risk reduction objectives
Services and protection objectives

2010: Objectives promoting healthy behaviors
Objectives promoting healthy and safe communities
Objectives to improve systems for personal
    and public health
Objectives to prevent and reduce diseases and
    disorders

Focus Areas

1990: 15 priority areas designated
2000: 22 priority areas designated
2010: 28 focus areas designated

Objectives

1990: 226 objectives identified
2000: 319 objectives identified
2010: 467 objectives identified

Progress Toward Achievement

1990: One third of objectives achieved by target date

2000: 15% of objectives achieved by target date
44% making progress toward achievement
18% moving away from the target
23% untracked

2010: Not applicable

Other Changes

1990: Not applicable

2000: Lead agencies responsible for monitoring
    progress identified
Emphasis placed on quality of life as well as longevity
Special attention given to high-risk groups
Emphasis given to access to health services
Baseline data provided where available

2010: Widespread input into the development of
    the objectives
Designation of leading health indicators
Included a single target for each measurable
    objective, identified as "better than the best"
Included developmental objectives
Development of a common structure for each
    focus area
Development of a standard data table for reporting
    progress toward achievement of objectives

Data from: U.S. Department of Health and Human Services. (2000). Healthy people 2010: Understanding and improving health *(2nd ed.). Washington, DC: Author.*

Case Study

Caring for Populations

1. Identify some of the neighborhoods in the area where your nursing program is located. What defines these neighborhoods—geographic boundaries, culture, or some other defining feature?
2. What kinds of neighborhoods make up the communities in the area? What similarities and differences are there among neighborhoods in a given community? What effects do differences among neighborhoods have on planning health

care services? Have these differences been taken into consideration in planning community health services?
3. What are some of the subpopulations or aggregates in your community? Select one of these aggregates and determine whether or not the health needs of that group are met within the community. If not, what health needs remain unmet? What could be done to meet the health needs of this aggregate?

Test Your Understanding

1. What is the difference between a neighborhood, a community, and an aggregate?

2. What is *population health*? What are some of the characteristics of healthy populations or healthy communities?

3. What changes have occurred in approaches to population health over time?

4. What are the three levels at which population health care occurs? Give an example of each in the care of an individual and the care of a population group.

5. Describe trends in national health objectives for 1990, 2000, and 2010. What are the overall goals of each document? What additional features have been added over time?

EXPLORE MediaLink

http://www.prenhall.com/clark
Resources for this chapter can be found on the Companion Website.

Audio Glossary
Exam Review Questions
Case Study: Seatbelt Safety

MediaLink Applications: The Ruth Freeman
    Population Nursing Award
Media Links

Challenge Your Knowledge
Advocacy Interviews

References

Adams, M. H., Sherrod, R. A., Packa, D. R., Forte, L., Lammon, C. A. B., Stover, L., et al. (2001). Levels of prevention: Restructuring a curriculum to meet future health care needs. *Nurse Educator, 26*(1), 6–8.

Awofeso, N. (2003). The Healthy Cities approach—reflections on a framework for improving global health. *Bulletin of the World Health Organization, 81,* 222–223.

Clark, M. J., Cary, S., Diemert, G., Ceballos, R., Sifuentes, M., Atteberry, I., Vue, F., & Trieu, S. (2003). Involving communities in community assessment. *Public Health Nursing, 20,* 456–463.

Coburn, D., Denny, K., Mykhalovskiy, E., McDonough, P., Robertson, A., & Love, R. (2003). Population health in Canada. *American Journal of Public Health, 93,* 392–396.

Davis, L. J., Okuboye, S., & Ferguson, S. L. (2000). Healthy people 2010: Examining a

decade of maternal & infant health. *AWHONN Lifelines, 4*(3), 26–33.

Drevdahl, D. (2002). Social justice or market justice? The paradoxes of public health partnerships with managed care. *Public Health Nursing, 19,* 161–169.

Duhl, L. J. (2000). A short history and some acknowledgments. (Healthy communities.) *Public Health Reports, 115,* 116–117.

Friedman, D. J., & Starfield, B. (2003). Models of population health: Their value for US public health practice, policy, and research. *American Journal of Public Health, 93,* 366–369.

Friedrich, M. J. (2000). More healthy people in the 21st century? *JAMA, 283,* 37–38.

Frisch, N. C., George, V., Govoni, A. L., Jennings-Sanders, A., & McCahon, C. P. (2003). Teaching nurses to focus on the health needs of populations: A master's

degree program in population health nursing. *Nurse Educator, 28,* 212–216.

Glouberman, S., & Millar, J. (2003). Evolution of the determinants of health, health policy, and health information systems in Canada. *American Journal of Public Health, 93,* 388–392.

Healthy Community Principles. (2000). *Public Health Reports, 115,* 122.

Huttlinger, K., Schaller-Ayers, J., & Lawson, T. (2004). Health care in Appalachia: A population-based approach. *Public Health Nursing, 21,* 103–110.

Keller, L. O., Strohschein, S., Lia-Hoagberg, B., & Schaffer, M. A. (2004). Population-based public health interventions: Practice-based and evidence-supported. *Public Health Nursing, 21,* 453–468.

Kesler, J. T. (2000). Healthy communities and civil discourse: A leadership opportunity for public health professionals. *Public Health Reports, 115,* 238–242.

Kickbusch, I. (2003). The contribution of the World Health Organization to a new public health and health promotion. *American Journal of Public Health, 93,* 383–387.

Kindig, D., & Stoddart, G. (2003). What is population health? *American Journal of Public Health, 93,* 380–383.

Leavell, H. R., & Clark, E. G. (1965). *Preventive medicine for the doctor in his community: An epidemiologic approach* (3rd ed.). New York: McGraw-Hill.

Lee, P. (2000). Healthy Communities: A young movement that can revolutionize public health. *Public Health Reports, 115,* 114–115.

MacQueen, K. M., McLellan, E., Metzger, D. S., Kegeles, S., Strauss, R. P., Scotti, R., et al. (2001). What is community? An evidence-based definition for participatory public health. *American Journal of Public Health, 91,* 1929–1938.

Matteson, P. S. (2000). Preparing nurses for the future. In P. S. Matteson (Ed.), *Community-based nursing education* (pp. 1–7). New York: Springer.

McAlearney, A. S. (2003). *Population health management: Strategies to improve outcomes.* Chicago: Health Administration Press.

McDowell, I., Spasoff, R. A., & Kristjansson, B. (2004). On the classification of population health measures. *American Journal of Public Health, 94,* 388–393.

National Center for Health Statistics. (1992). *Health United States, 1991.* Washington, DC: Government Printing Office.

Norris, T., & Pittman, M. (2000). The healthy communities movement and the Coalition for Healthier Cities and Communities. *Public Health Reports, 115,* 118–124.

Northridge, M. E., & Ellis, J. A. (2003). Applying population health models. *American Journal of Public Health, 93,* 365.

Porche, D. J. (2004). *Public and community health nursing practice: A population-based approach.* Thousand Oaks, CA: Sage.

Sakamoto, S. D., & Avila, M. (2004). The public health nursing practice manual: A tool for public health nurses. *Public Health Nursing, 21,* 179–182.

Smith, K., & Bazini-Barakat, N. (2003). A public health nursing model: Melding public health principles with the nursing process. *Public Health Nursing, 20,* 42–48.

Szreter, S. (2003). The population health approach in historical perspective. *American Journal of Public Health, 93,* 421–431.

U.S. Department of Health and Human Services. (1980). *Promoting health/preventing disease: Objectives for the nation.* Washington, DC: Government Printing Office.

U.S. Department of Health and Human Services. (1990). *Healthy people 2000: National health promotion and disease prevention objectives.* Washington, DC: Government Printing Office.

U.S. Department of Health and Human Services. (1996). *Healthy people 2000: Fact sheet.* Washington, DC: Author.

U.S. Department of Health and Human Services. (2000a). *Healthy people 2010* (Conference edition, in two volumes). Washington, DC: Author.

U.S. Department of Health and Human Services. (2000b). *Healthy people 2010: Understanding and improving health* (2nd ed.). Washington, DC: Author.

U.S. Department of Health and Human Services. (2000c). Healthy people 2010: Understanding and improving health. *Prevention Report, 14*(4), 1–2, 4.

Wilcox, R., & Knapp, A. (2000). Building communities that create health. *Public Health Reports, 115,* 139–143.

Meeting the Health Needs of Child and Adolescent Populations

Advocacy in Action

The Power of Research and Publication

As part of a capstone public health nursing course, senior nursing students in a Middle Eastern country conducted telephone interviews about the use of child safety seats. The students interviewed parents of children aged 1 to 13 months who lived in a geographically defined community. The community had relatively high income and educational levels, and most families had telephones and private automobiles. Students found that only 20% of parents reported transporting their children in child safety seats during the child's last car ride. The remainder reported that the child was held in someone's arms or transported in a baby carrier. Based on the data, the students planned educational interventions to be integrated into well-child care for this population.

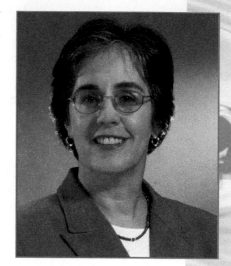

After the students graduated, the instructor thought that if wealthy and comparatively well-educated parents didn't transport their children in child safety seats, then the issue of safe transport of children would likely be an important one for the country at large. She urged the graduates to disseminate the findings of their study, but they were busy learning new skills and told the instructor to feel free to disseminate the findings herself. The instructor and a colleague developed a manuscript based on the students' findings that was published in a local nursing journal. This article was picked up by the local press, and multiple newspapers ran articles about the issue of safe transport of children in cars. The nursing instructor was interviewed by local media, helped legislators draft legislation requiring the use of safety seats, and testified before a legislative committee. Less than three years after the students completed their project, legislation was passed mandating the use of child safety seats in that country.

Derryl Block, PhD, MPH, RN

Professor and Chair Professional Program in Nursing

Director BSN-LINC

University of Wisconsin–Green Bay

Meeting the Health Needs of Child and Adolescent Populations

CHAPTER OBJECTIVES

After reading this chapter, you should be able to:

1. Identify factors affecting the health of children and adolescents.
2. Describe at least five primary prevention measures appropriate to the care of children and adolescents and analyze the role of the community health nurse with respect to each.
3. Identify at least three approaches to providing secondary preventive care for children and adolescents and give examples of community health nursing interventions related to each.
4. Describe three tertiary preventive considerations in the care of children and adolescents and analyze the role of the community health nurse with respect to each.

KEY TERMS

anticipatory guidance
attention deficit hyperactivity disorder (ADHD)
Denver Developmental Screening Test (DDST)
development
developmental milestones
fetal alcohol syndrome (FAS)
growth
herd immunity
menarche

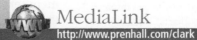

MediaLink
http://www.prenhall.com/clark

Additional interactive resources for this chapter can be found on the Companion Website. Click on Chapter 16 and "Begin" to select the activities for this chapter.

*A*ccording to the Federal Interagency Forum on Child Health and Family Statistics (2004), children under 18 years of age comprised 25% of the U.S. population. This figure encompassed nearly 73 million children and adolescents. By 2020, the proportion of the population under age 18 is expected to decrease slightly to 24%. Children and adolescents have specific health needs and problems that can be addressed by community health nurses. Community health nursing practice with children and adolescents involves assessing the health status and needs of these populations; deriving community health diagnoses; designing and implementing programs of care at primary, secondary, and tertiary levels of prevention to meet those needs; and evaluating the effectiveness of these programs.

THE EPIDEMIOLOGY OF CHILD AND ADOLESCENT HEALTH

Factors in each of the six dimensions of health influence the health of children and adolescents. We will briefly examine considerations related to the biophysical, psychological, physical environmental, sociocultural, behavioral, and health system dimensions as they affect the health of these populations.

Biophysical Considerations

Biophysical considerations related to the health of children and adolescents include the effects of maturation and aging and factors that affect both, genetic inheritance, and physiologic function. Factors contributing to health and illness among children and adolescents in each of these areas will be briefly addressed.

Age and Maturation

Areas to be assessed with respect to maturation and aging include growth and development. **Growth** is an increase in body size or change in the structure, function, and complexity of body cells until a point of maturity. Overweight and obesity are serious problems related to growth in the U.S. child and adolescent populations, whereas many children in other parts of the world are malnourished and exhibit growth retardation. In 2000, for example, 15% of 6- to 11-year olds and 16% of adolescents in the United States were overweight or obese (National Center for Health Statistics [NCHS], 2005b). At the same time, 8% of low-income children under 5 years of age exhibited growth retardation (Centers for Disease Control and Prevention [CDC], 2005a). Similarly, news reports in 2005 indicated that as many as one third of poor children in China were malnourished. There may also be significant disparities among subgroups within the population with respect to growth parameters. For example, refugee children are often below their age mates for height and weight due to malnutrition in their countries of origin. Obesity is also more prevalent in some child and adolescent populations than in others. For example, in 2000, 24% of Mexican American school-aged children in the United States were obese or overweight compared to 15% of the general population (CDC, 2005a). When rates of obesity among children and adolescents in the population are high, community health nurses can identify contributing factors and advocate for programs to prevent or treat obesity. For example, a nurse might advocate for more physical activity and healthier meals in school settings or for the development of recreational opportunities that encourage physical activity among children and adolescents.

Development is a process of patterned, orderly, and lifelong change in structure, thought, or behavior that occurs as a result of physical or emotional maturation. With the individual child or adolescent, the community health nurse would assess the extent to which specific developmental milestones have been met. **Developmental milestones** are critical behaviors expected at specific ages, and their assessment can be accomplished using a variety of tools addressed in your basic pediatric nursing text. Development from birth to 6 years of age is often assessed by means of the **Denver Developmental Screening Test (DDST)**, a test of age-specific development in four areas: fine motor, gross motor, personal-social, and language development. Failure to develop normally may result from a number of causes. At the population level, the community health nurse would focus on the extent of developmental delay in the population. The most common cause of delayed development is mental retardation, which will be discussed in more detail later in this chapter. Other causes of developmental delays are acute and chronic illness and lack of an environment that fosters development. When the latter is the case, the community health nurse can advocate with parents and other caretakers for conditions that stimulate appropriate development. For example, in some families, younger children do not develop language skills appropriate to their ages because family members anticipate and address their needs without the child having to voice them in understandable language. In such a case, the community health nurse would encourage parents and older siblings not to meet the child's needs until the child has indicated them verbally. Similarly, community health nurses may need to

EVIDENCE-BASED PRACTICE

*E*vidence-based practice requires that research be conducted with the same types of people to whom findings will be applied. For this reason, the federal government has ruled that all research receiving federal support include children as subjects, if relevant to the study. Why is such a ruling appropriate? What ethical dilemmas might this policy pose? In what types of studies would inclusion of children as subjects not be appropriate?

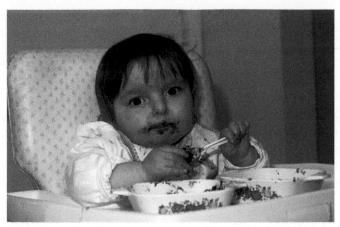

Children need opportunities to develop age-appropriate skills. (Molly Schlachter)

advocate for a balance between independence and supervision for adolescents so they gradually become independent from their parents. Nurses may also need to reassure parents that testing of family values is a normal part of adolescence, not evidence of rebellion.

Another maturational or developmental consideration for the adolescent population is the usual age at which adolescents become sexually mature, which may differ for different segments of the community. For example, African American adolescents may become sexually mature at an earlier age than their Caucasian or Asian counterparts.

Menarche, the first appearance of menstrual flow in the adolescent girl, usually occurs between 12 and 13 years of age. Menarche that occurs too early (age 8 or younger) is associated with precocious puberty, an anomaly of the endocrine system. Delayed menarche (after age 18) is also a signal that the endocrine system is not functioning properly. Either early or late onset of

menses is cause for referral for medical evaluation. Menarche may appear earlier or later than average in some ethnic populations, and the nurse should be familiar with population parameters for the onset of menstruation.

The physical and emotional changes that occur just prior to and with menarche have the potential to create physical or psychological problems for the adolescent girl. Assessment of preadolescent girls should include the extent of sexual changes, knowledge of menstruation, and preparation for the event. If menarche has occurred, other considerations related to menstruation may include menstrual regularity, extent and duration of flow, and the experience of dysmenorrhea, or painful menstruation. The nurse would also inquire about signs and symptoms of premenstrual distress (premenstrual syndrome) such as depression, irritability, nervousness, tension, inability to concentrate, breast tenderness, bloating, edema, fatigue, headache, and food cravings. Symptoms of premenstrual distress may be severe and require medical referral or may be less severe and respond to dietary changes and exercise. Menarche heralds the beginning potential for pregnancy, so the typical age of menarche in the population, or within certain subpopulations, can suggest the age at which sex education should be undertaken. Community health nurses also need to be aware of cultural attitudes to menarche within the population. Menarche in some societies is met with female genital mutilation, and community health nurses should be aware of the extent to which women in the community may have been subjected to this practice.

Physical sexual maturation in the male typically begins between ages 9.5 and 14 years and is completed between ages 14 and 18 years. Adolescent males are typically very concerned with sexual and physical development, often comparing themselves to other males and

Advocacy in Action

Developmental Delay

As both a pediatric nurse practitioner and a public health nurse working in a county health department, I had the opportunity to see clients in the child health clinic and to follow up with home visits as needed. One day in clinic I saw a 9-month-old child who was barely sitting and unable to accomplish most of the age-appropriate tasks of the Denver Developmental Screening Test (DDST). The child's mother seemed also to have a significant level of developmental delay, so I decided to make a home visit prior to making a referral for a complete diagnostic workup.

When I arrived at the home, I discovered the mother had been leaving the baby in her crib in a back bedroom except when she had to feed, bathe, or change her. The mother obviously took good physical care of the child. She knew

enough to feed the baby and keep her clean and dry, but, given her own limited mental capabilities, she had no idea that a baby required stimulation. There were no toys or other objects to interest the child, and she was left consistently without stimulation of any kind.

The father of the child lived in the home, but worked two jobs. When he arrived home at night, the baby was usually in bed, and he had no idea that his wife was not interacting with the baby other than to meet her physical needs. I encouraged him to make time to play with the baby and taught the mother how to talk to and play with the child. Once the mother realized the importance of interaction with the child, she was happy to comply. After 6 months or so of appropriate stimulation, the child was on track developmentally.

many times experiencing anxiety about the possibility that their development is delayed or inadequate. In some cases, this anxiety can be sufficient to cause social impairment or serious emotional distress, and the community health nurse should make a special effort to be supportive and accepting. The community health nurse can also assist adolescent male clients by offering information and reassurance about the normal patterns and variations in growth and development. In the majority of adolescent males, a degree of transient gynecomastia (enlargement of the breasts) occurs. This is variable in degree, but can be a source of significant concern to the adolescent; again, reassurance, explanation, and acceptance are of benefit.

During this period, adolescents become increasingly concerned with the values of peers and are increasingly focused on achieving acceptance from the peer group. They are prone to value the opinions of peers over those of parents, and attitudes are more reflective of peers than of family. Adolescent males often experience identity uncertainty, and may engage in a variety of behaviors that, although perhaps disconcerting to family or other adults, are necessary experiments in determining their self-concepts. Hormonal changes result in increased growth and libido, confronting adolescent males with the possibility of new (and perhaps anxiety-provoking) roles; these changes are also mirrored in the behavior of peers, on which the teenager tends to model his own behaviors and choices.

Adolescent males may feel embarrassed about the physical and emotional changes they experience. For example, they may have spontaneous and ill-timed erections or nocturnal emissions. Physical development and social circumstances, coupled with peer pressure and a desire to conform, may lead to varying degrees of sexual activity, presenting the risks of unwanted pregnancy and sexually transmitted diseases. It is not unusual for some of the adolescent male's sexual exploration to involve sexual contact with other males; approximately 50% of all males have had such contact at some point, and there is no correlation between such sexual activity and later sexual orientation (though the adolescent may again experience significant anxiety, guilt, or shame about this experimental behavior). Other adolescent males may begin to discover a same-sex orientation during these years and should be supported as well.

Over time, the adolescent male's preoccupation with sexual performance and activity as the major parameters of a relationship are increasingly replaced by romantic attributes and genuine caring; initially, these romantic views are often stereotypical and exaggerated, but this also changes as he progresses through early adulthood. Again, the nurse's role involves assessing the young male's development relative to existing norms; providing education about growth, development, sexuality, and related risks and safety precautions; and

providing reassurance and guidance relative to the changes experienced. Community health nurses can also advocate for appropriate sexuality education for adolescents to help them deal with the many issues surrounding sexual maturation.

Genetic Inheritance

Genetic inheritance is another biophysical consideration in the assessment of child and adolescent populations. Gender and racial or ethnic background are two intrinsic genetic factors that influence the health of children and adolescents. Male and female children and children of different racial and ethnic groups tend to experience different types of health problems. For example, the nurse might identify the prevalence of urinary tract infections in school-age girls as a community problem because urinary tract infections occur more frequently in girls than in boys in this age group. Similarly, screening tests for sickle cell disease should be routinely conducted on African American children and others at risk.

Physiologic Function

Considerations related to physiologic function include the incidence and prevalence of specific physical health problems in the child and adolescent populations. Information on the leading causes of child and adolescent deaths in the population provides an overview of the health status of these two groups. According to the U.S. Census Bureau (2004b), the leading causes of death for children 1 to 4 years of age in 2001 in descending order were accidents (contributing to more than a third of all deaths in this age group), congenital malformations, neoplasms, assault/homicide (a staggering 8% of deaths), and diseases of the heart. Accidents remained the leading cause of death for children aged 5 to 14 years (40% of deaths) and adolescents and young adults from 15 to 24 years (45%), with neoplasms, congenital malformations, homicide (4.5%), heart disease, and suicide (2.6% of deaths) following for 5- to 14-year-olds. Among 15- to 24-year-olds, causes of death after first-ranked accidents included homicide (16%), suicide (12%), malignant neoplasms, and diseases of the heart. The community health nurse would explore relevant mortality figures for the child and adolescent populations in his or her community.

Not all illnesses result in death, and assessment of the child and adolescent population may reveal high prevalence rates of other acute and chronic illnesses. For example, 45,000 new cases of epilepsy are diagnosed each year in children under 15 years of age (Epilepsy Foundation, 2005). Another one in every 400 to 500 children and adolescents has type 1 diabetes (American Diabetes Association, n.d.). Other acute and chronic conditions may also be found in this population. If acute and chronic diseases are prevalent among the child and adolescent population in the community, community health nurses may need to advocate for effective illness prevention programs or services to deal with existing illness. For example, if a large proportion of the school population has asthma, the community health nurse may advocate for creation of school-based asthma management programs. Similarly, if the prevalence of childhood cancers is high, community health nurses may initiate investigation of environmental factors that may be contributing to high prevalence.

Another aspect of physiologic function that should be explored with respect to the child and adolescent populations is immunization. Maintenance of high rates of immunization among children not only protects individual children from disease, but also serves to protect other members of the population via herd immunity. **Herd immunity** is the level of protection provided to unimmunized people when immunization rates are high among the rest of the population. If most children, for example, are immunized against varicella (chickenpox), the chances of an adult without immunity being exposed to the disease are considerably reduced. Recommended immunizations for children and adolescents are summarized in Table 1◆. The immunization schedule is updated by the Advisory Committee on Immunization Practices (ACIP) each year and published in a January issue of *Morbidity and Mortality Weekly Report*. Up-to-date information on recommended immunizations is also available from the National Immunization Program Web site at http:// www.cdc.gov/nip. When immunization levels within the population are low, community health nurses may need to advocate with parents for needed childhood immunizations for individual children or with health care delivery systems to make sure that immunizations are available. For example, the community health nurse might advocate for development of outreach immunization clinics for low-income families in underserved neighborhoods.

Psychological Considerations

A number of considerations related to the psychological dimension influence the health status of child and adolescent populations. These include family dynamics, parental coping and mental health, mental health problems in the child and adolescent population, and the potential for and extent of abuse.

Family Dynamics, Parental Expectations, and Discipline

Family dynamics affect the child's or adolescent's interactions with parents and other family members and influence the child's self-image and development of self-esteem. Children who are subjected to denigration, neglect, or harsh discipline may grow up considering themselves unworthy of love or esteem. Children may also internalize feelings and roles based on the dynamics of their families of origin. For example, children of divorced parents may experience feelings of guilt or emotional distress related to the dissolution of their family. Similarly, children in foster care have been shown to have twice the incidence of mental disorders as non-foster-care children receiving Supplemental Security Income through the Social Security program and 15 times the incidence among children receiving other forms of public aid (dos Rets, Zito, Safer, & Soeken, 2001). Research has also shown consistently that children exposed to hostility and aggressive behaviors by other family members are more likely to display these behaviors themselves.

TABLE 1	Recommended Child and Adolescent Immunizations									
Age	HBV	DTaP	Hib	IPV	PCV	MMR	Td	Var	Inf	MCV4
Birth	#1*									
1 month	#2*									
2 months		#1*	#1*	#1	#1					
4 months		#2	#2	#2	#2					
6 months	#3*	#3	#3	#3*	#3				☑*	
12 months			#4*		#4*	#1*		#1*	☑	
15 months		#4*								
24 months	†							†	☑	
4–6 years		#5		#4		#2*			☑	
11–12 years						#2†	#1		☑	#1
13–18 years							†		☑	

HBV, hepatitis B virus; DTaP, diphtheria and tetanus toxoids and acellular pertussis; Hib, *Hemophilus influenzae* type b; IPV, inactivated polio vaccine; PCV, pneumococcal conjugate vaccine; MMR, measles–mumps–rubella; Td, tetanus and diphtheria toxoids, adult type; Var, varicella; Inf, influenza (yearly), MCV4, meningococcal conjugate vaccine

* Indicates earliest acceptable time of dose; doses may be given within a window of time beginning at the time indicated

†Initiate series or give immunization if not given previously

☑ Given annually

Data from: Centers for Disease Control and Prevention. (2006). Recommended childhood and adolescent immunization schedule–United States, 2006. Morbidity and Mortality Weekly Report, 54(51–52), Q-1–Q-4.

Parental expectations of children shape children's expectations of themselves and others. Failure to meet parental expectations may contribute to guilt and depression, whereas unrealistic parental expectations may result in inappropriate discipline for behaviors that are normal for a child's or adolescent's developmental stage. For example, parents may expect a 3-year-old child to be toilet trained even at night and punish the child for bedwetting when this is still normal behavior at this age. Parental expectations may also stifle adolescent development. For example, in many Asian cultures, adolescents may be expected to choose an occupation that brings benefit or recognition to the family rather than one in which the adolescent may be personally interested. Such expectations may cause conflict within the family or psychological problems for the adolescent.

Parental Coping and Mental Health

Parental stress levels affect their ability to parent effectively. The number of women with small children in the population may provide indirect information on coping abilities, since child rearing has been found to contribute

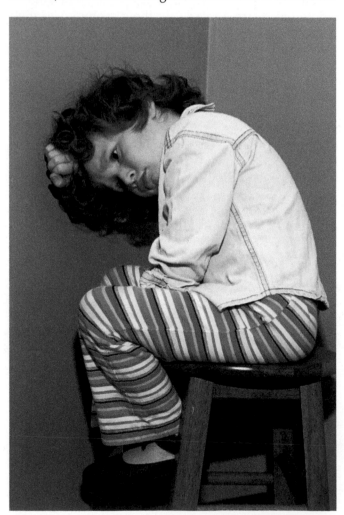

Discipline is frequently a thorny issue in raising children. (Molly Schlachter)

to cumulative stress, and the mental health of women with young children tends to be worse than those without children, particularly when accompanied by low resource levels (Jun, Subramanian, Gortmaker, & Kawachi, 2004). Similarly, the level of mental health problems in the adult population can affect parents' abilities to be effective in caring for their children.

Mental Health Problems Among Children and Adolescents

The frequency and types of mental health problems encountered in children and adolescents also provide information about the health status of these populations. According to the U.S. Department of Health and Human Services (2002), approximately 1 in 10 U.S. children and adolescents has some functional impairment due to mental illness. Only 20% of these children and adolescents receive needed mental health services, and many of them end up in jail. Depression is a significant problem, although depression may be difficult to diagnose in these age groups. Approximately 1 of every 33 children and 1 in 8 adolescents experience significant depression (Childers, 2004). High rates of mental illness in the child and adolescent population may necessitate community health nursing advocacy for effective treatment services. For example, a community health nurse may assist schoolteachers and counselors to set up a program that facilitates identification and referral of depressed students for treatment services.

Abuse

Physical, sexual, and psychological abuse and neglect are other problems that affect the psychological health of children and adolescents. The effects of childhood abuse are many and varied and may include future prostitution, drug and alcohol abuse, and more unprotected sexual activity (Dilorio, Hartwell, & Hansen, 2002). There were approximately 906,000 confirmed cases of child maltreatment in the United States in 2002. Most of these (61%) involved neglect, but physical, sexual, and psychological abuse were also reported. Abused children are at risk for adverse health effects as well as behavior problems as adults.

In 2002, there were 1,500 confirmed deaths due to abuse of U.S. children (National Center for Injury Prevention and Control, 2004a). The homicide rate in the first day of life is 10 times that of any other age period, and more than 9% of homicides occur in the first week of life (Epidemiology Program Office, 2002). Among adolescents 15 to 19 years of age, homicides account for 12.4% of all firearms-related deaths (Federal Interagency Forum on Child and Family Statistics, 2004). In addition, abuse of children and adolescents results in direct judicial, law enforcement, and medical costs of $24 billion a year in the United States. Indirect costs of abuse are estimated at $69 billion per year (National Center for Injury Prevention and Control, 2004a).

ETHICAL AWARENESS

You have encountered a 6-year-old boy who you suspect is being physically abused by his father. The family has come to the United States illegally from Central America. You know that as a nurse you are required by law to report instances of child abuse. You are afraid if you report the abuse, however, that the family will be deported and the child will be blamed for this outcome. In that event, he is likely to be subjected to even more abuse. What would you do in this situation?

Abuse of children is not just a problem in the United States or even in the developed world, but is a worldwide problem. For example, according to the United Nations Population Fund (2003) as many as 20% to 30% of young girls are sexually abused in India, Jamaica, Mali, Tanzania, and Zimbabwe, and 30% of young women in South Africa report that their first sexual experience was forced. In addition, an estimated 700,000 to 4 million women and children are forced into the international sex trade every year in response to conditions of poverty, low social status of women, lax border surveillance, and police collusion. In India, approximately 40% of sex workers are children under the age of 18.

Risk factors and protective factors for abuse are summarized in Table 2◆.

GLOBAL PERSPECTIVES

According to United Nations Population Fund (2003) figures, approximately 130 million girls and young women have been subjected to female genital cutting (FGC), also known as female genital mutilation (FGM) or female circumcision. FGC is a cultural practice in more than 28 countries throughout the world and is designed to control female sexuality. An estimated 6,000 incidents of FGC occur each day. Prevalence estimates range from 5% of young women in the Democratic Republic of Congo to 98% in Somalia. Figures for 1995 indicated that 97% of married women aged 15 to 49 years in Egypt had been subjected to FGC; 1998 figures for Mali were as high as 94%.

Although many countries have laws banning FGC, these laws are often poorly enforced. Recently several countries have begun initiatives to prevent FGC. For example, in Kenya, "circumcision with words" has been advocated. This program provides an alternative rite of passage that preserves positive elements of cultural practices but substitutes a week of seclusion, education, and counseling followed by a community celebration of girls' coming of age. Another program in Senegal, promoted by the organization Tostan, has resulted in agreements by 18% of registered villages to abandon FGC and early marriage.

What is the prevalence of FGC in your community? What cultural groups might promote FGC? What actions have been taken, if any, to prevent FGC? What additional actions are warranted and how could community health nurses be involved in these activities?

TABLE 2	Risk Factors and Protective Factors for Abuse of Children and Adolescents
Risk Factors	**Protective Factors**
▪ Disability or mental retardation among victims	▪ Supportive families
▪ Social isolation of families	▪ Nurturing parenting skills
▪ Parental lack of knowledge/ understanding of child needs and development	▪ Stable family relationships
	▪ Household rules and child monitoring
▪ Family history of domestic abuse	▪ Employment
▪ Poverty/unemployment	▪ Adequate housing
▪ Family disorganization/ intimate partner violence	▪ Access to health and social services
▪ Lack of family cohesion	▪ Adequate role models outside the family
▪ Substance abuse	▪ Supportive communities
▪ Young single-parenthood	
▪ Negative parent–child interactions	
▪ Parental stress or mental illness	
▪ Prevalence of community violence	

Data from: National Center for Injury Prevention and Control. (2004a). Child maltreatment: Fact sheet. Retrieved June 16, 2005, from http://www.cdc.gov/ncipc/factsheets/cmfacts.htm

Physical Environmental Considerations

Children are more susceptible than adults to a variety of environmental pollutants. For example, because their nervous systems are not yet fully developed, young children are more susceptible than adults or older children to the effects of lead poisoning. This may be even more apparent in some population groups. For instance, 30% of refugee children in one study developed elevated blood lead levels after resettlement due to living in older housing contaminated with lead-based paint and the effects of acute and chronic malnutrition due to economic conditions in their countries of origin (National Center for Environmental Health, 2005). Overall, however, the prevalence of elevated blood lead levels has declined significantly in recent years (Meyer et al., 2003).

Insecticide exposure and air pollution are other continuing problems for children and adolescents. From 1997 to 2000, for example, 52% of reported pesticide exposures in the United States occurred in children. An estimated 85% of families store and use pesticides with poisoning potential (Belson et al., 2003). In addition, more than one third of U.S. children in 2002 lived in areas that did not meet one or more National Ambient Air Quality Standards (Federal Interagency Forum on Child and Family Statistics, 2004). Community health nurses should be alert to the presence of environmental pollutants and other hazards and their effects on children.

Safety hazards are another major factor in the physical environment that influences the health of children of all ages. Safety concerns are related to children's physical surroundings and their ability to gain access to dangerous substances. Injuries accounted for 9% of all hospitalizations of children in 2000 (Wise, 2004), and the injury death rate among children aged 5 to 14 years was 17.3 per 100,000 population. Among 1- to 4-year-olds, the injury mortality rate was 33.3 per 100,000 children (Federal Interagency Forum on Child and Family Statistics, 2004). Motor vehicle accidents are, of course, the primary issue with respect to both child and adolescent safety. In 2003, for example, 6 children under 15 years of age were killed each day and 694 injured in motor vehicle accidents. In spite of evidence that use of seat-positioning booster seats results in a 59% decrease in the probability of injury of child passengers, only 22% of states and the District of Columbia have laws requiring booster seat use, and a recent telephone survey indicated that only 21% of 4- to 8-year-olds actually used booster seats (Centers for Disease Control and Prevention [CDC], 2005b). Approximately one fourth of motor vehicle accident deaths in children under 14 years of age involved alcohol use by the driver of the vehicle. In most cases, children riding with drivers who had been drinking were not restrained (Division of Unintentional Injury Prevention, 2004).

Young children are also injured as pedestrians and while riding on bicycles and tricycles. In 2003, for example, more than 7,000 children 1 to 14 years old were injured by a vehicle backing over them, and nearly half of deaths from back-over accidents in children occurred in their own driveways. Injury rates are six times higher for child pedestrians than for those riding bicycles and tricycles (National Center for Injury Prevention and Control, 2005).

Drowning is the second leading cause of death for children aged 1 to 14 years and the seventh cause of death for children of all ages (National Center for Injury Prevention and Control, 2004b). Children under 1 year of age most often drown in the bathtub, buckets, or toilet, whereas among children 1 to 4 years of age, residential swimming pools are the most common avenue for drowning deaths. Among adolescents, alcohol is involved in 25% to 50% of drownings. Approximately three times as many children and adolescents are seen in emergency departments for nonfatal submersion injuries as die (National Center for Injury Prevention and Control, n.d.d). Choking also accounts for significant morbidity in children. In 2001, more than 17,000 children were treated in emergency departments for choking incidents, and it is estimated that one death occurs for each 110 nonfatal episodes of choking (Division of Unintentional Injury Prevention, 2002). Advocacy for child and adolescent safety is an important aspect of community health nursing for this population. In carrying out this advocacy role, community health

nurses might campaign for effective enforcement of seat belt legislation or for gun safety education for local families and youth.

Sociocultural Considerations

A variety of sociocultural factors affect the health of children and adolescents. As we saw earlier, a number of these factors have implications for children's psychological health. In addition, factors such as employment, family income, and education levels affect access to health care services and knowledge of health care needs. For example, in the United States income is strongly associated with infant mortality (Rodwin & Neuberg, 2005) as well as effective control of chronic illness. In 2003, 17.6% of U.S. children were living in poverty, an increase from 16.7% in 2002, and the proportion of those in poverty is higher than for any other age group (U.S. Census Bureau, 2004a). In addition, half of poor children are in families that are considered "severely poor," those with incomes below 50% of the federal poverty level (Wise, 2004). In 2002, 0.8% of children under 18 years of age lived in households that were food insecure, where both adults and children experienced actual hunger at some times. This figure rises to 2.4% of households in poverty (Federal Interagency Forum on Child and Family Statistics, 2004).

Although significant proportions of both elderly and children are affected by poverty, current U.S. policy requires these two groups to compete for resources, with children and adolescents often coming out the losers. For example, the income for elderly persons has risen in recent years, whereas that for families with children has remained flat. In 1967, 37% of social welfare expenditures were directed to services for children. This figure declined to 25% in 1986, and expenditures for the elderly increased from 21% to 33% in the same time period. Actual per capita spending has increased for both groups, but grew 191% for the elderly from 1965 to 1986 compared to only 107% for children and adolescents. Health care providers have voiced concerns regarding allocation decisions that are prompted by political and economic conditions rather than the needs of the groups involved (Newacheck & Benjamin, 2004).

In addition to affecting family income, parental employment may also have other effects on the health of children and adolescents. Although 72% of U.S. children were living in two-parent families in 2003, in many of these families as well as in single-parent families, parents work. In 2002, for example, 55% of women who had given birth to a child in the last year were in the work force (U.S. Census Bureau, 2004b). Working parents may have less time and energy to interact effectively with their children, and children and adolescents may be less effectively supervised by working parents. For instance, in 2001, nearly 3% of children in kindergarten to third grade cared for themselves for at least some portion of the day. Self-care increases with age, with 25% of fourth to eighth graders caring for themselves (Federal Interagency Forum on Child and Family Statistics, 2004).

Parental work schedules have also been shown to affect child and adolescent health and welfare (Strazdins, Korda, Lim, Broom, & D'Souza, 2004). Many parents work nonstandard schedules precisely to allow them to arrange favorable childcare; however, childcare may be less available at nonscheduled times (e.g., during evening and night shifts). Nonstandard work hours also limit parent availability to children when children are home from school and diminish family time. Parents may be prevented from attending many family and community events involving their children, and nonstandard schedules may affect parental sleep and parenting capabilities. In one study, nonstandard parental work schedules were associated with increased likelihood of one or more behavioral or emotional problems in children of all ages. Among 2- to 3-year-olds, children whose parents worked nonstandard hours were more likely to exhibit hyperactivity/inattention, physical aggression, and separation anxiety than those whose parents worked regular hours. Similarly, among 4- to 11-year-olds, children with parents on nonstandard work schedules were more likely to display hyperactivity/inattention and physical aggression, but were also more likely to exhibit conduct disorder and commit property offenses.

Parental education level affects income and knowledge of effective parenting. These effects are compounded when one or more parents do not speak the dominant language of the community. In 2003, 15% of U.S. children had a parent without a high school education, and 20% had at least one foreign-born parent. In 1999, nearly 17% of children and adolescents in the United States spoke a language other than English in their homes, and 5% had difficulty speaking or understanding English (Federal Interagency Forum on Child and Family Statistics, 2004).

Legislation and media are two other important sociocultural factors that influence the health of child and adolescent populations. Legislation may have positive or negative effects. For example, legislation mandating graduated driver licensing requirements for adolescents have been shown to result in stricter limits on driving privileges for adolescents and fewer accidents (Simons-Morton, Hartos, Leaf, & Preusser, 2005). Similarly, legislation regarding immunization of middle

school students has been associated with increased immunity to measles, mumps, and rubella and hepatitis B (Averhoff et al., 2004).

Media coverage and role models are often associated with the assumption of risky behaviors such as smoking, drinking, and sexual activity by adolescents, but media may have beneficial effects as well. For instance, "truth" advertising campaigns that acquainted adolescents with tobacco company documents indicating specific plans to target adolescent markets were credited with a 22% decline in smoking prevalence among youth in one study (Farrelly, Davis, Haviland, Messeri, & Healton, 2005).

Prejudice in the social environment may also affect children. For instance, they may be subjected to ridicule by other children at school because of their dress, physical appearance, family culture, or religion. Family religious affiliation may provide social support, but can also lead to potential health problems. For example, children who receive exemption from immunization on the basis of religious beliefs are 22 times more likely to get measles and 6 times more likely to get pertussis than immunized children. When these children are in childcare or elementary school settings, their risk increases 62-fold and 16-fold, respectively (California Department of Health Services, 2001).

Behavioral Considerations

Several behavioral considerations also affect the health of children and adolescents. Behavioral considerations may relate to behaviors of children and adolescents themselves and those of their parents. Major areas for consideration in the behavioral dimension include nutrition, rest and exercise, and exposure to hazardous substances.

Nutrition

Earlier we noted the need for the community health nurse to assess the extent of poverty and hunger in the population. This is particularly important in developing countries, but should not be neglected in the United States and other areas of the developed world where poverty affects certain subgroups within the population. In the United States, however, nutritional deficits are more likely to reflect the lack of specific nutrients or caloric excess.

Community health nurses should be alert to child feeding practices in the community such as the extent to which newborns are breast-fed or bottle-fed, the availability of fast food in the community, and the extent to which families frequent fast food establishments. Exclusive breast-feeding for the first 6 months is the recommended dietary standard for infants. Based on data from the 1991–1994 National Health and Nutrition Examination Survey (NHANES), however, less than half of children (47%) were exclusively breast-fed at 7 days after birth. This figure declined to 10% at 6 months (Li, Ogden, Ballew, Gillespie, & Grummer-Strawn, 2002). Less exclusive breast-feeding has been associated with increased

CULTURAL COMPETENCE

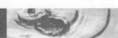

*C*hild-rearing practices can vary significantly from one cultural group to another. Differences in child-rearing practices can create problems when cultures interact with each other or when members of ethnic cultural groups interact with health care professionals. What are some examples of these types of cross-cultural difficulties involving ethnic groups in your area? How might they be addressed?

asthma and atopic conditions (e.g., atopic dermatitis) in children as well as other adverse effects (Oddy et al., 2004). Breast-feeding is strongly influenced by cultural beliefs and practices and with a family's degree of acculturation.

Dietary practices are also important among toddlers and older children and adolescents. Although the quality of diets improved slightly among preschool children in the United States from 1977 to 1998, there remains a need to increase consumption of fruits and vegetables and decrease total and saturated fat intake, juice, and sugar (Kranz, Siega-Riz, & Herring, 2004). In 1999–2000, approximately 20% of children aged 2 to 6 years consumed a healthy diet, compared to only 8% of those aged 7 to 12 years and 4% of adolescents. Conversely, 6%, 13%, and 19%, respectively, had poor diets. The vast majority of children at all age groups had diets that needed improvement in one or more areas (Federal Interagency Forum on Child and Family Statistics, 2004).

Obesity is a common problem related to diet and nutrition in the United States and worldwide. According to NHANES data, the prevalence of obesity in 6- to 11-year-olds increased threefold from 1960 to 2000 (Thorpe et al., 2004). The focused assessment provided below can be used to assess the nutritional status of individual children or can be adapted for use with groups of children in specific age ranges.

Rest and Exercise

Problems of obesity can be combated by adequate exercise as well as healthier diets, yet few children and adolescents engage in recommended levels of physical activity. In 2002, for example, the Youth Media Campaign Longitudinal Survey (YMCLS) found that 61.5% of U.S. children aged 9 to 13 years did not participate in any organized physical activity outside of school, and 22.6% did not engage in any free-time physical activity (National Center for Chronic Disease Prevention and Health Promotion, 2003). Many public health professionals have called for an increase in physical education in schools to promote physical activity among school-age children and adolescents (Datar & Sturm, 2004). Special attention should be given to the activity needs of children with chronic illness and handicapping disabilities. For example, children with asthma were found in one study to have higher basal metabolic indices due to reduced activity as a result of their reactive airway disease (Oddy et al., 2004). Again, community health nurses can advocate for age-appropriate physical activities for children and adolescents.

Exposure to Hazardous Substances

Exposure of children and adolescents to hazardous substances (e.g., lead) in the physical environment was addressed earlier; however, children and adolescents are exposed to other hazardous substances through

FOCUSED ASSESSMENT

Assessing the Nutritional Status of Children and Adolescents

Infant (birth–1 year)

- Is the infant breast- or bottle-fed?
  - If breast-fed,
    - How often does the infant nurse?
    - How long does the infant nurse?
    - Does the mother alternate breasts?
    - Is the mother's nutritional intake adequate?
    - Does the infant seem satisfied?
  - If bottle-fed,
    - How often does the infant eat?
    - How much formula is consumed in 24 hours?
    - What type of formula is used? Is it iron fortified?
    - Do caretakers prepare formula correctly?
    - Do caretakers use appropriate feeding techniques (e.g., not propping the bottle)?
    - Does the infant tolerate the formula well?
- Is the infant gaining weight?
- At what point did parents introduce solids?
- How much solid food does the infant eat?
- Do parents use individual foods rather than less nutritious combination foods (such as vegetable and beef combinations)?
- Is one new food introduced at a time? Over several days?
- Has the 1-year-old started eating table food?
- Is the child weaned from the bottle by 1 year?

Toddler, preschool, and school-age child (2–10 years)

- What foods is the child eating?
- How much food is the child eating?
- Is the child's diet well-balanced?
- Is the child eating the recommended number of daily servings of fruits, vegetables, and grains?
- Is the child's diet low in saturated fat and sodium?
- Is the child's calcium and iron intake adequate?
- Are any snacks provided nutritious?
- Is the child's growth pattern normal for his or her age?

Additional questions for preadolescent and adolescent (11–18 years)

- Is protein and calcium intake adequate to accommodate growth spurts?
- Is iron intake sufficient to accommodate blood loss in menstruating girls?
- Is the preadolescent/adolescent overweight or underweight for his or her height?
- Does the preadolescent/adolescent engage in food fads?
- Does the preadolescent/adolescent engage in binge eating or purging?
- Is the preadolescent/adolescent excessively concerned about body size?

their own behavior or that of parents and other family members. For example, in 2002, more than 11% of women giving birth in the United States smoked during their pregnancies (Division of Reproductive Health, 2004a). Although this represents a decline in maternal smoking of 38% from 1990 to 2002, many infants continue to be adversely affected by maternal smoking during pregnancy. Smoking during pregnancy is associated with poor birth outcomes and health problems such as increased gastric reflux, colic, sudden infant death syndrome (SIDS), and lower respiratory tract infections (Gaffney, 2001) as well as more than 900 infant deaths per year from 1997 to 2001 (Office on Smoking and Health, 2005a). In addition to the physical effects of fetal exposure to tobacco smoke, maternal smoking during pregnancy has been associated with behavioral problems in children (Wakschlag, Pickett, Cook, Benowitz, & Leventhal, 2002).

Maternal smoking during pregnancy also has significant economic effects on families and on society. In 1996 alone, smoking-attributable neonatal expenditures amounted to $366 million, roughly $704 for every woman who smoked during pregnancy (Division of Reproductive Health, 2004b). Smoking also has preconceptual effects and has been associated with infertility and delay in conception (Division of Reproductive Health, 2004a). Maternal smoking during pregnancy decreases with increasing levels of education. For example, fewer than 3% of college-educated women smoked during pregnancy, compared to 27% of those without a high school diploma. Lower rates of smoking cessation and higher rates of relapse are also associated with lower education levels (Jun et al., 2004).

Children and adolescents are not just exposed to the effects of smoking in utero. An estimated 30% to 60% of U.S. children under 5 years of age are exposed to tobacco smoke in the home (Gaffney, 2001), and in 1999, 19% of children under 7 years of age lived in a home with a regular smoker (Federal Interagency Forum on Child and Family Statistics, 2004). In addition, children and adolescents themselves may smoke or use other forms of tobacco. In 2004, for example, nearly 12% of middle school children and 28% of high school students reported tobacco use (Office on Smoking and Health, 2005b). In 2003, 5% of eighth graders, 9% of tenth graders, and 16% of twelfth graders smoked daily, and although these figures are not good, they are the lowest recorded since children in these grade levels began to be surveyed (Federal Interagency Forum on Child and Family Statistics, 2004).

Children and adolescents may also be exposed to alcohol and other drugs. **Fetal alcohol syndrome (FAS)** is a condition resulting from maternal alcohol consumption during pregnancy and is characterized by growth retardation, facial malformations, and central nervous system dysfunctions that may include mental retardation. FAS is also associated with spontaneous abortion, ectopic pregnancy, stillbirth, fetal death, low birth weight, preterm delivery, and intrauterine growth retardation. Other potential effects of FAS include placenta previa, abruptio placenta, premature rupture of membranes, and increased risk of SIDS in the infant (Beck, Morrow, Lipscomb, & Johnson, 2002).

FAS is a growing problem in many areas of the world. For example, although the rate of FAS in the United States is relatively low (0.3 to 1.5 per 1,000 live births), it is as high as 40.5 to 46.4 per 1,000 births in South Africa (National Center on Birth Defects and Developmental Disabilities, 2003). Even though U.S. rates of FAS are relatively low, approximately 5,000 infants each year are affected (CDC, 2004a), and its prevalence is likely to be underestimated due to failure to diagnose affected infants (Division of Birth Defects and Developmental Disabilities, 2002). The prevalence of alcohol use during pregnancy actually increased from 12.4% of pregnant women in 1991 to 16.3% in 1995 before dropping back down to 12.8% in 1999 (National Center on Birth Defects and Developmental Disabilities, 2002). Exposure to other drugs (e.g., cocaine) or infectious agents, such as herpes or HIV, may also occur during pregnancy, putting infants at risk for a variety of serious health consequences.

Alcohol-related neurodevelopmental disorders (ARNDs) and alcohol-related birth defects (ARBDs) are three times more common than FAS. Immediate effects of these perinatal exposures to alcohol include poor intrauterine growth, small stature, facial abnormalities, poor coordination, hyperactivity, and sleep and suck problems in infancy. Long-term consequences may include learning disabilities, speech and language delays, difficulties performing activities of daily living, and poor judgment and reasoning abilities. Perinatal alcohol exposure also places those affected at higher risk for psychiatric problems, crime, unemployment, and school dropout. FAS and other effects can be prevented by encouraging pregnant women to refrain from alcohol and drug use during pregnancy. For those children affected, early enrollment in special education programs can help mitigate the long-term effects of perinatal alcohol exposure (National Center on Birth Defects and Developmental Disabilities, 2004d).

As with tobacco, children and adolescents may expose themselves to alcohol and other drugs. In 2002, for example, nearly 12% of 12- to 17-year-olds reported being current users of illicit drugs (U.S. Census Bureau, 2004b). In 2003, 10% of eighth graders, 20% of tenth graders, and 24% of twelfth graders reported illicit drug use. Again, these are some of the lowest figures reported since 1993. Similar figures were noted for heavy drinking among children and adolescents—12% of eighth graders, 22% of tenth graders, and 28% of twelfth graders (Federal Interagency Forum on Child and Family Statistics, 2004).

Sexual Activity

Adolescent sexual activity can have a profound influence on health in this population group, particularly in terms of unwanted pregnancy and sexually transmitted diseases (STDs). Adolescent boys generally initiate sexual activity earlier than girls, with an average age of initiation of sexual intercourse by boys at 16.9 years and girls at 17.4 years (Alan Guttmacher Institute, 2002). According to the 2001 Youth Risk Behavior Surveillance System (YRBSS), 45.6% of U.S. high school students reported engaging in sexual intercourse. Boys were more likely to report intercourse than girls (48.5% versus 42.9%). Black and Hispanic students were more likely than White students to have had intercourse. A small percentage (6.6%) of students initiated sexual activity prior to 13 years of age, and boys were more than twice as likely as girls to initiate early sexual activity. Among those students who were sexually active at the time of the survey, only 57.9% reported condom use during their last episode of intercourse, and only 18% of respondents or their partners used oral contraceptives. Black students were more likely than White and Hispanic students to report condom use, but White students were more likely to report use of oral contraceptives. One fourth of the sexually active students reported that alcohol or drug use preceded their last sexual intercourse (Grunbaum et al., 2002).

Nearly 5% of high school students in the 2001 YRBSS reported having been pregnant or gotten someone else pregnant. Pregnancy was more likely among minority adolescents than their White counterparts (Grunbaum et al., 2002). In 2001, 18% of legal abortions occurred among girls 19 years of age and under. This amounted to a total of 138,000 abortions, more than 4,700 of which occurred in girls under 15 years of age. Abortions were performed in approximately three fourths of pregnancies in girls under age 15 and two thirds in girls 19 years of age or younger (Strauss et al., 2004).

Although one usually thinks of adolescent pregnancy as primarily affecting girls, boys are also involved. Approximately 2% of U.S. births and 5% of abortions involve boys 15 to 17 years of age, and another 5% and 8%, respectively, involve young men 18 to 19 years of age (Alan Guttmacher Institute, 2002). Pregnancy poses significant health risks for adolescent girls and may delay or impede educational and vocational plans for both boys and girls. Community health nurses may need to advocate for effective sexuality education for boys and girls as well as for access to condoms and contraceptive services for those who are sexually active.

Violence

Earlier we discussed the effects of abuse on children and adolescents, but these population groups are exposed to and may participate in other forms of violence as well.

For example, in 2003, 33% of high school students participating in the YRBSS reported being involved in a physical fight in the previous year. Boys were more likely than girls to report involvement in fighting (40.5% versus 25.1%). Fortunately, these figures have declined somewhat from 1991 reports (50.2% for boys and 34.4% for girls). Similarly, somewhat fewer students reported carrying weapons in 2003 (17%) than in 1991 (26%), but more students reported being threatened with a weapon in 2003 (9.2%) than in 1991 (7.3%), and more students did not attend school in 2003 than in 1991 because of safety concerns (5.4% versus 4.4%) (Division of Violence Prevention, 2004).

Health System Considerations

A number of factors in the health care delivery system influence the health of children and adolescents. Some of these factors include attitudes toward health and health care, usual sources of health care, and use of health care services. In 2002, only half of children with special health needs had a regular source of health care (Wise, 2004), and many well children do not have a regular source of care or a "medical home." A medical home is a regular source of health care that is characterized by access to preventive care, 24-hour availability of ambulatory and inpatient care, continuity, access to subspecialty referrals and interaction between providers and school and community agencies as needed, and maintenance of a central health record for the child.

Poor children, in particular, may lack a regular source of care, relying on emergency departments for care. This practice increases the costs of care and decreases opportunities for basic preventive and health-promotive services. Emergency departments have, however, been shown to be effective places for recruiting children who are eligible for the State Child Health Insurance Program (SCHIP) (Gordon, Emond, & Camargo, 2005). Having a regular source of care is impeded by reimbursement patterns of federal insurance programs for children. Welfare reform efforts have contributed to periods of uninsurance for low-income families including children (Holl, Slack, & Stevens, 2005).

In 2003, 8.4 million U.S. children (11.4%) had no health insurance coverage (U.S. Census Bureau, 2004a), another 5.8 million were enrolled in SCHIP, and slightly more than 17 million were insured by Medicaid (U.S. Census Bureau, 2004b). In 2002, Medicaid covered one fifth of all U.S. children and 40% of children in low-income families. In addition, Medicaid paid for the care of 70% of children with chronic disabilities (Klein, Stoll, & Bruce, 2004). By June 2004, SCHIP enrollment had declined to 3.7 million children due to state legislative changes limiting eligibility and enrollment and increasing premiums and cost-sharing provisions for children of low-income families (Blewett, Davern, & Rodin, 2004).

ASSESSING THE HEALTH STATUS OF CHILD AND ADOLESCENT POPULATIONS

Community health nurses provide services to individual children and adolescents and their families as well as to these populations as aggregates. Whether services are provided to individuals or population groups, community health nurses must first assess their health status and health needs. The focus of this chapter is on meeting the needs of children and adolescents as population groups. A tool for assessing the health of an individual child or adolescent is provided in Appendix H on the Companion Website and in the *Community Assessment Reference Guide* designed as a companion volume to this text. Here we will focus on the assessment of populations of children and adolescents using the dimensions of health as a framework.

In assessing the health of child and adolescent populations, the nurse would gather data on rates of growth and the prevalence of departures from normal growth. For example, the nurse might examine the records of school-aged children to determine the proportion of children above or below normal parameters for height and weight. The prevalence of obesity in these populations would also be determined. The incidence of maturational problems such as developmental retardation could be extrapolated from the number of children with these problems in schools or in interviews with physicians and others who provide health services to these children.

Information on sexual maturity, as well as on attitudes toward sexual maturity and sexual activity, has implications for the prevention of adolescent pregnancy and sexually transmitted diseases, and can be determined in interviews with community informants such as school officials and members of religious groups as well as in general community surveys. Community health nurses may also assess the knowledge of adults in the community with respect to normal maturation and development in children and adolescents. Armed with this information, community health nurses can design programs for parents that promote effective child and adolescent growth and development and provide anticipatory guidance for parents in dealing with developmental transitions experienced by their children. **Anticipatory guidance** involves providing information to parents and others regarding behavioral expectations of children and adolescents at a specific age, before they reach that age.

Community health nurses should also be familiar with the gender and ethnic composition of the child and adolescent populations in their communities. They would also obtain information on the prevalence of conditions with a tendency to genetic transmission (e.g., sickle cell disease or diabetes) in their communities in order to begin primary preventive services for conditions with high prevalence during childhood. Gender, racial, and ethnic composition of the child and adolescent population is available from census figures. The prevalence of some genetically transmitted conditions may be calculated by local health authorities, but may also be available from voluntary organizations specializing in these diseases.

Child and adolescent mortality data can be obtained from the local health department, which may also provide information on the incidence and prevalence of certain conditions in these populations. For example, the incidence of gonorrhea in the adolescent population would be available from health department sources. Data on other forms of morbidity for which official figures are not collected may be available from voluntary organizations or health care providers in the community. For example, information on the incidence and prevalence of diabetes in children and adolescents may be available from the local chapter of the American Diabetes Association. Similarly, school systems may have data on the number of school absences related to childhood asthma. Local hospitals and other health care agencies may have figures on the numbers of children and adolescents seen with specific conditions.

Information on the level of child and adolescent immunization in the population may be obtained from local health departments, schools, preschools, or clinics and physicians' offices that provide primary care services. Conversely, incidence rates for immunizable childhood diseases are available from local and state health departments. Assessment of biophysical factors affecting the health of children and adolescents can be guided by the focused assessment questions provided below.

Psychological dimension factors would also be assessed in determining the health status of the child

FOCUSED ASSESSMENT

Biophysical Considerations Influencing Child and Adolescent Health

- What is the age composition of the child and adolescent population?
- What is the gender composition of the child and adolescent population?
- What is the racial/ethnic composition of the child and adolescent population?
- What are the gender-specific attitudes and expectations regarding boys and girls in the population?
- What is the extent of growth retardation in the child and adolescent population?
- What is the extent of developmental delay in the child and adolescent population? What are the typical causes of delays?
- What are cause-specific child and adolescent mortality rates in the population?
- What are the rates of morbidity for specific acute and chronic health problems in the child and adolescent population?
- What is the level of immunization coverage in the child and adolescent population?

and adolescent populations. With the individual child or adolescent, the community health nurse would assess family dynamics. When assessing the health of children and adolescents as a population group, however, similar kinds of information about family dynamics (e.g., role structure, communication patterns, authority) are often not available. The nurse can, however, obtain information related to the sociocultural dimension, such as the prevalence of divorce and single-parent families, that may provide some insights into family dynamics that contribute to mental health or illness in children and adolescents.

In a similar vein, there will probably be no specific aggregate data available regarding parental expectations and discipline as there would be if a community health nurse were assessing an individual child or adolescent. However, the nurse can extrapolate inferences about parental expectations and discipline from knowledge of cultural attitudes, beliefs, and behaviors toward parenthood and child rearing among cultural and ethnic groups in the community. How are children generally viewed within the cultures represented in the population? How is discipline typically handled? Do disciplinary practices or typical parental expectations of children have any implications for the health of the child and adolescent populations in the community? The answers to these and other similar questions are best derived from observations in the community and through interviews with knowledgeable community informants.

Aggregate information is also unlikely to be available regarding the extent of coping among parents of children and adolescents in the population. The community health nurse can, however, make inferences based on data regarding stressors encountered by parents. For example, family size, the extent of single-parenthood, and other sociocultural factors faced by parents contribute to stress, which may tax coping abilities.

Community health nurses could obtain information on the extent of mental health problems in the child and adolescent population from psychiatric facilities in the area as well as from interviews with school counselors and other mental health service providers. Similar information can also be obtained with respect to mental health problems among adults in the community since many of these adults will be the parents of the child and adolescent populations.

Community health nurses should examine the incidence and prevalence of abuse of children and adolescents in their jurisdictions. Data on abuse will be available from local child protective service agencies as well as from police files. In addition, nurses should be alert to the presence of factors in the population that promote child and adolescent abuse and those that are protective against abuse, as indicated in Table 2◆. The focused assessment provided above right includes questions that can guide assessment of psychological factors affecting the health of the child and adolescent population.

FOCUSED ASSESSMENT

Psychological Considerations Influencing Child and Adolescent Health

- What is the extent of mental illness in the child and adolescent population? Among parents?
- What are the cultural expectations of children and adolescents in the population? To what extent do these expectations create stress for children and adolescents?
- What is the suicide rate among children and adolescents in the population?
- What are the typical approaches to discipline in the population?
- What is the extent of abuse in the child and adolescent population? What forms of abuse are prevalent? What factors contribute to abuse of children and adolescents? What is the attitude of the population to abuse of children and adolescents?

With respect to the physical environmental dimension, community health nurses should assess both the presence of hazardous conditions in the environment and public knowledge of safety-related behaviors. A tool to assess safety hazards in the environment of individual children is provided in the *Community Assessment Reference Guide* ▓ designed to accompany this text.

Community health nurses should obtain information on the morbidity and mortality resulting from child and adolescent safety hazards as well as the types of injuries occurring in their communities. Mortality data will be available from the local health department as well as from insurance departments. Both mortality data and information on nonfatal injuries among children and adolescents may be obtained from local emergency departments, poison control centers, and health care providers. Information on safety hazards present in the community can be derived from observations by community health nurses or in community surveys. A focused assessment for the physical environmental dimension is included below.

Community health nurses assessing the health of the child and adolescent populations would also obtain information related to the sociocultural dimension such as local income, employment, and education levels. Much of this information is available in census data or from local social service agencies. Employment figures

FOCUSED ASSESSMENT

Physical Environmental Considerations Influencing Child and Adolescent Health

- What safety hazards are present in the community? How do they affect the health of the child and adolescent population?
- How adequate is family housing in the community?
- What environmental pollutants are present in the community? How do they affect the health of the child and adolescent population?

may also be available from local government offices or employment agencies.

Parental education levels have implications for health knowledge and behaviors as well as for child performance in school and later success as adults, and community health nurses should assess the extent to which these factors exist in their communities and the effects they have on the health of children and adolescents in the community. Community health nurses should also examine high school completion rates among adolescents as well as the percentage of younger children held back in one or more grades. Such information can be obtained from local school officials or from state boards of education.

Community health nurses can also observe the quality of health-related messages provided through advertising, news coverage, and other media. Driving through the community or perusing magazines and newspapers read by children and adolescents in the community can provide some sense of the kind and level of negative advertising to which they are exposed as well as the presence of positive health-related messages. An overview of local television programming can provide similar information.

Information related to intergroup conflicts and discriminatory practices in the community that may affect the health of children and adolescents can be derived from a review of local news articles. School officials may also provide insight into racial or ethnic group conflicts that may affect the health of children and adolescents. The prevalence of fighting and other forms of violence involving children or adolescents may also be determined from school informants or local police data. Information on religious affiliations in the community can be suggested by perusal of the telephone directory. Insights into religious attitudes and practices that may influence the health of children and adolescents is best derived from interviews and other interactions with knowledgeable members of local groups and congregations. Community health nurses should also be aware of the extent of religious exemptions related to immunization and the potential effects of such exemptions. Assessment of sociocultural factors influencing child and adolescent health can be guided by the focused assessment questions provided at right.

With respect to the behavioral dimension of health, community health nurses would assess the nutritional status of children and adolescents in the community. Knowledge of basic dietary patterns of cultural subgroups in the population may be obtained from observation or interviews with knowledgeable community informants. Nurses can also assess the nutritional content of school lunch menus or observe purchases made in local grocery stores. Community health nurses should also assess the extent of dietary problems among children and adolescents, such as obesity or malnutrition, as well as the factors that contribute to those

 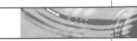
problems. Height and weight screening of children and adolescents in school settings can provide some of this data. Community health nurses should also be knowledgeable regarding infant feeding practices prevalent in the community and promote breast-feeding whenever possible. Again, this type of information may vary among cultural groups in the community and can best be obtained through observation or interviews with members of different ethnic groups.

Community health nurses will also assess the opportunities provided in the community for physical activity by children and adolescents as well as the actual levels of activity exhibited. School curricula can be examined for their inclusion of physical activities. The extent of participation in sports activities can also be determined. Other information on opportunities for recreational activities can be obtained from the telephone book and from observations of children at play in parks and neighborhoods.

Assessment of the health status of child and adolescent populations would also include information related to the incidence of hazardous substance exposures discussed earlier as well as types of exposures and their effects on the health of children and adolescents. Tobacco use by adolescents can be determined by observation in areas where they "hang out." Community surveys may also be used to provide information on tobacco, drug, and alcohol use. Police records may contain information on the number of adolescents arrested for crimes involving alcohol or drug use.

Community health nurses working with adolescent populations would also assess the extent of sexual activity and unsafe sexual practices (e.g., failure to protect against STDs or pregnancy) within the population. In addition, they would determine the rate of adolescent pregnancy and the availability of health and other services needed to meet the needs of pregnant adolescents and those who are sexually active. Adolescent pregnancy rates would be available from the local health department or from labor and delivery units of area hospitals. Data related to sexual practices would best be obtained by surveys of adolescent populations.

Rates of violence among children and adolescents are another aspect of assessing the health of these populations. Community health nurses might obtain data from local school officials regarding the extent of physical fighting on campuses. Police records might also indicate the extent to which children and adolescents are perpetrators or victims of violence in the local community. Behavioral considerations in child and adolescent health can be explored using the focused assessment questions provided below.

Community health nurses assessing the health status of child and adolescent populations will obtain information on the relative percentage of children without health insurance as well as those who have public or private sources of insurance coverage. Community health nurses can also determine the number of children seen for nonemergency purposes in emergency departments. Information on the use of health-promotive and illness-preventive services (e.g., utilization of immunization services, dental services, etc.) by children and adolescents can also be obtained from agencies and facilities that provide these services. Local Medicaid offices would have information on the number of children and adolescents with Medicaid coverage, and health care providers and emergency departments

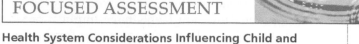

FOCUSED ASSESSMENT

Health System Considerations Influencing Child and Adolescent Health
- What percentage of the child and adolescent population has a regular source of health care?
- What is the extent of insurance coverage in the child and adolescent population?
- How adequate are available health services in meeting the needs of the child and adolescent population?
- To what extent do health care needs of the child and adolescent population go unmet?
- To what extent does the child and adolescent population make use of available health promotion and illness prevention services?

could provide information on the number of children seen who have no insurance coverage. The focused assessment provided above can guide the assessment of health system factors influencing child and adolescent health.

DIAGNOSTIC REASONING AND THE HEALTH OF CHILD AND ADOLESCENT POPULATIONS

Based on the data gathered in the assessment of the child or adolescent population, the community health nurse derives diagnoses or statements based on health status and health care needs. Both positive and problem-focused nursing diagnoses may be derived from the data obtained. Diagnoses may reflect the need for primary, secondary, or tertiary preventive measures. For example, a positive community nursing diagnosis related to primary prevention is "high immunization levels due to high parental motivation and access to immunization services." On the other hand, a problem-focused nursing diagnosis related to immunizations is "lack of appropriate immunizations for age due to lack of access to low-cost immunizations." Another problem-focused nursing diagnosis for the population related to primary prevention is "increased potential for child abuse due to widespread unemployment and increased community incidence of mental health problems."

Nursing diagnoses related to secondary prevention are necessarily problem focused because secondary prevention is warranted when actual health problems exist. An example of a nursing diagnosis for the child population might be "lack of services available in the community to meet the needs of children with developmental problems." For adolescents, a relevant nursing diagnosis might be "increased incidence of adolescent pregnancy due to widespread sexual activity, lack of effective sexuality education, and lack of access to contraceptive services." Nursing diagnoses at the population level might also reflect physical environmental, psychological, sociocultural, or behavioral

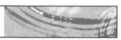

FOCUSED ASSESSMENT

Behavioral Considerations Influencing Child and Adolescent Health
- What are the dietary patterns typical of children and adolescents in the community?
- What are the physical activity patterns typical of children and adolescents in the community?
- What recreational activities are available to the child and adolescent population? What health benefits and hazards are posed by recreational activities?
- What are the effects of dietary and physical activity patterns on the health of the child and adolescent population?
- What is the extent of child and adolescent exposure to tobacco in the home? To use of other substances?
- What is the extent of tobacco, alcohol, and drug use among the child and adolescent population?
- What is the extent of sexual activity among children and adolescents?
- To what extent is safety instruction (including sexual safety) provided to children and adolescents?
- What is the extent, if any, of female genital mutilation among adolescent girls?
- To what extent do children and adolescents engage in effective safety practices (e.g., seat belt use, protective recreational equipment, condom use).

considerations affecting children's and adolescents' overall health status.

At the level of tertiary prevention, nursing diagnoses focus on the need to prevent complications of existing problems or to prevent the recurrence of problems. For example, the nurse might derive nursing diagnoses of "lack of respite for families of children with chronic health problems" or "barriers to effective participation in physical activity by children with handicapping conditions."

PLANNING AND IMPLEMENTING HEALTH CARE FOR CHILD AND ADOLESCENT POPULATIONS

Just as the nursing diagnoses derived from an assessment of child or adolescent health may reflect health problems at primary, secondary, and/or tertiary levels of prevention, interventions may be planned at each level to address identified health needs of children or adolescents.

Primary Prevention

A number of general interventions may be used to promote the health of children and adolescents or to prevent the development of health problems. These categories of intervention all reflect primary prevention and include assuring access to health care; preventing prematurity, low birth weight, and infant mortality; promoting growth and development; providing adequate nutrition; promoting physical activity; promoting safety; preventing communicable diseases; promoting dental care; supporting effective parenting; and other primary prevention activities.

Assuring Access to Health Care
One of the best means of promoting the health of children and adolescents is to ensure that they have access to needed health care services. Community health nurses can be instrumental in linking individual children and adolescents to needed services and in assuring that health services are available to these population groups. This can be accomplished by implementing several strategies that have been recommended for improving child health in general and reducing disparities in health status among subpopulations of children and adolescents. These strategies include the following:

- Assuring that all children and adolescents have a regular source of primary health care
- Eliminating copayments and cost sharing for primary care services
- Establishing disincentives for seeking health care directly from specialists
- Including assessment of the adequacy of primary care services in all quality assurance activities
- Supporting the education of primary care providers

- Developing information systems to monitor health activities and detect differences among subpopulations of children and adolescents (Starfield, 2004)

Implementing these strategies at the level of the individual child or adolescent will usually require referral to an effective source of primary health care. Implementation may also involve referral for public insurance programs such as SCHIP or Medicaid for those children and adolescents who are eligible for these programs. At the population level, implementing these strategies will most likely require community health nurses to be politically active in advocating and planning for services to meet identified child and adolescent health care needs.

Preventing Prematurity, Low Birth Weight, and Infant Mortality
Another approach to primary prevention with children and adolescents is action to reduce rates of prematurity, low birth weight, and infant mortality. Premature birth and low birth weight are two of the major contributors to infant mortality worldwide. In 2002, infant mortality was highest in Afghanistan at 189 deaths per 1,000 live births. Mortality among children under 5 years of age was greatest in Angola, with 262 deaths for every 1,000 live births (World Health Organization, 2004). In the United States, total infant mortality for that year was considerably lower, at 7 per 1,000 live births, but varied greatly among subpopulations. For example, the infant mortality rate was more than twice as high among non-Hispanic Blacks (13.9 per 1,000) as among non-Hispanic Whites (5.8 per 1,000). Higher rates were also seen among Hawaiian (9.6), Native American (8.6), and Puerto Rican infants (8.2). Lower infant mortality rates were noted among other ethnic populations, with the lowest seen among Chinese infants (3 per 1,000) (CDC, 2005b). In 2000, the United States ranked 25th among developed nations with respect to infant mortality and 33rd in relation to deaths among children under 5 years of age. The lower ratings of the United States when compared to other industrialized countries are thought to be a result of greater income disparities among U.S. families, the absence of universal health care, and the existence of policies inimical to effective primary health care (e.g., lack of regular source of care, frequent changes in insurance status among low-income families, etc.) (Starfield, 2004).

Although progress has been made in this area, with an 11% decrease in overall infant mortality in the United States from 1995 to 2001 (NCHS, 2005c), much remains to be done, both with respect to infant mortality and its primary underlying causes. In 2002, for example, low birth weight (LBW) babies accounted for 7.8% of all births in the United States. Adolescent mothers are more likely than older mothers to have a low birth weight baby. For example, in 2002, 13.8% of babies born to girls under 15 years of age and 9.9% of those born to girls aged 15 to 19 years were LBW compared to only 7.1% of mothers

25 to 29 years of age. Mothers who smoked during pregnancy also had a higher percentage of LBW babies than nonsmokers (12% vs. 7.5%). (U.S. Census Bureau, 2004b). Very low birth weight (VLBW) babies (those born weighing less than 3 pounds 4 ounces or 1,500 grams) have a 75% to 100% greater risk of death in the first month of life than normal weight babies (Regional Perinatal Programs of California, 2004). Although VLBW babies account for only 2% of all U.S. births, they contribute to 68% of neonatal deaths, and survivors have multiple problems throughout life (Wise, 2004).

Babies born prematurely are often of low or very low birth weight. In addition to contributing to death, prematurity and low birth weight start young children off at a disadvantage that may or may not be overcome in later years. For example, in one longitudinal study in New Zealand, babies born prior to 32 weeks gestation were found to make greater health care service demands and were six times more likely to be hospitalized in childhood than those born at term. In addition, 32% of these children required state-funded special education services (Olsen & Maslin-Prothero, 2001). In another study, extremely preterm infants had higher rates of cognitive impairment, mild to severe disability, and cerebral palsy than age mates born at full term (Marlow, Wolke, Bracewell, & Samara, 2005).

In spite of the overall decline in infant morality in the United States (45% from 1980 to 2000), the percentage of LBW babies has actually increased by nearly 12% and VLBW by more than 24% during the same period (Division of Reproductive Health, 2002). An estimated 200 VLBW babies are born each day in the United States (Nisbet, 2004). Both prematurity and low birth weight and subsequent infant mortality can be prevented by a group of community health nursing interventions including delayed pregnancy, early and effective prenatal care, adequate prenatal nutrition, and prevention of smoking during pregnancy. According to the Pregnancy Risk Assessment Monitoring System, in 1999 one third to one half of all pregnancies in the United States were unintended. These figures were even higher for women with lower educational levels. In 2002, 82% of legal abortions occurred among unmarried women, and slightly more than 18% occurred in girls younger than 19 years of age (Strauss et al., 2004). Each year approximately half a million teenage girls give birth in the United States. The direct societal costs of adolescent pregnancies for welfare, Medicaid, and foster care services are estimated at $6.9 billion per year (Koniak-Griffin, Anderson, Verzemnieks, & Brecht, 2000). Community health nurses can educate the public, particularly adolescents, regarding sexuality and contraception to prevent unintended pregnancies. In addition, they can advocate for effective and accessible contraceptive services for adolescents and other women of childbearing age. They may also need to ensure that services are available to provide care to pregnant teens and to support them in their role as parents. Particular attention is needed to see that adolescent mothers continue to meet their own personal developmental tasks as well as meeting those of their children. This may necessitate advocacy on the part of community health nurses for educational assistance and other support services for adolescent parents.

For women who carry their pregnancies to term, approximately 16% to 30% receive late or no prenatal care (Beck et al., 2002). Community health nurses can refer individual clients to prenatal services and engage in political advocacy to make sure that such services are available to all women of childbearing age. They can also educate the public regarding the need for adequate prenatal care.

In addition to promoting prenatal care, community health nurses can educate pregnant women regarding the need for good nutrition during pregnancy and make referrals for supplemental nutrition programs such as the Supplemental Nutrition Program for Women, Infants, and Children (WIC). WIC participation among pregnant women has been associated with a decreased incidence of low birth weight (Kowaleski-Jones & Duncan, 2002).

Promoting Growth and Development

To develop properly, children need an environment conducive to growth and development. Community health nurses can assist parents and communities in creating such environments. They can educate both the general public and specific families regarding developmental milestones children and adolescents need to accomplish. They can alert parents to the challenges posed by these milestones through anticipatory guidance, discussed earlier. Community health nurses can also advocate for community programs and environmental conditions that promote growth and development within safe parameters. For example, they can promote sports appropriate to children's abilities and developmental levels and foster the use of effective safety equipment in such programs. In addition, nurses can advocate for humanistic educational programs that

BUILDING OUR KNOWLEDGE BASE

A study by Koniak-Griffin, Anderson, Verzemnieks, and Brecht (2000) found that home visits by community health nurses to pregnant adolescents had no significant effects in terms of type of delivery (vaginal or caesarean) or birth weight among their infants, but did result in fewer days of birth-related hospitalizations and rehospitalizations for the infants. In addition, the group of adolescent mothers who were visited by community health nurses had better educational outcomes than those who were not visited. How might you replicate this study to provide sufficient evidence upon which to base routine community health nursing practice? Whom might you include as subjects? Would you want your subjects to be ethnically diverse or homogeneous? Why?

promote emotional and physical, as well as cognitive, development. A tool for assessing developmental levels in children and adolescents is provided in the *Community Assessment Reference Guide* 📋 designed to accompany this text.

Providing Adequate Nutrition

For infants, providing adequate nutrition can best be met by promoting breast-feeding. It is estimated that exclusive breast-feeding for the first 6 months could prevent 720 post-neonatal deaths (from 1 to 28 days of age) each year in the United States. Breast-fed infants have a 20% lower mortality risk than infants who are bottle-fed and also experience lower rates of infectious disease incidence (Regional Perinatal Programs of California, 2004). The effects of breast-feeding are also seen among VLBW infants, with one study indicating that exclusive breast-feeding saved $200 to $400 in health care costs per infant during the first year of life (Nisbet, 2004).

Good nutrition is also an issue for older children and adolescents. From 1999 to 2000, 15% of U.S. children were overweight, more than twice as many as in 1976 to 1980 (6%) (Federal Interagency Forum on Child and Family Statistics, 2004). Although children are overeating, they are not eating many of the nutrients needed for good physical health. For example, in one national survey, not quite 30% of girls and just over 45% of boys aged 11 to 18 years had diets that met the daily requirements for calcium intake. Similarly, the diets of large percentages of children and adolescents were deficient in fruits, vegetables, and grains, but overabundant with respect to fats (Neumark-Sztainer, Story, Hannan, & Croll, 2002).

Community health nurses can educate the public regarding the efficacy of breast-feeding and the need for and contents of an adequate diet for children and adolescents. In addition, they can advocate for nutritional supplementation programs and for adequate nutrition programs in schools and other institutional settings. Community health nurses can also promote policies that diminish access to "junk foods" for children and adolescents. For example, they can spearhead initiatives to remove candy and soft drink vending machines from schools and recreational areas and promote healthy fast food alternatives at popular chain restaurants. A tool for assessing the nutritional status of children and adolescents is provided in the *Community Assessment Reference Guide* 📋 designed as a companion volume for this text.

Promoting Physical Activity

Promoting physical activity among children and adolescents is another intervention aimed at promoting health and, in particular, preventing obesity. Based on 2003 data related to achievement of the *Healthy People 2010*◆ objectives for physical activity among high school students, much remains to be done in this area. For example, although the target is to increase the percentage of adolescents regularly engaged in moderate physical activity from a baseline of 27% in 1999 to 35% by 2010,

current figures (25% in 2003) actually indicate movement away from the target. Similar findings are noted for objectives related to vigorous physical activity and daily participation in physical education activities at school. Only for the objective related to decreasing television viewing to less than 2 hours per day do data indicate movement toward the 2010 goal of 75%, increasing from 57% in 1999 to 62% in 2003 (CDC, 2005a). Community health nurses can help to educate children and adolescents on the need for increased physical activity and advocate for the inclusion of physical activity in school curricula. They can also advocate for neighborhood environments that promote physical activity (e.g., schools within walking or biking distance of homes, bicycle paths, and safe activity areas).

Promoting Safety

Accidental injuries are a major cause of death and disability among children and adolescents, and community health nurses should be actively involved in promoting safety across the age spectrum. Again, parental and public education are the primary means for accomplishing this objective, but community health nurses can also campaign for safe conditions in play areas as well as the development and enforcement of safety regulations such as seat belt and helmet use, effective labeling and storage of household chemicals, and so on.

Community health nurses can promote the use of safety devices and equipment. For example, in 2003, 1,519 children under 14 years of age died in motor vehicle accidents and 220,000 were injured. This amounts to 4 deaths and 602 injuries per day. In half of the fatalities, children were riding in the car unrestrained. In one study, only 15% of child passengers were properly harnessed into correctly installed safety seats. Children are most often restrained when they are riding with a driver who also uses safety restraints. In fact, according to some figures, as many as 40% of children riding with unrestrained drivers did not use appropriate restraints

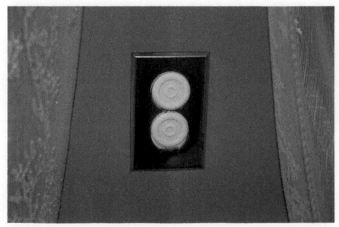

Child-proofing a home entails different strategies for children of different ages. (Patrick J. Watson)

(National Center for Injury Prevention and Control, n.d.a). Federal government figures indicate that use of appropriate child safety restraints decreases the risk of death by 50%, and placing children in the back seat of the vehicle reduces the risk of fatality by 30% (46% if the vehicle is equipped with front-seat air bags) (CDC, 2002a). Community health nurses educate individual families and their children, as well as the general public, regarding the need for effective restraint. In addition, they may campaign for strict enforcement of restraint legislation for all vehicle occupants.

Playground safety is another issue for children and adolescents. Each year, more than 205,000 preschool and elementary-age children are seen in emergency departments for injuries that occur on playgrounds (National Program for Playground Safety, 2005). In 1995, the treatment costs for these injuries amounted to $1.2 billion (National Center for Injury Prevention and Control, n.d.b). More than three fourths of these injuries (76%) occur on public play equipment, and nearly half (45%) occur at school. Although the majority of injuries occur in public settings, 70% of playground fatalities occur at home. The National Program for Playground Safety has developed recommendations for preventing playground injuries that can be used by community health nurses to educate parents and the general public regarding playground safety. These recommendations include:

- Adult supervision of children in play activities
- Choice of age- and developmentally appropriate play equipment
- Provision of safe surfacing below play equipment
- Regular maintenance of all equipment and play surfaces (National Program for Playground Safety, 2005)

Accidental and, among adolescents and preadolescents, intentional poisoning are other areas of concern for community health nurses caring for child and adolescent populations. More than 2.2 million poison

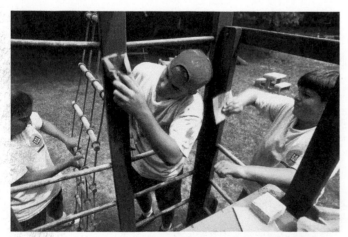

Playground safety is an important issue for child health. (Robert Harbison)

exposures were reported to poison control centers in the United States during 2000, nearly 53% involving children under 6 years of age (CDC, 2002c). Most of these incidents (90%) occurred in the home. Among adolescents, half of the poisoning incidents were intentional suicide attempts (National Center for Injury Prevention and Control, n.d.c). Community health nurses can actively promote safety education regarding the use and storage of poisonous materials among the general public. They may also be involved in efforts to promote effective labeling of hazardous substances and in suicide prevention activities with youth. Selected elements of an educational program to promote child and adolescent safety in the community are included in Table 3◆. The *Community Assessment Reference Guide* 📋 designed as a companion reference for this text contains an assessment tool that community health nurses can use to assess home safety for children and adolescents.

Preventing Communicable Diseases

The most effective means of preventing many communicable diseases among children and adolescents is, of course, immunization. Community health nurses may be actively involved in referring individual children and adolescents for immunizations and in assuring that immunization services are available to these populations. Community health nurses may also educate the public, particularly adolescents, regarding practices to prevent specific communicable diseases such as HIV/AIDS.

IMMUNIZATION Routine immunization of children has resulted in a 99% decline in the incidence of vaccine-preventable diseases (CDC, 2004b). Immunization is credited with preventing 10.5 million cases of disease and 33,000 deaths each year in the United States. In addition to the savings in lives and suffering, each dollar spent on immunizations saves an estimated $6.30 in direct medical expenses and $18.42 in indirect costs, for an annual savings to society of $42 billion (Trust for America's Health, 2004).

By 2 years of age, U.S. children should have received as many as 23 doses of vaccine to protect them against 12 communicable diseases. In 2003, 27.5% of children aged 19 to 35 months were deficient in one or more doses of the recommended vaccines (CDC, 2005c). By the end of 2004, immunization coverage in this age group for all vaccines except varicella had reached the *Healthy People 2010*◆ goal of 80% (Immunization Services Division, 2005b). Because of state and local regulations, immunization coverage is usually somewhat higher among school-aged children. During the 2003–2004 school year, for example, the extent of coverage for seven major vaccines (polio, DTP, measles, mumps, rubella, hepatitis B, and varicella) ranged from 93.3% for varicella to 96% for

TABLE 3	Educational Elements to Promote Child and Adolescent Safety
Age	**Safety Education**
Infant (birth–1 year)	Not leaving child unattended on elevated surfaces or in bath Use of car seat restraint Use of safety straps in high chairs, strollers, swings, infant seats, etc. Use of flame-retardant sleepwear Crib safety: Narrow spaces between slats, bumper pads, no plastic coverings, nontoxic paint, no soft pillows Toy safety: No sharp edges or small parts, no long strings, siblings' toys out of reach
Toddler (2–3 years)	Not leaving child unattended in bath or pool Use of car seat restraint Adequate adult supervision Home safety: Outlet covers, sharp and poisonous objects locked away, medications out of reach, child-resistant containers, gated stairs, bathroom doors closed, no dangling electrical cords Play equipment: Age-appropriate and in good repair, on appropriate surface Toy safety: Age-appropriate toys, no small parts Fenced yard/swimming pool
Preschool child (4–6 years)	Use of booster seat in vehicle Adequate adult supervision Home safety: Outlet covers, sharp and poisonous objects locked away, medications out of reach, child-resistant containers, gated stairs, bathroom doors closed, no dangling electrical cords Play equipment: Age-appropriate and in good repair, on appropriate surface Toy safety: Age-appropriate toys, no small parts, adult supervision with potentially hazardous toys Safety practices: Education regarding interaction with strangers, crossing the street, fire safety, water safety
School-age child (6–12 years)	Use of booster seat/adult seat belt based on height and weight Sports safety: Age-appropriate sports, use of safety equipment, adequate adult supervision Firearms: Locked separately from ammunition Safety practices: Education regarding stranger interactions, caring for self at home, sports, bicycling and helmet use, water safety, use of medications, swimming instruction
Adolescent (13–18 years)	Safe driving Use of seat belts Sports safety: Age-appropriate sports, use of safety equipment, adequate adult supervision Safety practices: Education regarding use of firearms, caring for self and others at home, use of medications, dangerous situations (e.g., alcohol and driving, fighting), stranger interactions Sexuality: Abstinence, safe sexual practices Use of drugs and alcohol

mumps (National Immunization Program, 2004). Hepatitis A coverage, however, lags rather far behind the other vaccines, with 51% of children in high-risk states, 25% in states with moderately high incidence, and only 1.4% of children in low-risk states being immunized (National Immunization Program, 2005). Similarly, influenza immunization in children and adolescents at high risk for complications was less than 35% during the 2004–2005 influenza season (Division of Adult and Community Health, 2005), and only 36% of 6- to 23-month-old children received the recommended influenza vaccine (Immunization Services Division, 2004).

In addition to the vaccines required by most states and local jurisdictions, the Advisory Committee on Immunization Practices has recommended routine immunization for meningococcal disease for all adolescents before high school entry. The goal is to provide routine immunization for all children at 11 years of age by 2008. Meningococcal vaccine is also recommended for previously unimmunized college students living in dormitories, military recruits, and travelers to endemic areas (Bilukha & Rosenstein, 2005).

Despite the benefits of immunization, there are still children in the United States and worldwide who remain unimmunized for one or more immunizable diseases. Periodic outbreaks of disease may occur in these populations. From 2001 to 2003, for example, the incidence rate for pertussis was 55.2 per 100,000 infants under 1 year of age. Incidence was nearly eight times higher for children under 6 months of age than for those 6 months to 1 year of age. Incidence among adolescents aged 10 to 19 years nearly doubled in the same period, suggesting waning immunity among previously immunized children (Epidemiology and Surveillance Division, 2005). Factors in poor immunization coverage include cost, lack of health insurance, inability to get appointments, parental lack of knowledge regarding the need for immunizations, and missed opportunities for immunization on the part of health care providers (O'Connor, Maddocks, Modie, & Pierce, 2001). Religious beliefs also play a part in outbreaks among groups that do not approve of immunization.

A number of interventions by community health nurses can improve immunization rates among children and adolescents. As mentioned earlier, nurses can refer individual clients and their families for available immunization services and educate parents and the public regarding the need for immunizations. They can also help to educate other providers to prevent missed opportunities for immunization. For example, they might campaign for providing initial hepatitis B immunizations at birth, which has been shown to increase the probability that the entire immunization series will be completed (CDC, 2002b). Community health nurses can also promote provider and client participation in immunization registries. Immunization registries are central databases used to record immunizations for all children in a jurisdiction. When they are regional in nature, they relieve the difficulty of immunization records scattered among many different providers. Registries also permit notification of needed immunizations and have been shown to increase immunization rates in participating populations (Kempe et al., 2004). Registries with additional capabilities for managing vaccines, reporting adverse vaccine events, storing lifespan immunization histories, and interacting with electronic medical records are called immunization information systems (IISs). Unfortunately, as of December 2003, only 44% of children under 6 years of age were enrolled in an IIS (Immunization Services Division, 2005a).

PREVENTING OTHER COMMUNICABLE DISEASES Because many communicable diseases are not immunizable conditions, community health nurses must engage in other activities to prevent these conditions in children and adolescents. HIV/AIDS and other sexually transmitted diseases are areas of concern for community health nurses working with child and adolescent populations. In 2002, for example, an estimated 2,292 children under age 13 and 732 adolescents 13 and 14 years of age were living with AIDS in the United States (U.S. Census Bureau, 2004b). Incidence rates are much higher for children in other parts of the world, particularly Africa. For most young children, HIV transmission occurs during pregnancy, the birth process, and via breast-feeding. Perinatal transmission of HIV infection, however, can be reduced from 25% to 2% with effective treatment of pregnant women (County of San Diego Health and Human Services Agency, 2004). Community health nurses can be actively involved in referring pregnant women for prenatal care and in promoting routine HIV screening during pregnancy. For those women who are infected, community health nurses can provide case management services for diagnosis and treatment as well as educating them and the general public about the dangers of breast-feeding in the presence of HIV infection. They can also arrange for screening of infants born to HIV-infected women and make referrals for treatment as needed. Prenatal treatment with zidovudine has been credited with a decrease in perinatal HIV transmission from 19% to 3% during 1993 to 2000 (National Center for HIV, STD, and TB Prevention, 2002). Prenatal care and screening can also help identify women with other sexually transmitted diseases (STDs) (e.g., syphilis, genital herpes, and hepatitis B) that can be transmitted perinatally to their infants.

Adolescents may also be at high risk for sexually transmitted diseases due to increased sexual activity. Community health nurses can educate this group regarding STD transmission and can promote use of condoms and safe sexual practices. In addition, community health nurses may need to advocate for condom availability to sexually active adolescents.

Hygiene and protection of food and water supplies are additional measures to prevent communicable diseases in children and adolescents, particularly in developing areas of the world. In the United States, acute gastroenteritis results in an estimated 300 deaths per year in children under 5 years of age. Worldwide mortality from these diseases approaches 1.5 to 2.5 million deaths each year (King, Glass, Bresee, & Duggan, 2003). Community health nurses can educate the public regarding hygiene and preventing contamination of food and water supplies. They can also advocate for safe water and food supplies at the societal level.

Promoting Dental Care

Dental hygiene should begin as soon as the child's first tooth erupts. At this time parents can be encouraged to rub teeth briskly with a dry washcloth. Later, parents can begin to brush the child's teeth with a soft toothbrush. Older children can be taught to brush and floss their own teeth with adult supervision. Use of fluoridated toothpaste should be encouraged in areas with unfluoridated water; parents can give fluoride-containing vitamins to infants in such areas. In addition to instructing parents about the need for preventive dental care, community health nurses can be actively involved in promoting fluoridation of community drinking water.

Community health nurses can educate the public about the need to wean infants from the bottle before a year of age to prevent bottle-mouth syndrome. The use of sugarless snacks and rinsing the mouth after eating—when brushing is not possible—can also be encouraged. Finally, community health nurses should encourage parents to obtain regular dental checkups for children and to get prompt attention for dental problems. Financial assistance may be needed for such services for low-income families. In such cases, the community health nurse should make a referral for Medicaid in those areas where dental care is covered or work to promote the availability of such services in the population.

Supporting Effective Parenting

Parenting has been described as one of the hardest jobs in the world and the one for which we receive the least preparation. In one study, both mothers and fathers described their first year as parents as overwhelming, with problems related to lack of confidence in the parental role, the demands of being parents, time for oneself, and feeling drained and fatigued (Nystrom & Ohrling, 2004). Other studies have shown that the availability of social support contributes to parental efficacy, the ability to "organize and execute a set of tasks related to parenting a child" (de Montigny & Lacharite, 2005, p. 387). In a review of related literature, the authors found four factors that contributed to efficacy: positive mastery experiences in past care of infants, vicarious experience obtained through parent training programs, verbal persuasion by significant others of one's capabilities, and an appropriate physical and affective state (e.g., not being fatigued or under stress).

Other studies have noted that both structural and functional elements of social support influence parenting abilities. Structural elements include formal and informal social networks and the people who make up those networks. Informal networks are comprised of family members and friends, whereas formal networks include health care professionals. Functional elements of social support address the kinds of support available to the parent and usually include informational, instrumental, emotional, and appraisal support (Warren, 2005). Each of these types of support can be provided by community health nurses to the parents of children and adolescents. For example, they may provide informational support by educating families regarding the needs of children and adolescents, or emotional support in dealing with the frustrations of parenthood. They may also provide appraisal support by giving parents both positive and negative feedback on their performance as parents. Less often, community health nurses may provide instrumental support by actually caring for a child, arranging respite services for a parent, or advocating the presence of such services in the community.

Support for parenting for parents of young children may frequently address issues of discipline. Table 4◆ provides several general principles of child and adolescent discipline that community health nurses can use to educate community members. The converse of promoting effective discipline of children and adolescents is preventing abuse of children and adolescents by their parents and other adults or older siblings. In the United States, the role of the community health nurse in identifying and reporting child abuse is quite clear cut. Community health nurses are part of a group of professionals, including health care providers, teachers, and others, who are required by law to report any suspicion of abuse of a child or adolescent. The role of the nurse is not as clearly defined in other countries, however. For example, one study in Scotland found considerable confusion among community health nurses regarding their responsibility with respect to child protection issues as well as the extent of activity by community health nurses in detecting cases of abuse. Many nurses in the study perceived detection and reporting of abuse as in conflict with their traditional role of support to families (Crisp & Lister, 2004). Contrary to these perceptions, however, identification and reporting of child abuse can foster effective parenting because it gives parents an opportunity to learn more appropriate ways to interact with their children.

Other Primary Prevention Activities

Additional primary preventive measures may be warranted for children with specific illnesses. For example, parents of children with AIDS and other immunosuppressive conditions should be taught to minimize exposure to opportunistic infections. Special intervention may also be warranted to create a healthy self-image in children with chronic conditions or disabilities. For

TABLE 4	Principles of Effective Discipline and Related Considerations
Principle	**Disciplinary Consideration**
Importance	Employ discipline for important matters Do not automatically say "no" to everything Determine what is unacceptable behavior
Consistency	Maintain consistency in what is considered unacceptable behavior Maintain consistency between and among authority figures If a behavior is acceptable in some situations and not in others, make sure children understand the difference and why it is so
Calm	Never act in anger Employ a "cooling off" period, if needed, and make sure children understand the need to deal with anger appropriately
Time	Allow time for compliance with directions before taking disciplinary action
Limits	Set rules and limits for behavior ahead of time and make sure children are aware of them Make sure limits are within the child's age and developmental capacity to comply Give a warning for unanticipated unacceptable behaviors the first time
Understanding	Make sure children understand the rules and the reasons for them
Prevention	Prevent unacceptable behavior rather than punish it whenever possible Remove sources of temptation from younger children Provide adequate adult supervision of children
Investigation	Ascertain the facts of the situation before taking disciplinary action Ask for the child's explanation of the situation and his or her behavior When the behavior is unacceptable but the child's reasons are appropriate, make sure he or she understands why the behavior should not be repeated
Meaningfulness	Make sure children understand the reason for disciplinary action Explain how the child can improve his or her behavior Use a form of discipline appropriate to the child and the situation

example, the physically handicapped child can be helped to develop skills such as artistic ability that contribute to a positive self-image. Primary preventive interventions employed by community health nurses in caring for children are summarized in Table 5◆.

Secondary Prevention

Secondary prevention is geared toward resolution of health problems currently experienced by children and adolescents. Activities are directed toward screening for conditions, care of minor illness, care of children and adolescents with chronic conditions, and care of those with terminal illnesses.

TABLE 5	Primary Prevention Interventions for Child and Adolescent Populations
Focus	Interventions
Assuring access to health care	Making referrals to sources of health care Promoting a regular source of health care for all children and adolescents Advocating health insurance coverage for children and adolescents
Reducing prematurity, low birth weight, and infant mortality	Sexuality education Promoting effective contraception to prevent unplanned pregnancies Promoting effective prenatal care and advocating for low-cost pregnancy services Promoting supplemental nutrition programs for pregnant women and children and making referrals to existing programs Promoting smoking cessation and alcohol abstinence during pregnancy
Promoting growth and development	Educating parents and the public regarding normal growth and development Advocating environments that promote adequate growth and development of children and adolescents Promoting continued development of adolescent parents as well as their children
Providing adequate nutrition	Promoting breast-feeding Educating parents, children, and the public regarding nutritional needs of children and adolescents Advocating healthy nutrition in schools and day care centers Advocating for healthier food choices in restaurants and other venues
Promoting physical activity	Educating children and adolescents regarding the need for physical activity Advocating for physical activity in school curricula Advocating for environments conducive to physical activity
Promoting safety	Encouraging provision of adequate supervision of children and adolescents Advocating for strong legislation and strict enforcement to protect children and adolescents Promoting use of effective safety devices Teaching children and adolescents regarding safety issues Advocating elimination of safety hazards in the environment
Preventing communicable diseases	Promoting immunization and referring for immunization services Modifying immunization practices or schedules for children with special needs Promoting prenatal care and screening for HIV and other STDs in pregnant women Promoting condom use and safe sexual practices among adolescents Educating the public and families with respect to good hygiene and protection of food and water supplies Advocating for effective sanitation and safe food and water supplies
Promoting dental care	Promoting dental hygiene Advocating access to dental care services
Supporting effective parenting	Providing support for parents Educating parents for care of children and adolescents Advocating for respite care as needed Assisting parents with discipline issues Educating parents for realistic expectations of their children Taking action to minimize parental sources of stress
Other primary prevention activities	Meeting the primary prevention needs of children with special needs

Screening for Health Problems

Screening for conditions at birth is usually employed when treatment soon after birth leads to improved health outcomes. Each state determines the panel of required screenings for newborns born in that state. In 2004, required newborn screening panels ranged from 4 tests to 40. Criteria for the selection of mandatory screening tests include the prevalence of the condition; the cost, feasibility, and accuracy of screening tests; the effectiveness of early intervention; and the availability of treatment. CDC recommends that newborn screening programs include follow-up treatment systems, parental education, and primary provider information systems (Grosse et al., 2004).

Routine screening for existing conditions takes place at other ages as well as at birth. Table 6◆ provides information about routine screening procedures for selected age groups. Other screening procedures may be warranted for children and adolescents in certain circumstances. For example, children with a family history of diabetes may be screened for this condition. Similarly, children or adolescents who have been exposed to traumatic events (e.g., school violence, natural disaster) should be screened for depression and other mental health problems. Community health nurses may be actively involved in providing routine and specialized screening services or may need to advocate for access to these services for the child and adolescent populations.

Caring for Minor Illness

Each year approximately 12 million children under the age of 5 years die of treatable conditions, mostly as a result of pneumonia, diarrhea, malaria, measles, and

TABLE 6	Routine Screening Procedures for Children and Adolescents
Age	**Screening Procedure**
Birth	Phenylketonuria (PKU), hypothyroidism, hearing, hemoglobinopathies, sickle cell disease, galactosemia, maple syrup urine disease, homocystinuria, biodatinase, congenital adrenal hyperplasia, cystic fibrosis
1 month	Lead, Denver Developmental Screening Test (DDST)
1–2 months	Head and chest circumference, height and weight (and periodically thereafter)
3 months	Blood pressure (and periodically thereafter)
3–4 months	Vision (and periodically thereafter)
6 months	Hematocrit or hemoglobin
9 months	Tuberculin skin test
1 year	DDST
2 years	DDST
3 years	Dental (and periodically thereafter)
5 years	School readiness, immunization status
6–12 years	Hearing, vision, school performance
11–18 years	Use of tobacco and alcohol and sexual activity (and periodically thereafter), immunization status, scoliosis, STDs and Papanicolaou smear (if sexually active)

Think Advocacy

Rowe, Onikpo, Lama, Cokou, and Deming (2001) conducted a study to examine the extent to which community health workers (CHWs) implemented WHO strategies for Integrated Management of Childhood Illness for children under the age of 5 years. They found that a significant portion of the community health workers failed to correctly implement the guidelines. Major areas of deficit included incomplete assessment, incorrect diagnosis and treatment, inappropriate drug therapy, missed opportunities for immunizations, and failure to refer children for professional care when needed. Qualitative data obtained from CHWs indicated reasons for these deficits included conflicts among health workers, overload, failure to use knowledge acquired in training, low morale and motivation, poor time management, lack of equipment, and lack of fluency in the local language. Other reasons given for poor implementation of guidelines were impatient parents or other caregivers, caregiver demands for medications, CHW perceptions that caregivers would report all of a child's symptoms without questioning or prompting or would be alarmed if told of a child's diagnosis, and CHW unwillingness to use charts or other diagnostic and treatment aids for fear of being thought incompetent. How might you address the factors contributing to poor implementation of guidelines by CHWs so that all the children seen receive adequate treatment for their illnesses?

malnutrition. The World Health Organization has established strategies for the Integrated Management of Childhood Illness for children 1 month to 5 years of age. These strategies include guidelines for assessing, diagnosing, treating, and referring ill children, counseling their caregivers, and immunizing them as needed (Rowe, Onikpo, Lama, Cokou, & Deming, 2001). Community health nurses can educate the public regarding appropriate home treatment for minor illness and when professional care is required.

Many minor illnesses and health care problems can be addressed effectively if parents or other caregivers know how to deal with them. For other problems, or when home care does not resolve the problem, professional care is required. Community health nurses can educate parents and the public on the signs of illness in children, appropriate measures to be taken at home, and when to seek medical intervention. Caretakers and the public should be acquainted with what is normal and what is abnormal, as well as what home remedies are appropriate and what might be harmful. In addition to providing such information, community health nurses frequently are called on to assess the health status of specific children and recommend appropriate interventions or make referrals for medical assistance.

Caring for Children and Adolescents with Chronic Illness

We most often think of chronic illness in the context of caring for elderly clients, but roughly 31% or 20 million U.S. children are affected in some way by chronic illness (Meleski, 2002). An estimated 400,000 of these children experience chronic, life-threatening conditions (Jennings, 2005). Chronic illness has been defined as "an incurable condition that interferes with long-term function and requires special assistance to manage" (Meleski, 2002, p. 48). Based on figures from the U.S. Federal Interagency Forum on Child and Family Statistics, 3% of children under 5 years of age and 7% of those aged 5 to 17 years have activity limitations due to chronic conditions. Approximately two thirds of these children experience only mild limitations, but 29% have moderate limitations and 5% are severely limited by their conditions (Meleski, 2002). The percentage of children who experience activity limitation due to chronic disease has more than tripled in the past four decades (Newacheck & Benjamin, 2004). Children with chronic conditions have three times as many physician contacts and hospitalizations and eight times as many hospital days as those without chronic illnesses. In fact, an estimated 80% of nontrauma spending in the care of children is allocated to chronic illness care (Wise, 2004). Chronic conditions may also affect children's performance or their interactions with others in the school setting.

Parental uncertainty has been shown to be a key feature of parental response to diagnosis of serious illness in their children. Uncertainty has been defined as the "inability to determine the meaning of illness related events" as a result of the inability to categorize an event due to a lack of understandable cues (Mu, 2005, p. 368). Four dimensions have been noted in the literature with regard to parental uncertainty in the face of serious illness in a child: ambiguity regarding the illness state; lack of information regarding the illness, its management, and its effects; the complexity of information and care systems; and the unpredictability of the child's prognosis, quality of life, and functional ability (Santacroce, 2003).

Parents of children and adolescents with chronic health problems have reported ongoing personal trauma throughout periods of diagnosis, treatment, and survivorship. Some of the traumas reported include having to approve or give painful treatments, watching their child's condition deteriorate, and being constantly alert for recurrent or subsequent health problems (Santacroce, 2003). Trauma and disequilibrium seem to center around five specific periods of transition in chronic illness: initial diagnosis, symptom exacerbation, movement to a new care setting (e.g., hospitalization), periods of parental absence (e.g., divorce or separation), and times when the child would be expected to experience a normal developmental transition such as learning to walk or talk, school entry, puberty, or a 21st birthday (Meleski, 2002). The approach of adulthood may be a particularly stressful time for families, as they are faced with the possible need for residential placement if children are not capable of living independently (Green, S., 2004). Coming of age may also make children ineligible for previously covered services, and each year half a million adolescents reach the age when they are ineligible for continued services (Wise, 2004).

Another period when disequilibrium may be experienced occurs when treatment regimens change, even if the change is not in response to the child's deteriorating condition. For example, parents of children with diabetes who were switched to insulin pumps reported having to rethink their disease management strategies with the advent of this technology. Changes required greater vigilance and more frequent glucose monitoring than they were accustomed to doing (Sullivan-Bolyai, Knafl, Tamborlane, & Grey, 2004).

Two models have been used to explain parental reaction to the presence of serious disease in their children. The first is a time-bound model in which parents are believed to adapt over time to the presence of the disease. In the chronic sorrow model, on the other hand, parents adapt, but may never accept the illness and experience continuing sorrow that fades and burgeons based on circumstances in the life of the child and the family. Perhaps the most appropriate model is one that integrates both perspectives: parents and families do adapt, but are apt to experience periods in which adaptation is more or less difficult (Meleski, 2002). Factors that may affect adaptation include family coping abilities, the availability of social support and appropriate services, respite, and the level of stigma attached to the child's condition, which may be influenced by cultural norms (Mu, 2005).

Many children and adolescents and their families need to learn to cope with the effects of chronic illness on a daily basis. Coping has been defined as the "specific cognitive and behavioral efforts by which an individual and family attempt to reduce or manage the demands placed upon them" (Mu, 2005, p. 368). McCubbin found three patterns of family coping in the presence of cystic fibrosis in a child that may have application for families dealing with other chronic illnesses. The first coping pattern involved maintenance of family integration, optimism, and cooperation. The second pattern addressed maintenance of self-esteem of family members and mobilizing social and psychological sources of support. The third pattern was understanding the disease and its effects through interactions with providers and with other parents whose children also were affected (Mu, 2005).

Much intervention with families with children experiencing chronic illness has focused on development of family resilience or hardiness. Hardiness "refers to the internal strengths and durability of the family, and is characterized by a sense of control over outcomes of life, a view of change as growth-producing, and an active rather than passive orientation in adapting to stressful situations" (Svavarsdottir & Rayens, 2005, p. 382). There is some evidence to suggest, however, that resilience may be associated with greater internalization of feelings such that negative effects of illness are just less visible rather than less real.

Research on families dealing with children and adolescents with chronic illnesses has identified a number of common themes that are relevant to community health nursing care of these population groups. Some of these themes address family interactions, and some deal with interactions with health care providers and the health care system. Others reflect the economic burden experienced by families. Families describe the need to live as normal a life as possible but being challenged by the need to be constantly alert to crises and the shift in perception of the home as a place of safety and refuge to one of providing care. The presence of a chronic illness in a child results in changes in family relationships with the affected child and among other family members. Families may also be at higher risk for social isolation due to the inability to find adequate care for the affected child. Parents describe ambiguity in their parental role and role conflict between the parental and formal caregiver roles, and frequently experience adverse health effects themselves related to fatigue, depression, fear, and panic (Wang & Barnard, 2004). Parents may also feel burdened by the need to provide emotional support to the child with a chronic illness as well as to his or her siblings, with limited emotional support for themselves (Svavarsdottir, 2005).

Health system factors that affect family response to chronic illness include fragmentation of care and lack of social support for parental caregivers. Parents may find themselves engaged in frequent battles to obtain needed health and education services for their children, and support programs for families of children with chronic illnesses are usually severely underfunded, if they exist at all. Parents also describe being unprepared for the demands of their new caregiver role and may view the presence of a community health nurse as both helpful and disruptive of family routine and privacy (Wang & Barnard, 2004).

Children and adolescents experience a wide variety of chronic health problems. A few of the major problems affecting these age groups will be addressed here.

HIV INFECTION AND AIDS Prevalence and prevention of HIV/AIDS in children and adolescents was addressed earlier in this chapter. Here we will concentrate on the role of the community health nurse in caring for children and adolescents with HIV infection or active AIDS. The primary aspect of this role lies in management of the disease and prevention of opportunistic infections. Community health nurses may refer children for diagnosis and treatment services, and may be involved in long-term follow-up for children with HIV/AIDS. In addition to halting the progression of the disease, highly active antiretroviral therapy (HAART) has been shown to reduce the incidence of opportunistic infections (OI) in children with AIDS. HAART is the most effective means of combating OI, since many protozoan, fungal, and viral infections are not amenable to antibiotic therapy (Mofenson, Oleske, Serchuck, Van Dyke, & Wilfert, 2004). Community health nurses monitor HAART therapy in children and observe for treatment effects and medication side effects. They can also educate clients and family members in dealing with side effects. In addition, they would also be alert to signs of OI in HIV-infected children and adolescents and refer them for treatment in keeping with new treatment guidelines published by CDC in 2004 (Mofenson et al., 2004).

ATTENTION DEFICIT HYPERACTIVITY DISORDER Attention deficit hyperactivity disorder is one of the three most common conditions in children (with asthma and otitis media) (Leslie & Stein, 2003) and the most common psychiatric disorder in the United States (Singh, 2004). **Attention deficit hyperactivity disorder (ADHD)** is a chronic condition characterized by poor attention span, impulsive behavior, and hyperactivity. Attention deficit with associated hyperactivity is frustrating for the children affected and for everyone who interacts with them.

Prevalence estimates for ADHD in the general population range from 4% to 12% (Leslie & Stein, 2003) with a 7% prevalence among children 6 to 11 years of age. More than three fourths of those affected are boys (Singh, 2004). Children with ADHD usually exhibit poor school performance and poor peer relationships and often have problems with family relationships (Leslie & Stein, 2003). Twenty to thirty percent of children with ADHD also have specific learning disabilities, including reading and spelling disabilities (e.g., dyslexia) and writing and arithmetic disorders. Other conditions that may occur in conjunction with ADHD include Tourette syndrome (a neurological disorder characterized by nervous tics and uncontrollable swearing), oppositional defiant disorder (stubborn, defiant, belligerent behavior), conduct disorder, anxiety and depression, and bipolar disorder (National Institutes of Mental Health [NIMH], 2003). Children with ADHD have also been shown to be at higher risk for injury due primarily to lack of attention to risk situations (National Center on Birth Defects and Developmental Disabilities, 2004a).

An additional 8 million adults are also affected by ADHD, which affects education and employment in adult life. Adults with ADHD also have higher rates of divorce, lower life satisfaction, and higher risks for substance abuse. Failure to complete their education is another common problem. Even those who manage to complete high school earn an average of $10,791 a year less than their counterparts who are not affected by ADHD, and college graduates earn on average $4,334 less than their nonaffected counterparts. Roughly one third of adults with ADHD are not diagnosed until after 18 years of age. Approximately half of adults with ADHD go on to have a child with the disorder, suggesting a genetic component to the disease (American Medical Association, 2004). Overall estimates of ADHD in the U.S. population stand at 5 million, with approximately half of those cases undiagnosed (Federwisch, 2005).

Only approximately 3% of school-age children with ADHD are receiving methylphenidate (Ritalin) therapy, and the prevalence of therapy has increased sixfold in the last decade (Singh, 2004). Ritalin is one of several medications used for the treatment of ADHD. Ritalin has been approved for use in children 6 years of age and older, but other drugs (e.g., Adderall and dextrostat) may be used with children as young as 3 (NIMH, 2003). Despite some controversy regarding the number of children on medication for ADHD, a recent NIMH study indicated that children on medication fared better than those without, whether or not they received behavioral therapy (Federwisch, 2005). For some children, particularly those with anxiety, poor academic performance or social skills, poor parent–child interaction, or oppositional defiant disorder, a combination therapy including medication management and behavioral treatment was more effective than either therapy alone (NIMH, 2003).

Treatment goals for children and adolescents with ADHD include the following:

- Decreasing symptoms through medication management and behavior modification
- Addressing co-existing medical conditions through medical management
- Addressing co-existing mental health problems through pharmacologic and behavioral therapies
- Addressing co-existing learning disabilities through special education services
- Addressing environmental and family stressors
- Promoting adequate development
- Promoting child and family competence (Leslie & Stein, 2003)

Community health nurses can be particularly helpful in assisting families with medication management and behavioral modification. They can also advocate for environments that minimize symptoms. For example, children with more green play areas have been shown to exhibit fewer ADHD symptoms than those without green play areas (Kuo & Taylor, 2004). Similarly, regular routines and organizing strategies can help students maintain focus and improve performance (NIMH, 2003). For example, a written schedule posted on the refrigerator can include activities such as homework, chores, and specific play activities (e.g., computer games or outdoor play). Community health nurses can also advocate for the necessary special education services as well as refer individual children and adolescents for diagnostic and treatment services. School nurses may be particularly helpful as case managers for children and adolescents with ADHD.

Community health nurses should also attend to the needs of those who care for children and adolescents with ADHD. Mothers, in particular, have been shown to blame themselves and to be blamed by others for their children's hyperactivity (Singh, 2004). These families may require a great deal of emotional support by the community health nurse.

OTHER CHRONIC AND DISABLING CONDITIONS Children and adolescents experience a variety of other chronic physical and mental conditions. For example, asthma is the leading cause of hospitalizations and emergency department visits among children (Nicholas et al., 2005) and the leading cause of school absence (Navaie-Waliser, Misener, Mersman, & Lincoln, 2004). The incidence of asthma in U.S. children nearly tripled from 3.7% of children in 1980 to 12.7% twenty years later (Wise, 2004). In 2003, an estimated 9 million U.S. children and adolescents had been diagnosed with asthma (NCHS, 2005a). Asthma is also a growing problem worldwide, with prevalence ranging from 10% to 50% of children in some countries (Huey, 2001).

Environmental modification may help control airway reactivity in children and adolescents with asthma.

For example, in one study, community health workers' efforts to assess home environments and educate families regarding elimination of asthma triggers resulted in fewer asthma symptom days, fewer asthma triggers in the home, less urgent care use, and increased quality of life for caregivers (Krieger, Takaro, Song, & Weaver, 2005). Removing pets from the homes of children with asthma has proven particularly effective in controlling symptoms (Shirai, Matsui, Suzuki, & Chida, 2005).

Seizure disorders are another type of chronic condition that may affect the health of children and adolescents. According to the Epilepsy Foundation (2005), each year approximately 300,000 people experience a first convulsion. More than one third of them (120,000) are children under 18 years of age, and 75,000 to 100,000 are children under 5 years of age who experience febrile seizures. Many of those who experience a first seizure, however, go on to develop chronic seizure disorder without any known cause. Overall, approximately 326,000 children under 14 years of age have diagnosed epilepsy, and roughly 1% of the U.S. population can be expected to develop epilepsy before the age of 20.

Medication is highly effective in the treatment of epilepsy, with approximately 70% of those treated remaining seizure-free for 5 or more years, at which time three fourths of them can discontinue medication without a return of seizures. Unfortunately, 10% of those with seizure disorders will be unable to gain control of them despite treatment (Epilepsy Foundation, 2005).

Caring for children and adolescents with seizure disorders involves assisting them to cope with the perceived or real stigma attached to the disease as well as encouraging compliance with medical therapy. Adolescents, in particular, may need to be referred for counseling if their condition contributes to a poor self-image or difficulty with interpersonal interactions, especially in the school setting. For children and adolescents whose disease is uncontrolled by medication, community health nurses may need to provide assistance in dealing with the limitations imposed by their condition. For example, the nurse might educate them about the inadvisability of swimming alone or help adolescents cope with their inability to obtain a driver's license. Both children and parents may need to be helped to cope with the fear and uncertainty caused by uncontrolled seizures. School nurses, in particular, may be in a position to educate others about seizure disorder and advocate for fair treatment of those affected.

Growing numbers of children are also affected by diabetes. Although children are most likely to develop type 1 diabetes, there are indications of growing incidence of type 2 diabetes among children as well, particularly among Native American, African American, and Hispanic youth (American Diabetes Association, n.d.). Overall, an estimated 210,000 people under 20 years of age have diabetes (National Diabetes Information Clearinghouse, n.d.).

Care of children and adolescents with diabetes is centered around controlling the disease while maintaining as normal a lifestyle as possible. Community health nurses will educate children and their parents regarding the need for dietary control, use of medication, exercise, and the need to monitor illness and injury carefully to prevent diabetic complications. Again, the community health nurse may need to function as an advocate for children with diabetes, particularly in the school setting. For example, in addition to educating others about the disease, the nurse may need to see that the school meal programs contain foods appropriate to a diabetic diet. The nurse can also assist older children and adolescents in designing their diet, so they can participate in activities enjoyed by their peers (e.g., a class picnic or an occasional trip to the local fast food restaurant).

Obesity is another chronic condition with increasing prevalence among children and adolescents. In 2000, for example, 15.3% of children were obese, compared to only 5.7% in 1980 (Wise, 2004). Community health nurses can be particularly effective in addressing the problem of obesity by promoting healthy diets and physical activity. Nurses can advocate for healthy school meal programs as well as healthy diets in the home setting. In addition, many community health nurses have been actively involved in local initiatives to remove vending machines or discontinue the sale of junk food on school premises. They can also make referrals to weight control programs for overweight and obese children and adolescents or establish such programs within school or recreational settings (e.g., a local Boys and Girls Club). In addition, they can attempt to decrease the stigma attached to being overweight or refer children and youth for counseling to improve self-image if needed.

Many children also experience congenital heart disease, hearing loss, and a variety of developmental disorders. Approximately 8 of every 1,000 babies are born with congenital heart disease. Children with congenital heart disease often exhibit delayed growth compared to normal children and have been shown to have increased exercise intolerance and risks for depression and anxiety disorders as adults (Chen, Li, & Wang, 2004; Green, A., 2004). Another 1 to 3 children per 1,000 live births have congenital hearing loss, yet, in 2001, only 65% of infants were screened for hearing loss (Division of Human Development and Disability, 2003).

Developmental disabilities encompass a variety of conditions "that initially manifest in persons ≤ 18 years and result in impairment of physical health, mental health, cognition, speech, language, or selfcare" (National Center on Birth Defects and Developmental Disabilities, 2004c). Mental retardation is the most common of these disabilities and affects 1% of U.S. children 3 to 10 years of age. Mental retardation may be caused by injury, disease, brain abnormality, genetic disorder, or fetal alcohol syndrome. The average lifetime costs for mental retardation in 2003 dollars were more than $1 million per person, with 76% of these costs going toward indirect support costs (National Center on Birth Defects and Developmental Disabilities, 2004e).

Cerebral palsy (CP) and autism are other developmental disabilities that affect children and adolescents. The overall prevalence of CP is 2.8 per 1,000 children aged 3 to 10 years. Average lifetime costs for a single person with CP in 2003 were $921,000 (National Center on Birth Defects and Developmental Disabilities, 2004b; 2005). Autism occurs less often, with an estimated prevalence of 2 to 6 per 1,000 children aged 3 to 10 years, and more than 500,000 people aged 10 to 21 years affected (National Center on Birth Defects and Developmental Disabilities, 2005).

The conditions described above and other chronic illnesses may result in disability for those affected. In the last two decades, perspectives on disability have been changing. In 1980, the WHO International Classification of Impairment, Disability, and Handicap (ICIDH) differentiated among these three effects of chronic conditions. Impairment was defined as a "loss or abnormality of psychological, physiological, or anatomical structure or function" (Kearny & Pryor, 2004, p. 164). Disability was defined as "any restriction or lack (resulting from impairment) of ability to perform an activity in the manner or within the range considered normal for a human being" (p. 164). Finally, a handicap was defined as "a disadvantage for a given individual, resulting from impairment or disability, that limits or prevents the fulfillment of a role that is normal (depending on age, sex and social and cultural factors) for that individual" (p. 164).

In 2001, WHO replaced this classification with the International Classification of Functioning, Disability, and Health (ICF), shifting from a personal-tragedy or consequences-of-disease perspective to a social-components-of-health perspective. In the social model, disability is not a property of the individual, but is a "multidimensional phenomenon resulting from the interaction between people and their physical and social environment" (WHO as quoted in Kearny & Pryor, 2004, p. 166). From this new perspective, functional ability and disability are not inherent in the individual and his or her health status, but are the product of the interaction between health status and contextual factors in the individual's environment. This perspective highlights the need to modify contextual factors such that disability is minimized to the extent possible. For example, community health nurses may work to remove asthma triggers from home and school environments to minimize airway reactivity in children with asthma. Similarly, they may be actively involved in environmental modifications that promote free access to educational, recreational, and service settings for people in wheelchairs. Although these kinds of modifications are often taken for granted in the United States, where compliance with the Americans with Disabilities Act is mandated for all public buildings, there are no such efforts underway in many other countries.

The interaction between health status and environment may lead to the creation of special needs in children with serious chronic conditions. Children with special needs have been defined by the U.S. federal government as "those who have or are at risk for a chronic physical, developmental, behavioral, or emotional condition, and who also require health and related services of a type or amount beyond that required by children generally" (Maternal and Child Health Bureau [MCHB], 2001, p. 2).

The Maternal and Child Health Bureau (2001) has established a plan to address the health of children with special needs. The plan includes six goals to be met in the care of all children with special needs. A similar set of eight goals has been established by the U.S. Department of Health and Human Services (2002) for dealing with chronic mental health problems in children and adolescents. Both sets of goals are presented in Table 7◆.

Community health nurses can educate both caregivers and the public regarding the mental health needs of children and adolescents and those of children with special needs. In addition, they can recognize signs of mental illness or other chronic health problems in children and refer them for screening, diagnosis, and treatment as needed. Community health nurses can assist children and adolescents with chronic illnesses and their families to cope with the day-to-day challenges of their conditions through education and emotional support. For example, they can educate the public and families regarding asthma self-management or diabetes control. They can also refer families to needed sources of support and advocate for the availability and accessibility of support and care services for children and adolescents in need of them. Finally, they can work to minimize the stigma attached to chronic illness through public education.

Caring for Children and Adolescents with Terminal Illness

Nearly 53,000 children die each year, approximately half of them from chronic disorders, and another 400,000 have life-threatening illnesses (Childers, 2005). The two primary functions of community health nurses in the care of children and adolescents are palliative care and assisting families with grieving. The World Health Organization has defined palliative care for children as "total care of the child's mind, body, and spirit" (quoted in Childers, p. 25). The goal of palliative care is to enhance the quality of life of the child and his or her family through control of symptoms and alleviation of other conditions (e.g., loneliness, depression) that may diminish quality of life. Palliative care also seeks to ensure continued effective functioning of the family unit (Jennings, 2005). Community health nurses may be involved in the provision of palliative care for individual children or adolescents or refer clients for palliative care services. At the aggregate level, they can work to assure the availability of palliative care services in the community and their accessibility to all those in need of them.

Family communication is another issue that can be addressed through palliative care. One communication issue that challenges families is whether to discuss the impending death with the child and with his or her siblings. Research has shown that impending death is harder on the child when it is not acknowledged by his or her parents (Childers, 2005) and that parents who discussed death with their seriously ill child did not regret having done so. On the other hand, parents who did not discuss the impending death with their child did regret not having done so and experienced more continuing depression and anxiety afterwards than parents who discussed death with their child (Kreicbergs, Valdimarsdottir, Onelov, Henter, & Steineck, 2004).

Some providers have noted the fine line between hope and realism that must be maintained to assist

TABLE 7	Goals for Addressing the Health Needs of Children and Adolescents with Special Needs and Those with Mental Health Problems
Children and Adolescents with Special Needs	**Children and Adolescents with Mental Health Problems**
Provide coordinated, ongoing, comprehensive care for all children with special needs within a medical home	Promote public awareness and reduce the stigma of mental illness
Provide adequate public or private insurance to pay for needed services	Study and promote effective treatment services
Provide early and continuing screening for special needs for all children	Improve recognition of mental health problems in children and adolescents
Incorporate families of children with special needs in decision making to improve satisfaction with care	Eliminate disparities in access to mental health care services
Develop easily used community-based systems of care for children with special needs	Improve the mental health care infrastructure
Provide services needed to make transitions to all aspects of adult life (e.g., health care, employment, independent living)	Increase access to and coordination of mental health services
	Educate providers to recognize and manage mental health problems in children and adolescents
	Monitor access to and coordinate mental health services

Data from: Maternal and Child Health Bureau, 2001; All aboard the 2010 express. Rockville, MD: Author; U.S. Department of Health and Human Services, 2002. Children's mental health is national priority. Prevention Report, 16 (2), 5–6.

families to deal with a terminal illness and the thought of the death of a child or adolescent. Providers may need to "plant the seeds of bereavement" even while parents are attempting every last effort to save their child. Providers may begin to discuss the possibility of death with the family when the child him- or herself expresses knowledge that something is very wrong, when parents begin to acknowledge the potential for death, or when siblings begin to question the possibility of death (Wolfe, 2004).

The grief of parents for a child may not follow the traditional pattern of grieving, which was based on research conducted with grieving widows or widowers. The death of an older person is considered a normal, albeit sad, event. The death of a child, however, is considered unnatural, at least in the developed world where child fatality rates are relatively low. Acceptance of death is more difficult since it is perceived as unnatural for parents to outlive their children. Unlike a dead spouse, who might eventually be replaced by a new love, a child is irreplaceable. Parents experience not only the loss of the child but also the loss of all of their hopes and dreams for that child. Traditional grief work usually involves the breaking of bonds with the deceased; however, research with bereaved parents has shown that they are often comforted by maintaining links with their deceased child through linking objects (e.g., a favorite toy), religious devotions, and rituals that evoke memories of the child. Parents often find that talking about the child with others who remember him or her helps, as does exploring the meaning of the child's life. On the other hand, parents may experience intense loneliness

and difficulty discussing the child with others who have not experienced similar losses (Davies, 2004).

Community health nurses can assist dying children and their families to deal with their feelings about an impending death and can make referrals for counseling, respite, and other services as needed. They may also provide information about the condition and palliative activities, help families create lasting memories of the child, or hold memorial events for groups of parents who have lost children (Childers, 2005). At the population level, community health nurses can initiate bereavement groups and advocate for the availability of both palliative and bereavement services for terminally ill children and their families. They can also advocate insurance coverage for both palliative and bereavement services. Community health nursing foci and interventions related to secondary prevention for children and adolescents are presented in Table 8◆.

Tertiary Prevention

Tertiary prevention is geared toward the particular health problems experienced by children or adolescents. Generally, there are three aspects to tertiary prevention with children and adolescents: preventing recurrence of problems, preventing further consequences, and, in the case of chronic illness or disability, promoting adjustment.

Preventing Problem Recurrence

Community health nurses may educate parents and children to prevent the recurrence of many health problems experienced by children. For example, the parent

TABLE 8	Secondary Prevention Interventions for Child and Adolescent Populations
Focus	Interventions
Screening for health problems	▪ Providing routine screening services for children and adolescents ▪ Interpreting screening test results for families and making referrals for follow-up diagnosis and treatment ▪ Advocating for available and accessible screening services
Caring for minor illness	▪ Educating families and the public to recognize signs of minor illness in children and adolescents ▪ Educating families and the public regarding home care of minor illness and how to know when professional care is needed ▪ Providing or referring for treatment for minor illness when needed ▪ Advocating available and accessible services for minor illness care
Caring for children and adolescents with chronic illnesses	▪ Educating families and the public regarding signs of chronic illness in children and adolescents ▪ Referring individual children and adolescents for diagnosis and treatment of chronic illness ▪ Providing case management services for children and adolescents with chronic illness ▪ Assisting families to adapt to the care needs of a child or adolescent with chronic illness ▪ Teaching children and adolescents and their families for self-management of chronic illness ▪ Referring caretakers of children and adolescents with chronic illnesses for respite services ▪ Promoting normal growth and development in children with chronic illness ▪ Advocating environmental changes to minimize disabilities due to chronic illness ▪ Advocating available and accessible diagnostic and treatment services for children and adolescents with chronic illness
Caring for children and adolescents with terminal illness	▪ Providing or referring families for palliative care ▪ Assisting families with the grief process ▪ Referring children and adolescents and their families for support services as needed ▪ Initiating bereavement care ▪ Advocating available and accessible palliative and bereavement care for children and adolescents and their families

may need information on the relationship of bottle propping to otitis media to prevent subsequent infections. Similarly, education about the need to change diapers frequently, to wash the skin with each diaper change, and to refrain from using harsh soaps to wash diapers may help prevent continued diaper rash. Preventing recurrence of conditions like lead poisoning may require environmental changes and political activity to promote those changes. For adolescents, tertiary prevention may focus on promoting use of contraceptives to prevent subsequent pregnancies, or condom use to prevent recurrent STDs.

Preventing Consequences

Tertiary prevention related to preventing further consequences of health problems is most often employed with children and adolescents who have chronic conditions. For example, the child with diabetes requires attention to diet, exercise, and medication to control the diabetes and prevent physical consequences of the disease itself. At the same time, attention must be given to promoting the child's adjustment to the condition and normalizing his or her life as much as possible. Nursing interventions would be geared toward convincing the child to stick to his or her diet and promoting social interactions with peers.

The nurse might also need to intervene to prevent or minimize the consequences of a child's condition for the rest of the family. For example, the nurse might need to point out to parents that in their concern for the child with a chronic heart condition, they are neglecting the needs of siblings. Tertiary prevention for an infant with AIDS may entail educating parents on the disposal of bodily fluids and excreta to prevent infection of other family members. Tertiary prevention may entail a wide variety of activities on the part of the nurse, from education on how to deal with specific conditions to referral for assistance with major medical expenses. Nurses may also need to act as advocates for children with chronic conditions. The example that most readily comes to mind is the need for advocacy for children with AIDS who are still well enough to attend school.

Emotional support by the nurse is a very important part of tertiary prevention for children with chronic conditions. Parents' and children's feelings about the condition need to be acknowledged and addressed. The nurse can also reinforce positive activities on the part of parent or child. Again, this support may need to be extended as families go through the grieving process. Grieving will probably occur with most chronic illnesses, even those that are not terminal, and the nurse should be prepared to reassure families that their feelings of grief are normal and to support them through this process.

Promoting Adjustment

The community health nurse may also engage in activities that are designed to return the child and family to a relatively normal state of existence. For children or adolescents with chronic illnesses or disabilities, this means restoring function as much as possible, preventing further loss of function, and assisting the child and his or her family to adapt lifestyles and behaviors to the presence of a chronic condition. The community health nurse might accomplish this by encouraging the family to discuss problems posed by the child's condition and to view the condition in the most positive light possible. The nurse should also encourage the family to normalize family life as much as possible. For example, if the Little League activities of a sibling have been curtailed because of an exacerbation of the child's illness, parents should make an attempt to reinstitute those activities as soon as the youngster's condition is stable, or the family can be encouraged to call on members of their support network to take the sibling to baseball practice and games.

With the advent of information technology, adjustment may be fostered by computer-mediated parent support groups. Parents of children with special needs or specific chronic illnesses can find support from parents who experience similar problems. Computer-mediated support groups have been shown to assist parents to find needed assistance and to improve parent–child interactions. In addition, computer-mediated groups have the advantage of eliminating the problem of finding appropriate childcare for a child with special needs that exists with participation in face-to-face support groups (Baum, 2004). Interventions that might be used by community health nurses in tertiary prevention with children and adolescents and their families are presented in Table 9◆.

EVALUATING HEALTH CARE FOR CHILD AND ADOLESCENT POPULATIONS

The effectiveness of nursing interventions for the individual child or adolescent is assessed in the same manner that care of any specific client is evaluated. Has intervention fostered the child's growth and development? Is the child's nutrition adequate for normal needs? Is the child up to date on his or her immunizations? Have physical or psychological hazards been eliminated from the child's environment? Is the child receiving health care as needed? Have acute health care problems been resolved?

The community health nurse would also examine the extent to which care has contributed to the adjustment of the child and family to an existing chronic disease or disability. Are parents comfortable and adequately prepared to parent a child with special needs? Do they perform this role adequately? Have complications of the child's condition been prevented?

The community health nurse may also be involved in evaluating the effects of interventions at the aggregate level. This might entail evaluating the extent to

TABLE 9	Tertiary Prevention Interventions for Child and Adolescent Populations
Focus	Interventions
Preventing recurrence	■ Educating children, adolescents, their families, and the public to prevent recurrence of health problems ■ Advocating societal and environmental changes needed to prevent recurrence of health problems
Preventing consequences	■ Monitoring and promoting effective disease management for children and adolescents with chronic conditions ■ Advocating for support services for children and adolescents with chronic conditions ■ Promoting development of children and adolescents with chronic conditions ■ Providing or referring for counseling for children and adolescents and their families as needed ■ Providing emotional support for children, adolescents, and their families ■ Referring caretakers for respite care as needed
Promoting adjustment	■ Promoting lifestyle changes consistent with effective disease management ■ Promoting normal family life as much as possible ■ Promoting communication within the family and between the family and health care providers ■ Initiating or referring families to existing support groups ■ Advocating for societal and environmental changes necessary for effective adjustment to a chronic illness

which national objectives for the health of children and adolescents have been achieved. Evaluative data regarding the status of several of these objectives are summarized below. For the most part, data are derived from the *Healthy People 2010*◆ Web site. As can be seen from the table, a few of the objectives (e.g., those related to low birth weight, preterm birth, and visual impairment) are actually moving away from the targeted levels. Community health nurses might be involved in gathering data related to the status of these objectives in their own communities to evaluate the effectiveness of child and adolescent care.

Community health nursing services for children and adolescents are one of the most effective means of enhancing the health of the population. Community health nurses can educate the public, parents, and children on health-promoting behaviors and provide early intervention for existing health problems to minimize their effects on the health of individual children and on the population during childhood and adolescence and on into adulthood.

HEALTHY PEOPLE 2010

Goals for Population Health◆

OBJECTIVE	BASELINE	MOST RECENT DATA	TARGET
■ 1-4b. Increase the proportion of children and youth aged 17 years and under who have a specific source of ongoing care	93%	94%	97%
■ 1-9a. Reduce pediatric hospitalizations for asthma (per 100,000 children)	23.0	21.4	17.3
■ 6-9. Increase inclusion of children with disabilities in regular education programs	45%	47%	60%
■ 8-11. Eliminate elevated blood lead levels in children 1 to 5 years of age	4.4%	NDA	0
■ 9-3. Increase the proportion of females at risk of unintended pregnancy who use contraceptives (age 15 to 19 years)	93%	NDA	100%
■ 9-7. Reduce pregnancies among adolescent females (per 1,000 girls 15 to 17 years of age)	68	NDA	43
■ 9-10. Increase the proportion of sexually active girls who use effective barrier contraception	68%	NDA	75%
■ 14-24. Increase the proportion of young children (19 to 35 months) who receive all vaccines that have been recommended for universal administration for at least five years	73%	80.9%	80%
■ 14-26. Increase the proportion of children who participate in fully operational population-based immunization registers	21%	45%	95%
■ 15-20. Increase use of child restraints	92%	95%	100%
■ 15-33. Reduce maltreatment and maltreatment fatalities of children (per 1,000 children)	12.6	12.4	10.3
■ 15-38. Reduce physical fighting among adolescents	36%	33%	32%
■ 15-39. Reduce weapon carrying by adolescents on school property	6.9%	6.1%	4.9%
■ 16-1c. Reduce infant deaths (per 1,000 live births)	7.2	7.0	4.5
■ 16-2. Reduce child death rates (per 100,000 children)			
a. 1 to 4 years	34.1	31.2	18.6
b. 5 to 9 years	17.2	15.2	13.3

Continued on next page

HEALTHY PEOPLE 2010 *continued*

■ 16-3. Reduce deaths of adolescents (per 100,000)			
a. 10 to 14 years	21.5	19.5	16.8
b. 15 to 19 years	69.5	67.8	39.8
■ 16-10. Reduce			
a. low birth weight	7.6%	7.8%#	5%
b. very low birth weight	1.4%	1.5%#	0.9%
■ 16-11. Reduce preterm births	11.6%	12.1%#	7.6%
■ 16-17. Increase abstinence among pregnant women			
a. alcohol	86%	NDA	94%
b. cigarette smoking	87%	87%	98%
c. illicit drugs	98%	NDA	100%
■ 16-19. Increase the proportion of mothers who breast-feed their babies (at 6 months)	29%	33%	50%
■ 18-2. Reduce the rate of suicide attempts by adolescents (12-month average)	2.6%	2.9%#	1%
■ 19-3. Reduce the proportion of children and adolescents who are overweight or obese (6 to 19 years)	11%	15%#	5%
■ 19-4. Reduce growth retardation in low-income children	8%	8%#	5%
■ 21-2. Reduce untreated dental decay in			
a. 2 to 4 years	16%	NDA	9%
b. 6 to 8 years	29%	NDA	21%
c. adolescents	20%	NDA	15%
■ 22-6. Increase the proportion of physically active adolescents	27%	25%#	30%
■ 26-9. Increase in high school seniors never using			
a. alcohol	19%	23%	29%
b. illicit drugs	46%	49%	56%
■ 27-2. Reduce tobacco use by adolescents (past month)	40%	27%	21%
■ 27-9. Reduce child tobacco exposure at home	20%	NDA	10%
■ 28-4. Reduce blindness and visual impairment in children and adolescents (per 1,000 children)	24	25	20
■ 28-12. Reduce otitis media in children and adolescents (visits per 1,000 children)	344.7	302.9	294

 # Objectives moving away from the 2010 target

NDA = No data available for this objective

Data from: Centers for Disease Control and Prevention. (2005). Healthy People Data 2010. Retrieved August 3, 2005, from http://wonder.cdc.gov/data2010

Case Study

Promoting Child Health

You have received a referral to visit Mrs. Kwon, a 24-year-old mother with a newborn baby. There is also another child in the family, Mandy, who is 3. Mrs. Kwon's pregnancy and delivery were uneventful, and mother and baby were discharged after 2 days in the hospital. When you make your home visit, Mrs. Kwon tells you that the baby is spitting up an ounce or so of formula after each feeding but had gained almost a pound at her 2-week visit to the pediatrician yesterday. Otherwise, the baby is doing well.

When you first arrive in the home, Mandy is sitting with her back to you watching cartoons on television. The TV is rather loud, and she does not seem to be aware that a visitor has arrived. While you are talking to Mrs. Kwon, Mandy turns around and sees you. She picks up her rag doll and comes to lean against her mother's knee with her thumb in her mouth. She seems to be rather pale compared with her mother's coloring.

Mandy pulls at her mother's sleeve to get her attention. When Mrs. Kwon continues to tell you about the baby spitting up, Mandy hits the infant with her doll. Mrs. Kwon scolds her and then tells you that Mandy used to be a very good girl, but ever since they brought the new baby home, she has been throwing tantrums and sucking her thumb.

1. What biophysical, psychological, sociocultural, behavioral, and health care system factors are influencing the health of these two children? Based on Mandy's pallor, what environmental factor may be present in this situation?
2. What screening tests and immunizations should these two children have had?

3. Based on the data presented above, what are your nursing diagnoses?
4. How could you involve members of the family in planning to resolve the problems identified?
5. What primary, secondary, and/or tertiary preventive measures might you employ with this family?

6. What community resources for child health would be helpful to this family? How would you go about locating them?
7. How would you go about evaluating the effectiveness of your nursing interventions?

Test Your Understanding

1. What is the difference between growth and development? How would you go about assessing each?

2. What are some safety considerations in the care of children and adolescents?

3. Describe at least five primary prevention measures appropriate to all children and adolescents. What modifications might be needed in these measures when caring for a child or adolescent with a chronic or terminal illness or a disability?

4. What are four areas in providing secondary prevention services to children and adolescents? Give an example of a community health nursing intervention related to each.

5. What are the three considerations in tertiary prevention for children and adolescents with existing health problems? Give an example of a community health nursing intervention related to each consideration.

EXPLORE MediaLink

http://www.prenhall.com/clark
Resources for this chapter can be found on the Companion Website.

Audio Glossary
Appendix C: Nursing Interventions for Common Health Problems in Children
Appendix H: Child and Adolescent Health Assessment and Intervention Guide

Exam Review Questions
Case Study: Promoting Children's Health and Safety
MediaLink Application: Adolescent Risk-Taking (video)

Media Links
Challenge Your Knowledge
Update *Healthy People 2010*
Advocacy Interviews

References

Alan Guttmacher Institute. (2002). *Sexual and reproductive health: Women and men.* Retrieved September 18, 2005, from http://www.guttmacher.org/pubs/fb_10-02.html

American Diabetes Association. (n.d.). *National diabetes fact sheet.* Retrieved March 8, 2006, from http://www.diabetes.org/diabetes-statistics/national-diabetes-fact-sheet.jsp

American Medical Association. (2004). *Breaking news: The social and economic impact of ADHD.* Retrieved June 7, 2005, from http://www.ama-assn.org/ama/pub/category/print/12869.html

Averhoff, F., Linton, L., Peddlecord, K. M., Edwards, C., Wang, W., & Fishbein, D. (2004). A middle school immunization law rapidly and substantially increases immunization coverage among adolescents. *American Journal of Public Health, 94,* 978–984.

Baum, L. S. (2004). Internet support groups for primary caregivers of a child with special health care needs. *Pediatric Nursing, 30,* 381–390.

Beck, L. F., Morrow, B., Lipscomb, L. E., & Johnson, C. H. (2002). Prevalence of selected maternal behaviors and experiences, Pregnancy Risk Assessment Monitoring System (PRAMS), 1999. *Morbidity and Mortality Weekly Report, 51*(SS-2), 1–27.

Belson, M., Kieszak, S., Watson, W., Blindauer, K. M., Phan, K., Backer, L., et al. (2003). Childhood pesticide exposures on the Texas-Mexico border: Clinical manifestations and poison center use. *American Journal of Public Health, 93,* 1310–1315.

Bilukha, O., & Rosenstein, N. (2005). Prevention and control of meningococcal disease: Recommendations of the Advisory Committee on Immunization Practices. *Morbidity and Mortality Weekly Report, 54*(RR-7), 1–21.

Blewett, L. A., Davern, M., & Rodin, H. (2004). Covering kids: Variation in health insurance coverage trends by state, 1996–2002; Despite nationwide improvements, variation persists in levels of children's coverage among states. *Health Affairs, 23,* 170–180.

California Department of Health Services. (2001, February 14). *Miniupdate,* 1.

Centers for Disease Control and Prevention. (2002a). Child passenger safety week, February 10–16, 2002. *Morbidity and Mortality Report, 51,* 104.

Centers for Disease Control and Prevention. (2002b). Hepatitis B vaccine. *Morbidity and Mortality Weekly Report, 51,* 33.

Centers for Disease Control and Prevention. (2002c). National poison prevention week, March 17–23, 2002. *Morbidity and Mortality Weekly Report, 51,* 215.

Centers for Disease Control and Prevention. (2004a). Indicators for Chronic Disease Surveillance. *Morbidity and Mortality Weekly Report, 53*(RR-11), 1–114.

Centers for Disease Control and Prevention. (2004b). National Infant Immunization Week, April 25–May 1, 2004. *Morbidity and Mortality Weekly Report, 53,* 290.

Centers for Disease Control and Prevention. (2005a). *Healthy People Data 2010.* Retrieved

August 3, 2005, from http://wonder.cdc.gov/data2010

Centers for Disease Control and Prevention. (2005b). Infant mortality rates, by selected ethnic populations—United States, 2002. *Morbidity and Mortality Weekly Report, 54,* 126.

Centers for Disease Control and Prevention. (2005c). National Infant Immunization Week, April 24–30, 2005. *Morbidity and Mortality Weekly Report, 54,* 361–362.

Centers for Disease Control and Prevention. (2006). Recommended childhood and adolescent immunization schedule—United States, 2006. *Morbidity and Mortality Weekly Report, 54*(51–52), Q-1–Q-4.

Chen, C.-W., Li, C.-Y., & Wang, J.-K. (2004). Growth and development of children with congenital heart disease. *Journal of Advanced Nursing, 47,* 260–269.

Childers, L. (2004). Baby blues. *Nurseweek, 17*(21), 24.

Childers, L. (2005). Caring to the end. *Nurseweek, 18*(11), 14–15.

County of San Diego Health and Human Services Agency. (2004). *Standards of care for the prevention of perinatal HIV transmission in San Diego County.* San Diego: Author.

Crisp, B. R., & Lister, P. G. (2004). Child protection and public health: Nurses' responsibilities. *Journal of Advanced Nursing, 47,* 656–663.

Datar, A., & Sturm, R. (2004). Physical education in elementary school and body mass index: Evidence from the Early Childhood Longitudinal Study. *American Journal of Public Health, 94,* 1501–1506.

Davies, R. (2004). New understandings of parental grief: Literature review. *Journal of Advanced Nursing, 46,* 506–513.

de Montigny, F., & Lacharite, C. (2005). Perceived parental efficacy: Concept analysis. *Journal of Advanced Nursing, 49,* 387–396.

Dilorio, C., Hartwell, T., & Hansen, N. (2002). Childhood sexual abuse and risk behaviors among men at high risk for HIV infection. *American Journal of Public Health, 92,* 214–219.

Division of Adult and Community Health. (2005). Estimated influenza vaccination coverage among adults and children—United States, September 1, 2004–January 31, 2005. *Morbidity and Mortality Weekly Report, 54,* 304–307.

Division of Birth Defects and Developmental Disabilities. (2002). Fetal alcohol syndrome—Alaska, Arizona, Colorado, and New York, 1995–1997. *Morbidity and Mortality Weekly Report, 51,* 433–435.

Division of Human Development and Disability, National Center on Birth Defects and Developmental Disabilities. (2003). Infants tested for hearing loss—United States, 1999–2001. *Morbidity and Mortality Weekly Report, 52,* 981–984.

Division of Reproductive Health. (2002). Infant mortality and low birth weight among black and white infants—United States, 1980–2000. *Morbidity and Mortality Weekly Report, 51,* 589–592.

Division of Reproductive Health. (2004a). Smoking during pregnancy—United States, 1990–2002. *Morbidity and Mortality Weekly Report, 53,* 911–915.

Division of Reproductive Health. (2004b). State estimates of neonatal health-care costs associated with maternal smoking—United States, 1996. *Morbidity and Mortality Weekly Report, 53,* 915–917.

Division of Unintentional Injury Prevention, National Center for Injury Prevention and Control. (2002). Nonfatal choking-related episodes among children—United States, 2001. *Morbidity and Mortality Weekly Report, 51,* 945–948.

Division of Unintentional Injury Prevention, National Center for Injury Prevention and Control. (2004). Child passenger deaths involving drinking drivers—United States, 1997–2002. *Morbidity and Mortality Weekly Report, 53,* 77–79.

Division of Violence Prevention. (2004). Violence-related behaviors among high school students—United States, 1991–2003. *Morbidity and Mortality Weekly Report, 53,* 651–655.

dos Rets, S., Zito, J. M., Safer, D. J., & Soeken, K. L. (2001). Mental health services for youths in foster care and disabled youths. *American Journal of Public Health, 91,* 1094–1099.

Epidemiology and Surveillance Division, National Immunization Program. (2005). Pertussis—United States, 2002–2003. *Morbidity and Mortality Weekly Report, 54,* 1283–1286.

Epidemiology Program Office. (2002). Variation in homicide risk during infancy—United States, 1989–1998. *Morbidity and Mortality Weekly Report, 51,* 187–189.

Epilepsy Foundation. (2005). *Epilepsy and seizure statistics.* Retrieved March 8, 2006, from http://www.efa.org/answerplace/statistics.cfm

Farrelly, M. C., Davis, K. C., Haviland, L., Messeri, P., & Healton, C. G. (2005). Evidence of a dose-response relationship between "truth" antismoking ads and youth smoking prevalence. *American Journal of Public Health, 95,* 425–431.

Federal Interagency Forum on Child and Family Statistics. (2004). *America's Children 2004.* Retrieved June 16, 2005, from http://www.childstats.gov/ac2004

Federwisch, A. (2005). Paying attention: Helping families cope with ADHD. *Nurseweek, 18*(21), 10–12.

Gaffney, K. F. (2001). Infant exposure to environmental tobacco smoke. *Journal of Nursing Scholarship, 33,* 343–347.

Gordon, J. A., Emond, J. A., & Camargo, C. A. Jr. (2005). The State Children's Health Insurance Program: A multicenter trial of outreach through the emergency department. *American Journal of Public Health, 95,* 250–253.

Green, A. (2004). Outcomes of congenital heart disease: A review. *Pediatric Nursing, 30,* 280–284.

Green, S. (2004). The impact of stigma on maternal attitudes toward placement of children with disabilities in residential life care facilities. *Social Science & Medicine, 59,* 799–812.

Grosse, S. D., Boyle, C. A., Botkin, J. R., Comeau, A. M., Kharrazi, M., Rosenfeld, M., et al., (2004). Newborn screening for cystic fibrosis: Evaluation of benefits and risks and recommendations for state newborn screening programs. *Morbidity and Mortality Weekly Report, 53*(RR-13), 1–37.

Grunbaum, J. A., Kann, L., Kinchen, S. A., Williams, B., Ross, J. G., Lowry, R., et al. (2002). Youth Risk Behavior Surveillance—United States, 2001. *Morbidity and Mortality Weekly Report, 51*(SS-4), 1–62.

Holl, J. L., Slack, K. S., & Stevens, A. B. (2005). Welfare reform and health insurance: Consequences for parents. *American Journal of Public Health, 95,* 279–285.

Huey, F. L. (Ed.). (2001). *Global impact of innovations on chronic disease in the genomics era.* New York: Pfizer.

Immunization Services Division, National Immunization Program. (2004). Estimated influenza vaccination coverage among adults and children—United States, September 1–November 30, 2004. *Morbidity and Mortality Weekly Report, 53,* 1147–1153.

Immunization Services Division, National Immunization Program. (2005a). Immunization Information System progress—United States, 2003. *Morbidity and Mortality Weekly Report, 54,* 722–724.

Immunization Services Division, National Immunization Program. (2005b). National, state, and urban area vaccination coverage among children aged 19–35 months—United States, 2004. *Morbidity and Mortality Weekly Report, 54,* 717–721.

Jennings, P. D. (2005). Providing pediatric palliative care through a pediatric supportive care team. *Pediatric Nursing, 31,* 195–200.

Jun, H.-J., Subramanian, S. V., Gortmaker, S., & Kawachi, I. (2004). Socioeconomic disadvantage, parenting responsibility, and women's smoking in the United States. *American Journal of Public Health, 94,* 2170–2176.

Kearney, P. M., & Pryor, J. (2004). The International Classification of Functioning, Disability, and Health (ICF) and nursing. *Journal of Advanced Nursing, 46,* 162–170.

Kempe, A., Beaty, B. L., Steiner, J. F., Pearson, K. A., Lowery, N. D., Daley, M. F., et al. (2004). The regional immunization registry as a public health tool for improving clinical practice and guiding immunization delivery policy. *American Journal of Public Health, 94,* 967–972.

King, C. K., Glass, R., Bresee, J. S., & Duggan, C. (2003). Managing acute gastroenteritis among children: Oral rehydration, maintenance, and nutritional therapy. *Morbidity and Mortality Weekly Report, 52*(RR-16), 1–16.

Klein, R., Stoll, K., & Bruce, A. (2004). *Medicaid: Good medicine for state economies, 2004 update.* Retrieved August 30, 2004, from http://www.families.org

Koniak-Griffin, D., Anderson, N. L. R., Verzemnieks, I., & Brecht, M.-L. (2000). A public health nursing early intervention program for adolescent mothers: Outcomes from pregnancy through 6 weeks postpartum. *Nursing Research, 49,* 130–138.

Kowaleski-Jones, L., & Duncan, G. J. (2002). Effects of participation in the WIC program on birthweight: Evidence from the National Longitudinal Survey of Youth. *American Journal of Public Health, 92,* 799–804.

Kranz, S., Siega-Riz, A. M., & Herring, A. H. (2004). Changes in diet quality of American preschoolers between 1977 and 1998. *American Journal of Public Health, 94,* 1525–1530.

Kreicbergs, U., Valdimarsdottir, U., Onelov, E., Henter, J.-I., & Steineck, G. (2004). Talking about death with children who have severe malignant disease. *New England Journal of Medicine, 351*, 1175–1186.

Krieger, J. W., Takaro, T. K., Song, L., & Weaver, M. (2005). The Seattle-King County Healthy Homes project: A randomized, controlled trial of a community health worker intervention to decrease exposure to indoor asthma triggers. *American Journal of Public Health, 95*, 652–659.

Kuo, F. E., & Taylor, A. F. (2004). A potential natural treatment for attention-deficit/hyperactivity disorder: Evidence from a national study. *American Journal of Public Health, 94*, 1580–1586.

Leslie, L. K., & Stein, M. T. (2003). Attention-deficit hyperactivity disorder. In H. M. Wallace, G. Green, & K. J. Jaros (Eds.), *Health and welfare for families in the 21st century* (2nd ed., pp. 407–421). Sudbury, MA: Jones and Bartlett.

Li, R., Ogden, C., Ballew, C., Gillespie, C., & Grummer-Strawn, L. (2002). Prevalence of exclusive breastfeeding among US infants: The Third National Health and Nutrition Examination Survey (Phase II, 1991–1994). *American Journal of Public Health, 92*, 1107–1112.

Marlow, N., Wolke, D., Bracewell, M. A., & Samara, M. (2005). Neurological and developmental disability at six years of age after extremely preterm birth. *New England Journal of Medicine, 352*, 9–19.

Maternal and Child Health Bureau. (2001). *All aboard the 2010 express*. Rockville, MD: Author.

Meleski, D. D. (2002). Families with chronically ill children: A literature review examines approaches to helping them cope. *American Journal of Nursing, 102*(5), 47–54.

Meyer, P. A., Pivetz, T., Dignam, T. A., Homa, D. M., Schoonover, J., & Brody, D. (2003). Surveillance for elevated blood lead levels among children—United States, 1997–2001. *Morbidity and Mortality Weekly Report, 52*(SS-10), 1–21.

Mofenson, L. M., Oleske, J., Serchuck, L., Van Dyke, R., & Wilfert, C. (2004). Treating opportunistic infections among HIV-exposed and infected children: Recommendations from CDC, the National Institutes of Health, and the Infectious Diseases Society of America. *Morbidity and Mortality Weekly Report, 53*(RR-14), 1–92.

Mu, P.-F. (2005). Paternal reactions to a child with epilepsy: Uncertainty, coping strategies, and depression. *Journal of Advanced Nursing, 49*, 367–376.

National Center for Chronic Disease Prevention and Health Promotion. (2003). Physical activity levels among children aged 9–13 years—United States, 2002. *Morbidity and Mortality Weekly Report, 52*, 785–788.

National Center for Environmental Health. (2005). Elevated blood lead levels in refugee children—New Hampshire, 2003–2004. *Morbidity and Mortality Weekly Report, 54*, 42–46.

National Center for Health Statistics. (2005a). Percentage of children aged < 18 years who have ever had asthma diagnosed by age group—United States, 2003. *Morbidity and Mortality Weekly Report, 54*, 312.

National Center for Health Statistics. (2005b). Prevalence of overweight among children and teenagers by age group and selected period—United States, 1963–2002. *Morbidity and Mortality Weekly Report, 54*, 203.

National Center for Health Statistics. (2005c). Racial/ethnic disparities in infant mortality—United States, 1995–2002. *Morbidity and Mortality Weekly Report, 54*, 553–556.

National Center for HIV, STD, and TB Prevention. (2002). Progress toward elimination of perinatal HIV infection—Michigan, 1993–2000. *Morbidity and Mortality Weekly Report, 51*, 93–97.

National Center for Injury Prevention and Control. (n.d.a). *Child passenger safety: Fact sheet*. Retrieved June 16, 2005, from http://www.cdc.gov/ncipc/factsheets/childpas.htm

National Center for Injury Prevention and Control. (n.d.b). *Playground injuries: Fact sheet*. Retrieved June 16, 2005, from http://www.cdc.gov/ncipc/factsheets/playgr.htm

National Center for Injury Prevention and Control. (n.d.c). *Poisonings: Fact sheet*. Retrieved June 16, 2005, from http://www.cdc.gov/ncipc/factsheets/poisoning.htm

National Center for Injury Prevention and Control. (n.d.d). *Water-related injuries: Fact sheet*. Retrieved June 16, 2005, from http://www.cdc.gov/ncipc/factsheets/drown.htm

National Center for Injury Prevention and Control. (2004a). *Child maltreatment: Fact sheet*. Retrieved June 16, 2005, from http://www.cdc.gov/ncipc/factsheets/cmfacts.htm

National Center for Injury Prevention and Control. (2004b). Nonfatal and fatal drownings in recreational water settings—United States, 2001–2002. *Morbidity and Mortality Weekly Report, 53*, 447–452.

National Center for Injury Prevention and Control. (2005). Nonfatal motor-vehicle-related backover injuries among children—United States, 2001–2003. *Morbidity and Mortality Weekly Report, 54*, 144–146.

National Center on Birth Defects and Developmental Disabilities. (2002). Alcohol use among women of childbearing age—United States, 1991–1999. *Morbidity and Mortality Weekly Report, 51*, 273–276.

National Center on Birth Defects and Developmental Disabilities. (2003). Fetal alcohol syndrome—South Africa, 2001. *Morbidity and Mortality Weekly Report, 52*, 660–662.

National Center on Birth Defects and Developmental Disabilities. (2004a). *ADHD: Attention-deficit/hyperactivity disorder*. Retrieved June 16, 2005, from http://www/cdc.gov/ncbddd/adhd/injury.htm

National Center on Birth Defects and Developmental Disabilities. (2004b). *Cerebral palsy*. Retrieved June 16, 2005, from http://www/cdc.gov/ncbddd/dd.ddcp.htm

National Center on Birth Defects and Developmental Disabilities. (2004c). Economic costs associated with mental retardation, cerebral palsy, hearing loss, and vision impairment—United States, 2003. *Morbidity and Mortality Weekly Report, 53*, 57–59.

National Center on Birth Defects and Developmental Disabilities. (2004d). *Fetal alcohol syndrome*. Retrieved June 16, 2005, from http://www/cdc.gov/ncbddd/fas/fasask.htm

National Center on Birth Defects and Developmental Disabilities. (2004e). *Mental retardation*. Retrieved June 16, 2005, from http://www/cdc.gov/ncbddd/dd/ddmr.htm

National Center on Birth Defects and Developmental Disabilities. (2005). *Autism*. Retrieved June 16, 2005, from http://www/cdc.gov/ncbddd/autism/asd_common.htm

National Diabetes Information Clearinghouse. (n.d.) *National diabetes statistics*. Retrieved June 16, 2005, from http://diabetes.niddk.nih.gov/dm/pubs/statistics/index.htm

National Immunization Program. (2004). Vaccination coverage among children entering school—United States, 2003–2004 school year. *Morbidity and Mortality Weekly Report, 53*, 1041–1044.

National Immunization Program. (2005). Hepatitis A vaccination coverage among children aged 24–35 months—United States, 2003. *Morbidity and Mortality Weekly Report, 54*, 141–144.

National Institutes for Mental Health. (2003). *Attention deficit hyperactivity disorder*. Retrieved March 8, 2006, from http://www.nimh.nih.gov/publications/NIMHadhdpub.pdf

National Program for Playground Safety. (2005). *Playground-related statistics*. Retrieved June 16, 2005, from http://www.playgroundsafety.org/resources/statistics.htm

Navaie-Waliser, M., Misener, M., Mersman, C., & Lincoln, P. (2004). Evaluating the needs of children with asthma in home care: The vital role of nurses as caregivers and educators. *Public Health Nursing, 21*, 306–315.

Neumark-Sztainer, D., Story, M., Hannan, P. J., & Croll, J. (2002). Overweight status and eating patterns among adolescents: Where do youths stand in comparison with the *Healthy People 2010* objectives? *American Journal of Public Health, 92*, 844–851.

Newacheck, P. W., & Benjamin, A. E. (2004). Intergenerational equity and public spending; The United States should embrace a new doctrine of fairness to ensure that vulnerable populations are not forced to compete for resources. *Health Affairs, 23*, 142–146.

Nicholas, S. W., Jean-Louis, B., Ortiz, B., Northridge, M., Shoemaker, K., Vaughan, R., et al. (2005). Addressing the childhood asthma crisis in Harlem: The Harlem Children's Zone Asthma Initiative. *American Journal of Public Health, 95*, 245–249.

Nisbet, C. (2004, Summer). Human milk for the very low birthweight infant. *Perinatal Care Matters*, pp. 1–2.

Nystrom, K., & Ohrling, K. (2004). Parenthood experiences during the child's first year: Literature review. *Journal of Advanced Nursing, 46*, 319–330.

O'Connor, M. E., Maddocks, B., Modie, C., & Pierce, H. (2001). The effect of different definitions of a patient on immunization assessment. *American Journal of Public Health, 91*, 1273–1275.

Oddy, W. H., Sherriff, J. L., de Klerk, N. H., Kendall, G. E., Sly, P. D., Beilin, L. J., et al. (2004). The relation of breastfeeding and body mass index to asthma and atopy in children: A prospective cohort study to age 6 years. *American Journal of Public Health, 94,* 1531–1537.

Office on Smoking and Health, National Center for Health Promotion and Disease Prevention. (2005a). Annual smoking-attributable mortality, years of potential life lost, and productivity losses—United States, 1997–2002. *Morbidity and Mortality Weekly Report, 54*(RR-7), 1–21.

Office on Smoking and Health, National Center for Health Promotion and Disease Prevention. (2005b). Tobacco use, access, and exposure to tobacco in media among middle and high school students—United States, 2004. *Morbidity and Mortality Weekly Report, 54,* 297–301.

Olsen, R., & Maslin-Prothero, P. (2001). Dilemmas in the provision of own-home respite support for parents of young children with complex health care needs: Evidence from an evaluation. *Journal of Advanced Nursing, 34,* 603–610.

Regional Perinatal Programs of California. (2004, Summer). Breastfeeding decreases infant mortality. *Perinatal Care Matters,* p. 2.

Rodwin, V. G., & Neuberg, L. G. (2005). Infant mortality and income in 4 world cities: New York, London, Paris, and Tokyo. *American Journal of Public Health, 95,* 86–90.

Rowe, A. K., Onikpo, F., Lama, M., Cokou, F., & Deming, M. S. (2001). Management of childhood illness at health facilities in Benin: Problems and their causes. *American Journal of Public Health, 91,* 1625–1635.

Santacroce, S. J. (2003). Parental uncertainty and posttraumatic stress in serious childhood illness. *Journal of Nursing Scholarship, 35,* 45–51.

Shirai, T., Matsui, T., Suzuki, K., & Chida, K. (2005). Effect of pet removal on pet allergic asthma. *Chest, 127,* 1565–1571.

Simons-Morton, B. G., Hartos, J. L., Leaf, W. A., & Preusser, D. F. (2005). Persistence of effects of the checkpoints program on parental restrictions of teen driving privileges. *American Journal of Public Health, 95,* 447–452.

Singh, I. (2004). Doing their jobs: Mothering with Ritalin in a culture of mother-blame. *Social Science & Medicine, 59,* 1193–1205.

Starfield, B. (2004). U.S. child health: What's amiss, and what should be done about it?; A strong primary care infrastructure is key to improving and reducing disparities in children's health. *Health Affairs, 23,* 165–170.

Strauss, L. T., Herndon, J., Chang, J., Parker, W. Y., Bowens, S. V., Zane, S. B., et al. (2004). Abortion surveillance—United States, 2001. *Morbidity and Mortality Weekly Report, 53*(SS-9), 1–32.

Strazdins, L., Korda, R. J., Lim, L. L.-Y., Broom, D. H., & D'Souza, R. M. (2004). Around-the-clock: Parent work schedules and children's well-being in a 24-h economy. *Social Science & Medicine, 59,* 1517–1527.

Sullivan-Bolyai, S., Knafl, K., Tamborlane, W., & Grey, M. (2004). Parents' reflections on managing their children's diabetes with insulin pumps. *Journal of Nursing Scholarship, 36,* 316–323.

Svavarsdottir, E. K. (2005). Caring for a child with cancer. *Journal of Advanced Nursing, 50,* 153–161.

Svavarsdottir, E. K., & Rayens, M. K. (2005). Hardiness in families of young children with asthma. *Journal of Advanced Nursing, 50,* 381–390.

Thorpe, L. E., List, D. G., Marx, T., May, L., Helgerson, S. D., & Frieden, T. R. (2004). Childhood obesity in New York City elementary school students. *American Journal of Public Health, 94,* 1496–1500.

Trust for America's Health. (2004). *Closing the vaccination gap: A shot in the arm for childhood immunization programs.* Retrieved September 28, 2004, from http://www.healthyamericans.org

United Nations Population Fund. (2003). *State of world population 2003: Making 1 billion count: Investing in adolescents' health and rights.* Geneva, Switzerland: Author.

U.S. Census Bureau. (2004a). *Poverty: 2003 highlights.* Retrieved September 30, 2004, from http://www.census.gov

U.S. Census Bureau. (2004b). *Statistical abstract of the United States: 2004–2005.* Retrieved May 12, 2005, from http://www.census.gov/prod/2004pubs/04statab

U.S. Department of Health and Human Services. (2002). Children's mental health is national priority. *Prevention Report, 16*(2), 5–6.

Wakschlag, L. S., Pickett, K. E., Cook, E. Jr., Benowitz, N. L., & Leventhal, B. L. (2002). Maternal smoking during pregnancy and severe antisocial behavior in offspring: An overview. *American Journal of Public Health, 92,* 966–974.

Wang, K.-W. K, & Barnard, A. (2004). Technology-dependent children and their families: A review. *Journal of Advanced Nursing, 45,* 36–46.

Warren, P. L. (2005). First-time mothers: Social support and confidence in infant care. *Journal of Advanced Nursing, 50,* 479–488.

Wise, P. (2004). The transformation of child health in the United States; Social disparities in child health persist despite dramatic improvements in child health overall. *Health Affairs, 23,* 9–25.

Wolfe, L. (2004). Should parents speak with a dying child about impending death? *New England Journal of Medicine, 351,* 1251–1253.

World Health Organization. (2004). *The world health report.* Geneva, Switzerland: Author.

Meeting the Health Needs of Men

CHAPTER OBJECTIVES

After reading this chapter, you should be able to:

1. Describe major considerations in assessing the biophysical, psychological, physical environmental, sociocultural, behavioral, and health care system factors affecting men's health.
2. Describe factors that contribute to adverse health effects for gay, bisexual, and transgender men.
3. Identify major considerations in primary prevention for men and analyze the role of the community health nurse with respect to each.
4. Describe secondary prevention considerations for men and related community health nursing roles.
5. Identify areas of emphasis in tertiary prevention for men and analyze the role of the community health nurse in each.

KEY TERMS

disclosure
erectile dysfunction (ED)
gender dysphoria
heterosexism
joblessness
reframing
unemployment

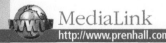

MediaLink
http://www.prenhall.com/clark

Additional interactive resources for this chapter can be found on the Companion Website. Click on Chapter 18 and "Begin" to select the activities for this chapter.

Advocacy in Action

Juan

Juan was a Spanish-speaking man in his 70's who had recently moved to the area from Puerto Rico with his family. He had problems with high blood pressure, which we were treating at St. Agnes Nurses Center. Over the course of a couple of weeks, we noticed that Juan appeared depressed. After exploring this further, we discovered that he was unhappy because in his native land he was used to working to support his family and was very upset by his inability to work here.

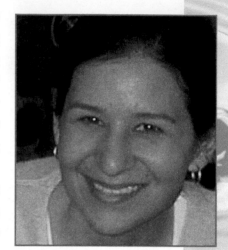

The nurses put their heads together, and within a week or so I accompanied Juan to the local grocery store. I spoke with the manager about Juan and told Juan about the job opportunity that was available. After I helped Juan complete the application, he was hired.

I occasionally ran into Juan at the grocery store and was always greeted with a big smile as well as an exuberant "Hola, mi amiga!"

Vienna Tomesheski, BA, BSN, RN

Med-Surg Staff Nurse, Paoli Hospital, PA

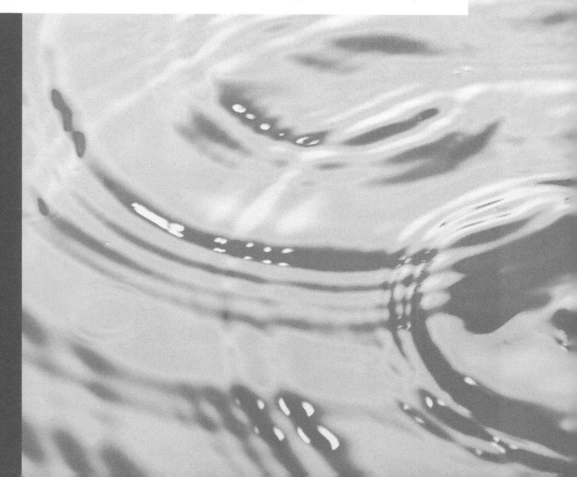

*I*n 2003, men between the ages of 20 and 64 years constituted roughly 30% of the U.S. population. This amounted to 87.8 million men in age groups that are more likely than any other segment of the population to lack access to health care services. By 2030, although the proportion is expected to remain stable, the actual number of men in this age group is expected to increase by 4.3 million to more than 92 million men (U.S. Census Bureau, 2005). Although health care services have traditionally been built around men's health care needs, U.S. men die an average of 7 years earlier than women (Huey, 2001), and mortality rates for all but one of the top 15 causes of death are higher for men than women (Williams, 2003). Only since the late 1990s has men's health been considered a separate and specific area of health care endeavor (White & Banks, 2004).

Men differ from women in their patterns of physical health disorders and health-related needs. These differences are attributable to (a) physiologic differences between men and women, (b) differences in health-related habits and health-seeking behavior, and (c) differences in social roles, stress, and coping. A great deal of health-related literature has been written about specific problems that influence men's health status (e.g., cardiovascular disease, lung cancer, etc.). Very little, however, is written about the overall health needs of men. The health care of men has been fragmented, approached from an episodic perspective. Little effort has been made to provide comprehensive, holistic health services.

Lack of emphasis on holistic health for men is evident in previous versions of the national health objectives. Women, children, and the elderly are among the populations that have been specifically targeted in previous sets of objectives; men have not. Only in the most recent objectives is prostate cancer addressed (U.S. Department of Health and Human Services [USDHHS], 2000)◆. Many of the past and current objectives will benefit men. The lack of attention to the total health of men, however, is a justifiable concern of community health nurses. The focus of this chapter is on preparing community health nurses to provide holistic care to men as a population group.

THE EPIDEMIOLOGY OF MEN'S HEALTH

Factors in each of the six dimensions of health affect men's health status. We will briefly consider major factors in the biophysical, psychological, physical environmental, sociocultural, behavioral, and health system dimensions and their influence on the health of the male population.

Biophysical Considerations

Men experience a variety of physical health conditions, many of which can be prevented or their effects ameliorated by effective community health nursing interven-

tion. In 2002, the leading causes of death for men were (a) heart disease, (b) malignant neoplasms, (c) unintentional injuries, (d) cerebrovascular disease, (e) chronic lower respiratory diseases, (f) diabetes mellitus, (g) influenza and pneumonia, (h) suicide, (i) nephritis, nephrotic syndrome, and nephrosis, and (j) chronic liver disease and cirrhosis. The overall age-adjusted male mortality rate for 2002 was 1,013 deaths per 100,000 men, compared to only 715.2 per 100,000 women (Centers for Disease Control and Prevention [CDC], 2004a). Men are twice as likely as women to die from heart disease, bronchitis, and accidental injuries, and three times more likely to commit suicide (Donaldson, 2004). Table 1◆ provides a comparison of male and female mortality for selected causes of death in the United States. Worldwide, the most frequent cause of death in young and middle adult men is traffic accidents. Other significant causes of male mortality and morbidity in developing regions are depression and bipolar disorder, alcohol use, violence, tuberculosis, the effects of war, suicide, schizophrenia, and anemia (Huey, 2001).

Men also experience higher levels of morbidity for many health problems than do women (Table 2◆). For example, cancer diagnoses occur 1.3 times more often in men than women (Williams, 2003), and one half of men will have a diagnosis of cancer at some time in their lives compared to only one third of women (CDC, 2004b). Men are also more likely to die from cancers than women, primarily because the major site for cancer in men is the lung, with poor prognosis for recovery. Women, on the other hand, often have more highly detectable and treatable cancers (Division of Cancer Prevention and Control, 2004). Much of the difference in cancer mortality between men and women is attributable to malignant melanoma, one of the most virulent

TABLE 1	Age-adjusted Male and Female Mortality from Selected Causes, United States, 2002 (per 100,000 population)		
Cause of Mortality	Men	Women	Ratio Men to Women
Overall	1,013.7	715.2	1.4 to 1
Heart disease	297.4	197.2	1.5 to 1
Cerebrovascular disease	56.5	55.2	ca. 1 to 1
Malignant neoplasms	238.9	163.1	1.5 to 1
Cancer of lungs, trachea, bronchus	73.2	41.6	1.75 to 1
Lower respiratory diseases	53.5	37.4	1.4 to 1
HIV/AIDS	7.4	2.5	2.9 to 1
Homicide	9.4	2.8	3.4 to 1

Data from: Centers for Disease Control and Prevention. (2004). Health, United States, 2004. Retrieved August 9, 2005, from http://www.cdc.gov/nchs/data/hus/hus04.pdf

TABLE 2	Age-adjusted Male and Female Morbidity from Selected Causes, United States, 2002		
Cause of Morbidity	Men	Women	Ratio Men to Women
AIDS (per 100,000 population)	27.4	9.0	3 to 1
Lung cancer (per 100,000 population)	73.6	46.4	1.6 to 1
Colorectal cancer (per 100,000 population)	59.5	44.1	1.3 to 1
Prostate cancer (per 100,000 population)	171.4	N/A	N/A
Cancer of oral cavity and pharynx (per 100,000 population)	14.6	6.2	2.3 to 1
Stomach cancer (per 100,000 population)	11.5	5.6	2 to 1
Pancreatic cancer (per 100,000 population)	12	9.2	1.3 to 1
Bladder cancer (per 100,000 population)	35.5	8.8	4 to 1
Arthritis	17.8%	23.7%	
Activity limitation due to chronic conditions	12.3%	12.3%	
Elevated blood cholesterol	16.9%	17%	
Hypertension	25.1%	25.7%	
Overweight	68.8%	61.7%	
Obesity	28.1%	34.0%	
Injury (per 100,000 population)	92.9	77.2	1.2 to 1

Data from: Centers for Disease Control and Prevention. (2004). Health, United States, 2004. Retrieved August 9, 2005, from http://www.cdc.gov/nchs/data/hus/hus04.pdf; Division of Adult and Community Health. (2005c). Racial/ethnic disparities in the prevalence and impact of doctor-diagnosed arthritis—United States, 2002. Morbidity and Mortality Weekly Report, 54, 119–123; U.S. Census Bureau. (2005). Statistical abstract of the United States: 2004–2005. Retrieved August 16, 2005, from http://www.census.gov/prod/2004pubs/04statab

forms of skin cancer. Melanoma mortality increased 66% among U.S. men from 1969 to 1999. It has subsequently declined in younger men due to earlier age at diagnosis, but continues to be high in men over 65 years of age (Culpepper & McKee, 2004). Differences in melanoma mortality between men and women most likely arise from differential exposure to sunlight in occupational and recreational activities.

Men develop heart disease at earlier ages and die earlier than women, and gender differences in traditional risk factors for heart disease have been found to explain only approximately 40% to 50% of the difference in mortality (Purcell, Daly, & Petersen, 2004; Weidner & Cain, 2003). On average, one in four men will die from myocardial infarction, compared to one in six women (Purcell et al., 2004).

Although the prevalence of self-reported emphysema or chronic bronchitis has been found to be lower in men than in women (45.5% and 73.2%) and women make slightly more total visits to providers for these conditions, the annual rate of visits per 1,000 men is higher than that for women (46.8 visits per 1,000 men and 43.4 for women). In addition, men are more likely to be hospitalized for chronic obstructive pulmonary disease (COPD) than women at 42.4 hospitalizations per 1,000 men compared to only 40.2 per 1,000 women. Men are also more likely than women to die as a result of COPD, with mortality rates of 82.6 per 100,000 for men in 2000 versus 56.7 per 100,000 for women (Mannino, Homa, Akinbami, Ford, & Redd, 2002).

Breast cancer and osteoporosis, often considered diseases of women, can also be found in men. In 2001, for example, an estimated 1,400 to 1,600 men received a diagnosis of breast cancer and an estimated 400 deaths occurred. Breast cancer incidence in the United States increased by 50% from 1995 to 2000. Risk factors for male breast cancer include a family history of the disease (in male or female relatives), age 50 to 60 years, Klinefelter's syndrome with its extra X chromosome, gynecomastia, a history of radiation therapy as a child, and cirrhosis or parasitic liver disease. Breast cancer diagnosis for a man brings feelings of isolation, embarrassment, and loss of self-image (Banks, 2002).

Osteoporosis, which is a frequent occurrence in postmenopausal women, also occurs in men. The World Health Organization has defined osteoporosis as a bone matter density 2.5 standard deviations below the mean for young adults (Lim & Fitzpatrick, 2004). As many as 2 million American men are affected by osteoporosis, with as many as 3 million more at risk for the disease (Curry & Hogstel, 2002). An estimated one in every eight men will experience an osteoporotic fracture at some point in their lives. Men account for approximately 30% of hip fractures and 20% of vertebral fractures due to osteoporosis (Lim & Fitzpatrick, 2004). Age-related bone loss begins for both men and women after age 40 and progresses at 0.5% to 1% loss in bone density per year. Although men do not experience the accelerated bone loss suffered by women at menopause, a 60-year-old man has a 25% chance of an osteoporotic fracture at some point in his life (Shepherd, 2004). Most risk factors for osteoporosis are similar for men and women, but men have higher levels of some risk factors (e.g., smoking, alcohol use) than women. Other predisposing factors include long-term corticosteroid use, hypogonadism, organ transplantation, gastrointestinal conditions such as celiac disease and pancreatic insufficiency, chronic liver disease, diabetes, and a variety of medications, such as anticonvulsants, psychotropic drugs, and immunosuppressants (Lim & Fitzpatrick, 2004).

Men also have higher rates of sexually transmitted diseases (STDs) than women. For example, the incidence of gonorrhea among men in their early 20s is 500 to 600 cases per 100,000 population. Similar incidence is also seen for *Chlamydia trachomatis*, a sexually transmitted disease often thought to occur primarily in women. In 2002, men had incidence rates for primary and secondary syphilis three times those for women (CDC, 2005). Men often have very little knowledge of STDs beyond HIV infection, gonorrhea, and syphilis and less knowledge of STD prevention (Alan Guttmacher Institute, 2004). Approximately 80% of U.S. adults with AIDS are men, and genital herpes affects one in every six men (Pinkelman, 2002a).

In addition to experiencing conditions that occur in women, but at frequently lower rates of incidence, men are subject to some unique biophysical conditions. Among these are prostate and testicular cancers and erectile dysfunction. An estimated 230,000 new cases of prostate cancer were expected to be diagnosed in U.S. men in 2004 (Johnson, 2004). Prostate cancer is the second leading cause of cancer deaths in men and contributes to 10% of all deaths in men. One in every six men will develop prostate cancer in his lifetime and one in 32 men will die of this disease despite increasing survival rates with treatment (Pinkelman, 2002b). Prostate cancer may result in feelings of inadequacy that lead to changes in relationships, feelings of lost manhood, and changes in sexual feelings, as well as to erectile dysfunction (Johnson, 2004). Although prostate cancer is frequently not life threatening, its implications for men's quality of life cannot be underestimated. Prostate cancer and benign prostatic hyperplasia (BPH) may both obstruct urinary flow, resulting in reduced urinary flow, increasing frequency, and nocturia. Approximately 43% of middle-aged and older men experience BPH (Kirby & Kirby, 2004). An additional 2% to 6% of men at any given time may experience prostatitis, an inflammation of the prostate gland and the most common urological diagnosis in men over age 50. Prostatitis may cause pain, difficulty voiding, and sexual dysfunction, all symptoms that can significantly alter quality of life (Nickel, 2004).

Testicular cancer is the most common cancer in men 15 to 44 years of age and causes 2% of all cancers in men. Overall incidence of testicular cancer in men under 50 years of age is 2 per 1,000 men. Men with a history of cryptorchism (an undescended testicle) account for 10% of testicular cancers, and the risk increases sixfold for testes that remain in the abdominal cavity. Even normally situated testes are affected in 20% of cases of one maldescended testicle. Surgical removal of the undescended testicle is recommended if the testicle cannot be effectively placed and maintained in the scrotal sac. Trauma is another contributing factor in testicular cancer, as is intrauterine exposure to hormones such as diethylstilbestrol or radiation (Hendry & Christmas, 2004).

In addition to its life-threatening potential, testicular cancer has profound psychological implications for men in terms of sexuality, self-identity, and fertility. Five-year survival rates for testicular cancer are high at 90%, but sexuality concerns may delay seeking treatment and contribute to greater potential for death. Anywhere from 15% to 30% of men with testicular cancer have long-term sexual dysfunction after treatment, and a diagnosis of testicular cancer may lead to feelings of inadequacy, hopelessness, and depression (Gurevich, Bishop, Bower, Malka, & Nyhof-Young, 2003).

Erectile dysfunction (ED), formerly called impotence, occurs when a man cannot achieve or maintain an erection sufficient for satisfactory sexual activity (Carson, 2004). The relatively high prevalence of ED was not recognized until a landmark study in Massachusetts in 1994 indicated that 52% of men between 40 and 60 years of age experienced some level of difficulty (Solomon & Jackson, 2004). Approximately 20% to 30% of U.S. men (approximately 30 million) have erectile dysfunction, but only 5% to 10% seek treatment for this problem (Chua & Bakris, 2004; Johnson, 2004). Worldwide prevalence of ED is estimated at more than 150 million men and is expected to double by 2025 (Kirby, 2004). The incidence of ED increases with age, with approximately 39% of men aged 40 to 50 years affected compared to 70% of those over age 70 (Johnson, 2004). Research has indicated that both age and atherosclerotic processes contribute to the development of ED, but that diminished blood flow due to atherosclerosis has a greater effect on its development than age (Solomon & Jackson, 2004).

An estimated 35% of men 40 to 70 years of age experience moderate to severe ED that may be due to a number of factors. Some of the common contributing factors are chronic diseases such as diabetes, hypertension, and arteriosclerosis; medications used to treat these and other conditions; and anxiety. For example, 39% to 64% of men with cardiovascular disease also experience ED, and the presence of erectile dysfunction may suggest coronary heart disease or a worsening of an existing cardiac condition. In addition, 44% to 64% of men who have had myocardial infarction develop ED. Similarly, more than 68% of men with hypertension develop ED, and the prevalence increases in men with both hypertension and diabetes. Over half of men with diabetes will experience erectile dysfunction at some point (Kirby, 2004), and men with diabetes are four times more likely than other

MediaLink

Prostate Cancer (video)

men to experience complete ED (Solomon & Jackson, 2004).

Obesity has also been linked to erectile dysfunction; a man with a 42-inch waist is 50% more likely to have erectile difficulties than one with a 32-inch waist (Calandra, 2004). Renal failure and alcohol use are additional contributing factors in erectile dysfunction (Johnson, 2004). Smoking appears to be another risk factor, and pharmacologic treatment for many of the conditions that cause ED may also contribute to erectile dysfunction. For example, statin therapies for cardiovascular disease may exacerbate ED, and sexual dysfunction is a common side effect of many antihypertensive medications (Solomon & Jackson, 2004).

Infertility is another condition that poses significant threats to men's self-image. Male infertility is implicated in approximately half of couples unable to conceive, either independently or in conjunction with female fertility factors. Approximately 25% of male infertility arises from unknown causes. Possible causes of infertility include prior surgeries, pelvic trauma, sexually transmitted disease, genetic causes such as Klinefelter's syndrome, medication use, and toxic exposures. One relatively common and treatable cause of male infertility is varicocele, a dilatation of spermatic veins, which can be addressed with surgical intervention. Hormone therapies or in vitro fertilization may be effective for other forms of infertility (Alam, Niederberger, & Meacham, 2004).

Another area to be addressed in assessing men's physiologic function is the presence of adverse effects related to accidental injury. Males at all ages have higher rates of unintentional injuries than females. This is particularly true for motor vehicle accidents. In the 2001–2002 period, for example, men accounted for 17% more emergency department visits than women (CDC, 2004a). Unintentional firearms mortality among men from 1993 to 1998 was eight times higher than among women (Gotsch, Annest, Mercy, & Ryan, 2001). As we will see later in this chapter, many of these differences arise from risk behaviors engaged in by men. Other factors that may contribute to accidental injuries and should be assessed by the community health nurse are sensory impairments. These impairments, if undetected and uncorrected, may contribute to a variety of physical and psychological health problems.

The last aspect of physiologic function to be considered in assessing the health status of men is immunization levels. Men, as well as women, should be immunized against tetanus and diphtheria (Td), influenza, and pneumococcal disease, and susceptible men should also receive varicella vaccine. Although men are more likely than women to have received tetanus vaccines in the last 10 years, they are less likely to have received influenza vaccine in the past year or to ever have received pneumococcal vaccine (Singleton, Greby, Wooten, Walker, & Strikas, 2000).

GLOBAL PERSEPECTIVES

Around the world, men fare worse than women in many health-related venues. For example, in 2003, differences in life expectancy at birth varied from 2 years less for men than women in the African Region of the World Health Organization (WHO) to 9 years less in the European Region. Similarly, health life expectancy varied from 1 to 6 years, with men having a shorter expectation of a healthy life span. In fact, men in the African Region, on average, can expect only 40 years of healthy life before dying at the relatively young age of 46 years (WHO, 2005). In part, these differences are due to differences in disease and injury incidence and behavioral risk factors and would be even worse if not for the relatively high rates of maternal mortality in much of the developing world.

Mean systolic blood pressure is consistently higher among men than women in each of the six WHO regions. Similarly, tobacco use among adolescent boys is nearly twice that of girls in all WHO regions except the Americas (WHO, 2005). Men also have higher levels of alcohol consumption and greater risk of accidental injury than women. Poverty and poor employment opportunities can threaten men's mental and physical health status, particularly in areas where gender socialization casts men as the primary bread-winner in the family. In addition, growing urbanization and movement of young men to large cities to find employment separates them from the support of extended families, contributing to depression and substance abuse (Alan Guttmacher Institute, 2005a; Monts, 2002a).

What other factors may contribute to the global lower health status of men than women? To what extent do these factors contribute to differences in your own community?

Psychological Considerations

Several related elements of the psychological dimension are of concern to community health nurses caring for men. These elements include socialization, stress, and coping abilities, as well as suicide as an outcome of ineffective coping.

Men, like women, have several basic psychological needs. These include the needs to know and be known to others, to be mutually interdependent, to love and be loved, and to live meaningful lives. Society, however, has socialized both men and women to accept a stereotypical male role that makes it difficult to meet these needs. General dimensions of this stereotyped role include a need to actively differentiate oneself from women and refrain from behaviors ascribed to women (such as demonstrating affection or seeking help) and a need to see oneself as superior to others. Other dimensions include the need to be strong and self-reliant and to be more powerful than others, even if this means resorting to violence to demonstrate one's power.

Because of this stereotyped view of the masculine role, men experience social pressures to conform that sometimes conflict with health. Socialized to view the male role as strong or invulnerable, a man may have difficulty admitting health-related frailties to a community health nurse. Similarly, men who believe that taking physical risks is fundamental to their masculinity may experience more frequent health impairment from trauma. Pressure to assert one's manliness also contributes to early initiation of sexual activity by young men, putting them at risk for STDs and unintended fatherhood (Alan Guttmacher Institute, 2005a). In addition, internalization of the typical male gender role has been shown to be associated with less attention to routine screenings such as testicular self-examination (Gurevich et al., 2003). As can be seen in these examples, when societal messages about male roles are internalized by men, they become psychological factors influencing health-related behaviors.

Men may also have a stronger psychological need than women to see themselves as healthy and even invulnerable. Because men tend to value strength and endurance more than women, they are more likely to conceal or suppress pain and other perceived indicators of frailty. An example of this state of mind can be seen in the male post–myocardial infarction client who resumes shoveling snow against the recommendations of health care professionals and his family, and who continues the activity despite the return of the now-familiar angina. As a result of this need for strength in his self-image, the male client minimizes the importance of the problem. Consequently, when shoveling snow causes further angina, he may seek health care less readily and use it less effectively than would a female client in a similar situation.

Similar responses may occur with mental health problems. Traditional American culture prohibits men from expressing emotions other than anger and aggression, and men may be unable to express grief, sadness, or powerlessness, allowing these emotions to fester and contributing to depression (Calandra, 2004). Gendered communication styles are another aspect of gender socialization that may make it difficult for men to express needs and feelings (Marston, 2004).

Based on data from 1993 to 2001, men less frequently reported frequent mental distress than women (7.2% versus 10.3%) (National Center for Chronic Disease Prevention and Health Promotion, 2004). Men are also less likely than women to report depression, but still account for 20% of diagnoses of clinical depression. Physicians are also less likely to diagnose depression in men than women (Monts, 2002b). Men are less willing to acknowledge depression and deal with it less well than women, contributing to a variety of health problems (Weidner & Cain, 2003). For example, depression is more often associated with coronary heart disease in men than in women (Monts, 2002b).

Conversely, male values of strength and endurance do not always adversely affect a male client's health. Some men who value strength actually may be more motivated to exercise and maintain a higher level of general fitness and to seek preventive health care to preserve their sense of themselves as strong and invulnerable.

Another psychological barrier to men's health is the male client's conflicting response to feelings regarding a health problem. For example, a man who values strength may exercise regularly, but he may avoid having a swelling in his groin examined because he cannot cope effectively with the fear that the swelling may represent a threat to his sexuality. This is particularly true with respect to problems like testicular growths, because testicular integrity is closely linked to perceptions of manliness, sexual attractiveness, and desirability (Gurevich et al., 2003).

Men and women are exposed to different types of stress and cope with stress in different ways. For example, men are more likely than women to engage in avoidant coping strategies (Weidner & Cain, 2003). Similarly, post-traumatic stress disorder (PTSD) arises from different types of events and manifests differently in men and women. One frequent cause of PTSD in men is combat exposure, which contributes to approximately 28% of PTSD in men. In one study, PTSD was found to contribute to 7.4% of depression, 8% of substance abuse disorder, 12% of job loss, 9% of current unemployment and divorce or separation, and 21% of partner or spouse abuse in combat veterans (Prigerson, Maciejewski, & Rosenheck, 2002).

PTSD and other mental health problems may contribute to suicide. Although women make more suicide attempts, rates of completed suicide are four times higher in U.S. men than women (Monts, 2002b). Suicide mortality is highest among White men, at 19.1 per 100,000 population, compared to 4.3 per 100,000 among White women. Similar gender differences are noted for Black men (10.0 per 100,000) and women (1.8 per 100,000) (U.S. Census Bureau, 2005).

Suicide claims more lives among men annually than many of the diseases that health care professionals combat so effectively. Because suicide is such a frequent cause of mortality for men, it is important that community health nurses assess the male population for the presence of suicide risk factors:

- Significant portions of the population 15 to 24 years of age or older than 65 years
- High rates of chronic physical or mental disorders (particularly those that are progressively debilitating or that lead to deterioration in function)
- High rates of depression
- High rates of substance abuse

Physical Environmental Considerations

With the exception of the occupational environment, which is addressed in the discussion of the sociocultural dimension, the effects of the physical environment on

59

men's health are much the same as they are on women's health. Pollution, overcrowding, and safety hazards adversely affect both. Men, however, may have increased exposure to environmental hazards due to occupational and leisure activity choices.

Sociocultural Considerations

Many influences on men's health arise from the sociocultural dimension. We have already discussed the influences of gender socialization, a sociocultural factor, on men's psychological health. Other considerations in the sociocultural dimension affecting men's health include family interactions, economic and occupational issues, and issues related to violence.

Family Interactions

By far, the largest proportion of men live within a family situation, which may create both positive and negative health effects. Worldwide, most men are married by the time they are in their 30s, but delayed marriage is associated with higher educational levels. By their 40s to mid-50s, most men have been married, some of them several times (Alan Guttmacher Institute, 2005a). Approximately 27% of American men marry in their early 20s, and this figure doubles by the late 20s. White and Hispanic men tend to marry earlier than Black men. About 70% of men in their 30s are married and 80% of men in their 40s are married or cohabiting (Alan Guttmacher Institute, 2004). In 2003, 61% of adult men were married, 28% had never married, nearly 3% were widowed, and close to 9% were divorced (U.S. Census Bureau, 2005).

Marriage has been shown to have a protective health effect for men and less so for women; however, because of socialization to a stereotyped male role and gender communication styles discussed earlier, men may have difficulty interacting within the family in ways that effectively meet their psychological needs. Differing role expectations between husband and wife may lead to marital conflicts and, in some cases, spouse or child abuse. It is important for the community health nurse dealing with male clients to assess the marital status of the male population.

Parenting is another aspect of family interaction that may affect men's health. Approximately one fourth of U.S. men have had a child by 20 years of age and 50% by age 30. Early parenthood is more likely among minority men and those with lower educational levels. Younger men are often involved in pregnancies that end in abortion. In fact, in the United States, 13% of pregnancies that result in abortion involve adolescent fathers, and 53% involve men in their 20s. Half of all live births in the U.S. involve men in their 20s (Alan Guttmacher Institute, 2002), and 80% of births involving men in their early 20s and 50% in the late 20s occur

outside of marriage. Thus, men may have children who do not live with them. Divorce may also separate many men from their children. Sixty-seven percent of U.S. men in their 30s and 85% of men in their 40s have one or more children who may or may not be living with them (Alan Guttmacher Institute, 2002). In fact, an estimated 11% of U.S. men in their 30s have biological children who do not live with them (Alan Guttmacher Institute, 2004).

Because of typical male socialization, many men have little or no childcare experience, yet the increase in the number of working women has led to greater assumption of childcare duties by men. Married women with children have been shown to spend 50% more time with them than their fathers do, although the amount of time men spend with their children increased about one hour per day between 1965 and 1995 (Alan Guttmacher Institute, 2002). Many men may find themselves single parents as a result of divorce or the death of their wives. Others may have partial custody of children as a result of divorce. In 2003, 19% of single-parent households were headed by men, an increase from 17% in 2000. Four percent of these single male-headed households included three or more children (U.S. Census Bureau, 2005).

Although stressful, parenthood, like marriage and particularly in the context of marriage, may have a protective health effect for men. In one study, for example, married men with children had lower overall mortality rates and lower rates of death due to ischemic heart disease, accidents, and addictions than single childless men and fathers who did not live with their children. Single parenthood by men was also associated with lower mortality rates than childlessness or noncustodial parenthood, but differences were not as great as for married men with children (Weitoft, Burstrom, & Rosen, 2004).

Divorce is one of the most significant stressors a person can experience, and it frequently has a profound effect on physical and psychological health. Divorced men, in particular, have been shown to experience increased morbidity and mortality as compared with married men. Men may respond to divorce or its

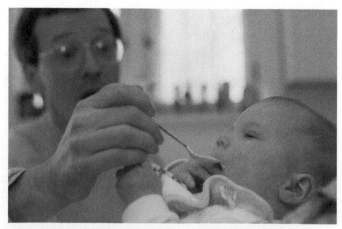

More men are raising children as single parents. (Patrick J. Watson)

aftermath with intense anger, a profound sense of loss, or significant depression. Suicidal behavior occasionally occurs as the man reacts to the divorce as an assault against his self-image and self-worth, or homicidal behavior if he directs his anger toward his ex-spouse. Widowed men also fare less well than widowed women (Weitoft et al., 2004). Although women are more likely than men to experience divorce, separation, or widowhood in their 40s, men tend to have greater health effects due to the loss of a spouse (Alan Guttmacher Institute, 2002; Weitoft et al., 2004).

Economic and Occupational Issues

In most cultures, men are the primary breadwinners for the family, although more and more women throughout the world can be found in the workforce. Worldwide poverty and poor employment prospects undermine men's ability to fulfill their provider roles. Unemployment may be high in many developing countries and urbanization may lead young men to leave their families for extended periods of time to seek employment where it can be found (Alan Guttmacher Institute, 2005a). In the United States, men fare better than women in terms of their economic status, yet economic influences can have profound effects on their health status.

Economic status is closely linked to employment and unemployment. Some authors make a distinction between the societal experience of unemployment and the individual experience of "joblessness." From this perspective, **unemployment** is the proportion of the workforce that is not employed at a specific point in time and is a statistical measure reflecting the general state of the economy. **Joblessness**, on the other hand, is the personalized experience of being out of work when one desires employment. Joblessness can have significant implications for both physical and mental health among men since "most men in America gain at least part of their sense of manhood from their participation in the workforce" (Cooke, 2004, p. 156). Although joblessness affects the mental health of both men and women, its mental health effects seem to be worse for men than women (Artazcoz, Benach, Borrell, & Cortes, 2004).

In 2003, nearly 69% of U.S. men over 16 years of age were employed, and employment rates are expected to rise to 73% by 2012. Slightly more than 5% of employed men hold more than one job. Another 6% of men were unemployed in 2003, 62% of them due to job loss. The median hourly wage for all men was $13.25, but more than 1% of male workers over age 25 received minimum wage or less. Similarly, the median family income for families headed by a man without a spouse present was $41,711, but 483,000 of these families have annual incomes less than $15,000. Nearly 15 million men (11.2% of all U.S. men) had incomes below poverty level in 1999, only slightly less than women at 13.5% (U.S. Census Bureau, 2005). In 2003, 13.5% of male-headed households had incomes below poverty level (U.S. Census

Bureau, 2004b). Poverty is one of several reasons that men are more likely than women to be homeless. Despite the differences in the incidence of homelessness among men and women, homeless shelter systems are often better designed to meet the needs of women and children than those of men (Archambault, 2002).

Men are more likely than women to be employed in jobs that entail physical health risks. In 2002, for example, the rate of occupational injury deaths was nearly 10 times higher for men (6.8 per 100,000 employed workers) than women (0.7 per 100,000). The highest rates of death occurred in agriculture, forestry, fishing, mining, and construction, enterprises less likely to employ women (CDC, 2004a). In addition, a higher percentage of men (4%) than women (3.8%) have work-related disabilities (U.S. Census Bureau, 2005).

Economic status is also associated with educational levels. Men are more likely to drop out of high school than women and less likely to attend college. In 2002, for example, only 62% of men aged 16 to 24 years were enrolled in college, compared to 68% of women (U.S. Census Bureau, 2005).

Violence and Trauma

Earlier, we discussed the implications of PTSD for men's psychological health. PTSD and other health problems arise from exposure to a variety of forms of violence and trauma. Men are more likely than women to be exposed to societal violence in many forms. For example, in 2002 men constituted 78% of homicide victims over 18 years of age. In 2002, the homicide rate for men was 9.4 per 100,000 men, down from 13.6 in 1976, but still more than three times the rate for women (2.8 per 100,000) (CDC, 2004a; U.S. Census Bureau, 2005). Men are also exposed to higher rates of physical assault than women. In 2002, the assault victimization rate for men was 23.9 per 1,000 men compared to 19.8 for women (CDC, 2005).

Violence also occurs in families, and men, as well as women, are subjected to intimate partner violence (IPV). Men, however, are less likely to be injured as a result of IPV. In one study of IPV in rural settings, more men than women (4.7% versus 2.9%) reported being the victim of at least one episode of severe physical violence by their partner. Men were less likely than women, however, to report emotional abuse (30.2% and 46.7%, respectively). Interestingly, men engaged in farm work reported more physical abuse and controlling abuse than other men, possibly related to the greater stress and economic uncertainty experienced in agriculture than in other areas of employment (Murty et al., 2003). Overall, men report considerably less IPV than women, with rates of 4.2 per 1,000 women in 2000 compared with only 0.8 per 1,000 men (CDC, 2005). In part, however, these differences may be related to men's reluctance to report being victims of IPV because of threats to their self-image.

Trauma also results from unintentional injury. In 2002, men experienced six times as many firearms-related deaths as women and nearly twice as many deaths related to poisoning. The unintentional injury mortality rate for men was similarly nearly twice that for women. Men also experience high rates of injury requiring emergency department services. For example, the rate of emergency department visits for men in 2002 was 154 per 1,000 men compared to 123 per 1,000 women (CDC, 2005).

Behavioral Considerations

Behavioral factors seem to make a greater contribution to men's health status than to that of women, probably because men are generally more likely than women to engage in high-risk behaviors (Denton, Prus, & Walters, 2004). Because of their gender socialization, men are more inclined to engage in high-risk behaviors and less apt to perform healthful behaviors (Griffiths, 2004). Some behavioral considerations to be addressed in assessing men's health include consumption patterns, exercise and leisure, sexual activity, and other behavioral risk factors.

Consumption Patterns

Consumption patterns include diet as well as substance use and abuse. As we saw earlier, U.S. men are more likely than women to be overweight, but less likely to be obese. In the United Kingdom, 21% of men are considered obese and an additional 40% are overweight. Healthy weight involves 10% to 20% of body weight as fat. Less than 10% body fat is considered underweight and unhealthful, 20% to 25% is considered overweight, and greater than 25% is considered obese (Campbell, 2004). As of 2000, only 32% of U.S. men over 20 years of age had achieved a healthy diet, compared to 35% of women (CDC, 2005). With respect to specific nutrients, men are less likely than women to consume the recommended five or more servings of fruits and vegetables per day (CDC, 2004b), but more likely to eat six or more servings of grains. Based on baseline data for the *Healthy People 2010*◆ objectives, only 32% of men restricted their fat intake to less than 10% of their daily calories. Men were more likely than women (63% versus 39%) to have sufficient calcium in their diets, but women were five times more likely than men to restrict their sodium intake to recommended dietary limits (CDC, 2005).

With respect to substance use and abuse, men are involved in more than three times more alcohol-related motor vehicle accidents than women, and men are more likely to engage in binge drinking. For example, 51% of college-age men report binge drinking, compared to 33% of women, and similar differences occur with older age groups. In addition, men are twice as likely as women to die of cirrhosis, a major consequence of alcohol consumption, and nearly twice as likely to experience a drug-induced death (CDC, 2005). Men are more

likely than women to smoke (25% and 20%, respectively), and women smokers are slightly more likely than men to attempt to quit smoking (CDC, 2005).

Exercise and Leisure

Men are more likely than women to engage in leisure-time physical activity, but in 2002, 35% of U.S. men did not engage in any leisure-time physical activity at all. Another 35% of men engaged in moderate physical activity and 27% in vigorous activity (CDC, 2005). Higher levels of physical activity have been shown to be associated with decreased risk of hip fracture (Mussolino, Looker, & Orwoll, 2001), as well as improved cardiovascular health.

Men and women increasingly share similar leisure patterns in American culture. Nevertheless, men still tend to be more active in competitive contact sports and, more often than women, to choose leisure activities involving some degree of physical risk (skydiving, white-water rafting, rock climbing). Participation in athletic sports is closely linked with images of masculinity and reinforces tendencies to aggressiveness and violence, increasing the potential for injury. Expectations of masculinity may also lead men to downplay the severity of injuries, delay treatment, and take insufficient time for healing. Men also tend to choose leisure activities associated with alcohol consumption. For these reasons, men experience relatively greater incidence of recreation-related trauma.

Sexual Activity

On average, men are sexually active for approximately 10 years prior to marriage, and the average age for initiating sexual activity in the United States is 16.9 years (Alan Guttmacher Institute, 2002; 2005b). Less than 10% of boys are sexually active at age 15, but approximately 90% have initiated sexual activity by age 20 (Pinkelman, 2002a). Worldwide, most men have initiated sexual activity prior to their 20th birthday. In various populations, anywhere from 15% to 65% of single men report more than one sexual partner, and 7% to 36% of married men report extramarital partners. More than twice as many men as women report multiple partners, although men may exaggerate the number of partners and women may underreport due to gender socialization expectations for male and female behavior (Nnko, Boerma, Urassa, Mwaluko, & Zaba, 2003). Men are often unaware of measures to prevent STDs, and knowledge of condom use to prevent STDs ranges from a low of 6% of men in Bangladesh to 82% of men in Brazil (Alan Guttmacher Institute, 2005a). Most men with multiple sexual partners do not use condoms, and those that do tend to use them for contraceptive purposes rather than STD prevention (Alan Guttmacher Institute, 2004; 2005a). In the United States, condom use is relatively high at first intercourse (close to two thirds) but declines with increased age, with only 16% of sexually active men using condoms by age 35 to 39 years (Alan Guttmacher Institute, 2002).

Other Behavioral Risk Factors

Use of seat belts and other safety devices is another behavior that can significantly affect men's health. Because of masculine socialization to risk as an element of manliness, men are less likely than women to engage in a variety of safety practices, including seat belt or helmet use. They are also more likely to engage in high-risk recreational activities, particularly in the context of alcohol or drug use.

Another relatively recent phenomenon that may affect men's health is the increase in genital piercing. Piercing is not a new phenomenon, and historical texts refer to various forms of piercing. Similarly, anthropologists have found evidence of genital piercing in some ancient cultures. In men, piercing may involve the pubis just above the penis, the glans, the foreskin, frenum, body of the penis, or the scrotum, as well as the nipples. Piercings may be singular or multiple. Piercing is not regulated in any way in most countries, and there are no data regarding complications resulting from piercing. There have been cases of hepatitis B and C and HIV transmission associated with piercing, but it is difficult to ascribe causality since many men who engage in piercing have other risk factors for these diseases. Localized bleeding, infection, and cellulitis are other possible complications. Urethral fistulas have also been noted in some cases. Allergic reactions to metal rings and studs and difficulty with hygiene have also been reported. Piercings have also occasionally proved hazardous to sexual partners in terms of injury and choking hazards (Anderson & Holmes, 2004). Community health nurses should be alert to the extent of a "piercing culture" among the male population and its possible implications for health.

Health System Considerations

Generally speaking, men define health as the ability to be employed and to be economically independent, and, in some cases, to have adequate sexual function (Hjelm, Bard, Nyberg, & Apelqvist, 2005). Despite unhealthy lifestyles and shorter lives than women, 70% of men consider themselves to be in good health. As noted earlier, on average, women live 7 years longer than men, and White women live an average of 14 years longer than Black men. Gender socialization leads men to "tough out" pain and not seek help until conditions interfere with their ability to work. In addition, media portrayals of men engaged in unhealthy behaviors contribute to risk taking and negative health effects in men (Monts & Smith, 2002).

All of these factors combine to make men less likely than women to seek health care services. Each year, men make 130 million fewer visits to health care providers than women, and in any given year, approximately 37 million men have not seen a provider in the last year (Monts & Smith, 2002). In addition, only 14% of men 15 to 49 years of age make reproductive health visits in any given year, and reproductive health needs of men are largely ignored (Alan Guttmacher Institute, 2004, 2005b). Even in the face of symptoms, men may delay seeking care. For example, men who perceive themselves to be in "good" health may wait as long as 3 years before seeking assistance for recognizable symptoms of testicular cancer. Physicians may also succumb to genderized perspectives in delaying referrals for specialist care. Young men are not supposed to present with possible life-threatening illness (Griffiths, 2004).

Factors other than gender socialization may also prohibit men from seeking health care. Some of these factors include lack of trust in providers, language barriers, lack of health insurance, financial difficulties, and difficulty relating to providers. Lack of health insurance is a particularly salient factor in men's failure to access health care services. In 2003, only 84% of U.S. men had health insurance, 61% through employment, 11% through Medicaid, and 12% under Medicare. Another 17% had no coverage at all (U.S. Census Bureau, 2004a). During the previous year, men constituted 53.5% of those who were without health insurance for the entire year (U.S. Census Bureau, 2005). Lack of health insurance is even more prevalent among young adult men; 40% of men 20 to 24 years of age are uninsured, compared to only 30% of women in the same age group (Alan Guttmacher Institute, 2002).

CULTURAL COMPETENCE

*I*n many cultural groups, men and women do not interact with or touch each other unless they are family members. This may make some men uncomfortable interacting with female nurses. In addition, in some cultural groups, women have lower social status than men, and men are the authority figures. These cultural perspectives may make men less willing to see female nurses as knowledgeable and make them hesitant to act on health-related information presented by women. How might you go about counteracting these cultural perspectives in planning health education offerings designed to improve men's health in the community?

U.S. men and women have similar levels of coverage under employment-based health insurance. Many government services, however, are designed to meet the needs of women and children rather than men, and women are more likely than men to have coverage under Medicaid (Alan Guttmacher Institute, 2002). It is often difficult for men to obtain Medicaid coverage, but a depressed economy leads to greater unemployment or employment in jobs that do not provide health insurance benefits and less employment-based coverage. Section 1115 of the Social Security Act permits states to request waivers to provide care to groups of people (including men) who would not ordinarily be eligible for Medicaid services. Unfortunately, few states have done so. A few programs have been developed to provide primary care services for nondisabled men 50 to 64 years of age with incomes at or below 50% of the federal poverty level. Even with these few programs, however, it is sometimes difficult to find providers willing to accept Medicaid reimbursement (Bufalini, 2002). A few additional programs have been set up to meet the needs of homeless clients, who are primarily men, and in 2002, 154 such Health Care for Homeless Centers existed throughout the United States (Archambault, 2002).

Another factor in men's failure to use health care services on a level commensurate with women is their perceived lack of a need for health care. Women routinely enter the health care system through services related to pregnancy, contraception, and routine screenings (e.g., Papanicolaou smears). These services serve as avenues for other health promotion activities as well as for detection of illness. Men do not routinely access any health-promotive services that would provide a similar door to other needed health care. Health care services are not crafted to target men, nor are many providers educated specifically to address the health care needs and motivations (or lack thereof) of men (White & Banks, 2004).

THE EPIDEMIOLOGY OF HEALTH FOR GAY, BISEXUAL, AND TRANSGENDER MEN

Homosexuality has been present throughout recorded human history, but, until recently, it has rarely been considered in terms of its effects on men's health status and health behaviors (Savage, Harley, & Nowak, 2005). An estimated 2.8% to 9% of U.S. men are believed to be homosexual in their sexual orientation (Meyer, Silenzio, Wolfe, & Dunn, 2000). This figure includes both gay men (those who have a primary sexual or affectional orientation to members of the same sex) and bisexual men (those who may interact sexually with both men and women). Transgenderism is relatively rare, occurring in approximately one in 30,000 U.S. men. Rates of transgenderism are somewhat higher in countries like the Netherlands with policies that support sexual

reassignment surgery or so-called sex change operations (Sember, 2000). Although no specific number of gay, bisexual, or transgender men is available, approximately 5% of unmarried partner households in United States in 2000 were comprised of two men (U.S. Census Bureau, 2005). Many other gay, bisexual, or transgender men may not live in partnered arrangements.

There is no general consensus on the use of the terms *heterosexual, homosexual*, and so on, primarily because the terms are defined differently by different groups. Homosexuality is culturally defined, and what is considered homosexual in one culture may not be in another, even if it involves same-sex sexual activity (Murray, 2000). For example, 24% of African American men and 15% of Latino men who had sex with other men identified themselves as heterosexual (Scout & Robinson, 2000). Similar lack of clarity occurs in definitions of bisexuality. For instance, in one study, 82% of men who self-identified as gay also had sexual interactions with women, yet did not consider themselves bisexual (Taylor, 1999). Definitions may incorporate one or more of three dimensions: one's sexual identity orientation, sexual behavior, and/or sexual attraction (Sell, 2000). For the purposes of this text, self-identification as a gay, bisexual, or transgender individual will be used as the primary means of distinguishing membership in these groups. Readers should be aware, however, that different definitions have been used in some of the research that will be reported here. Where relevant, the term "men who have sex with men" (MSM) will be used since it encompasses both gay and bisexual men as well as some men who self-identify as heterosexual despite occasional same-sex sexual activity.

Biophysical Considerations

Biophysical considerations related to gay, bisexual, and transgender men's health include maturation and aging and the presence of physical illnesses. Although gay culture emphasizes youth, there is a significant older population among both gays and lesbians. Gay men and lesbians are estimated to constitute approximately 6% of the older population of the United States (Heath, 2002), with 1 million to 3 million gay men over 65 years of age. This number is expected to rise to 4 million by 2030 (Hawke, 2002). An additional 545,000 to 872,000 lesbians and gay men over 65 are estimated in the United Kingdom (Price, 2005). Because of their marginal status in society, older gay men and lesbians may have more difficulty than others in obtaining assistance in old age (Hawke, 2002), creating a population of particular concern to community health nurses.

Gay, bisexual, and transgender men tend to be at greater risk for a number of physical health problems than their heterosexual counterparts. In part, this is due to the greater prevalence of high-risk behaviors in this population, as well as to their reluctance to seek medical care. Much of the attention given to health issues among gay, bisexual, and transgender men to date has focused on the extent of sexually transmitted diseases in this population. From 2000 to 2001, for example, the number of cases of syphilis in the United States increased by more than 15% in men; most of this increase occurred among men who have sex with men (Natinsky, 2002). Since 2001, approximately 60% of all cases of primary and secondary syphilis have occurred in MSM, and half of MSM with primary and secondary syphilis are co-infected with HIV (Division of STD Prevention, 2004b). MSM also contribute greatly to the incidence of HIV infection in cities considered "AIDS epicenters," U.S. cities with unusually high rates of HIV infection. HIV incidence ranged from 14% to 31% of MSM in Chicago, Los Angeles, San Francisco, and South Beach, Florida (Webster et al., 2005). Many MSM, particularly Black MSM, do not perceive themselves to be at risk for HIV infection. For example, in a 1994–1998 Young Men's Survey in six U.S. cities, 93% of HIV-infected Black MSM did not know they were infected and 71% stated that there was "no chance" or it was "very unlikely" that they were infected. Forty-two percent also perceived themselves at low risk of ever being infected (Division of HIV/AIDS Prevention–Intervention, Research, and Support, 2002).

MSM are also at risk for other STDs. For example, they are at increased risk for lymphogranuloma venereum (LGV), a sexually transmitted disease rarely seen in the general U.S. population. Risk of LGV is increased with sexual contact with European gay, bisexual, and transgender men. Because of the presence of ulcerative lesions, LGV increases one's susceptibility to HIV infection and other STDs (Division of STD Prevention, 2004a). Because of anal insertive sexual activity, many MSM are also at risk for sexual transmission of enteric diseases such as *Shigella flexneri, Entamoeba histolytica, Giardia lamblia, Campylobacter, Shigella,* and hepatitis A (Division of Bacterial and Mycotic Diseases, 2005). They may also be at increased risk for "gay bowel syndrome," an intestinal infection due to anal intercourse, as well as for anal carcinoma. Due to their frequent lack of interaction with health care providers, MSM may also have undetected prostate cancer. In addition, low levels of testosterone may lead to erectile dysfunction at higher rates than in the general population (Hawke, 2002).

There is some evidence to suggest that gay, bisexual, and transgender men may also be at increased risk for certain forms of cancer. In part, this increased risk may relate to the effects of stress on the immune system, with clients who don't disclose their sexual orientation at even higher risk than other gay, bisexual, and transgender men. Among gay and bisexual men with HIV infection, rates of Kaposi's sarcoma are thousands of times higher than in the general population. Incidence of Kaposi's sarcoma among gay and bisexual men has declined with the advent of more effective treatments for AIDS. The incidence of AIDS-related non-Hodgkin's lymphoma is also higher among MSM than among heterosexual groups. Gay and bisexual men also appear to be at increased risk for anal cancers, though not for cancers at other sites, than the heterosexual male population. This increased risk is thought to be due to the increased prevalence of human papillomavirus infection and smoking as risk factors among gay men. In addition, survival rates for gay men with cancer are lower than in the general population, probably due to HIV/AIDS comorbidity and delay in disease detection and treatment (Meyer & Bowen, 2000).

Immunity is another consideration in the biophysical dimension. In addition to routine immunizations suggested for adults, gay, bisexual, and transgender men should also receive immunization for hepatitis A and B. Unfortunately, figures indicate low immunization rates for these diseases among the homosexual population (3%) (Silenzio, 2000). Community health nurses should assess immunity among individual clients as well as levels of immunity in the gay, bisexual, and transgender population at large.

Homosexual males are also vulnerable to other physiologic conditions found among their heterosexual counterparts. Due to discriminatory attitudes among some health care professionals and prior unpleasant experiences with the health care system, however, many homosexuals may not volunteer information about health problems or seek assistance. These barriers to care help to explain the lower cancer survival rates among this population. For this reason, community health nurses should carefully assess homosexual clients for evidence of physical illness.

Psychological Considerations

Homosexuality was considered a psychiatric disease by the American Psychiatric Association until 1993 (Savage et al., 2005), and the "gender dysphoria" experienced by some transgender individuals is still considered a mental illness. **Gender dysphoria** is a sense of incongruity between one's physical gender and one's self-perceptions (Sember, 2000). The American Psychiatric Association has retained the diagnosis of gender identity disorder in its *Diagnostic and Statistical Manual of Mental Disorders IV-TR,* but is moving to a consideration of pathology only in those individuals who exhibit significant levels of distress over their transgender identity (McLeer, 2004; Meyer, Rothblum, & Bradford, 2000). These individuals may be at particular risk for suicide, auto-castration, or substance abuse. Psychological well-being seems to increase and gender dysphoria to disappear in most individuals who experience sexual reassignment surgery (Sember, 2000). In the interim, however, community health nurses may need to be particularly alert to suicidal ideation in these individuals.

Although gay, bisexual, and transgender men do not appear to be any more intrinsically susceptible to mental illness than their heterosexual counterparts, there is some evidence to suggest that they have a slightly higher prevalence of mental illness, possibly as a result of perceptions of discrimination (Mays & Cochran, 2001). MSM have been shown in some studies to have higher prevalences of substance abuse, partner violence, depression, and childhood sexual abuse than the heterosexual population. In addition, increased numbers of psychosocial problems have been linked to greater prevalence of high-risk sexual behaviors and HIV infection in MSM (Stall et al., 2003). Same-sex attraction has also been linked to the incidence of depression, anxiety, conduct disorder, suicide ideation and suicide attempts, and other disorders (Ridge, Hulme, & Peasley, 2003).

Suicide is a particular problem among gay, bisexual, and transgender men, particularly among youth, and the link between same-sex attraction and suicide attempts is stronger for boys than for girls, particularly when both partners were of the same ethnic group (Pinhey & Millman, 2004). The lifetime prevalence of suicide ideation for adult gay men and lesbians is estimated at 24% to 41%, with 7% to 20% of gay men and lesbians actually attempting suicide sometime in their lives. Among gay and lesbian youth, 20% to 40% attempt suicide. In one study, MSM attempted suicide over five times more often than men who had only female partners (Paul et al., 2002). Other studies have noted a link between sexual orientation and suicide mediated by depression, hopelessness, alcohol abuse, and victimization (Russell & Joyner, 2001).

Psychological factors also seem to influence sexual risk behaviors among MSM. For example, MSM who have been found to have high relationship needs are more likely than others to maintain steady partner relationships. Conversely, those whose sexual behavior is motivated by pleasure seeking are more likely to have a number of casual relationships; they are also more likely than those in steady relationships to engage in unprotected anal intercourse (UAI) (Craft, Smith, Serovich, & Bautista, 2005).

Sociocultural Considerations

Factors in the sociocultural dimension have a profound impact on the health status and health-related behaviors of gay, bisexual, and transgender men. Gay men and lesbians have been described as a "sociological minority," which is defined as "any segment of the population subjected to negative acts and behaviors inflicted by the rest of society" (Savage et al., 2005, p. 134). Discrimination against gay men and lesbians has been attributed to homophobia, a "fear of lesbian and gay male individuals or of homosexual feelings within oneself leading to hatred, loathing, prejudice, and possible discrimination toward individuals known or perceived to be lesbian or gay" (Savage et al., 2005, p. 135). Some authors note, however, that the use of the term *homophobia* restricts responses to gay men and lesbians to an individual phenomenon, when it is evident that it is in reality a societally constructed entity that influences many

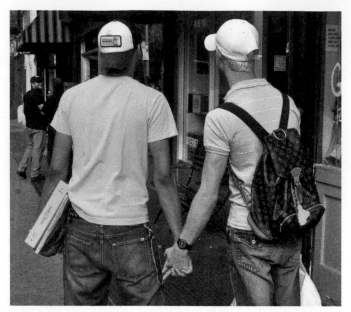

Gay men may experience discrimination in health care settings as well as in the wider society. (© Lee Snider/ The Image Works)

aspects of the sociocultural environment. For that reason, many authors prefer the term **heterosexism**, which is defined as an "ideological system that denies, denigrates, and stigmatizes any non-heterosexual form of behavior, identity, relationship, or community" (Herek, as quoted in Savage et al., 2005, p. 135).

Heterosexism results in oppression through force or imposition or by deprivation (Savage et al., 2005). Oppression by force is seen in physical abuse and victimization of MSM, whereas oppression by deprivation is reflected in failure to afford same-sex partners in long-term relationships the same benefits accorded to heterosexual married couples. Oppression may occur in a variety of forms, including language, assumptions of heterosexuality, simultaneous support and denial of civil rights, criminalization of same-sex sexual behavior, and failure to educate health care professionals and counselors regarding the health needs of nonheterosexual clients (Savage et al., 2005).

MSM who are members of cultural minority groups may be faced with even more conflict. For example, some authors have noted that Latino gay and bisexual men in Southern California are simultaneously exposed to more relaxed attitudes to homosexual behavior in the majority culture and strict cultural attitudes. Community programs, such as SOLAAR (Superacion, Orgullo y Lucha Atraves de Amor en Relaciones), are designed to enhance self-understanding within this cultural conflict and to promote long-term monogamous relationships among Latino MSM to reduce the risk of HIV exposure (Conner et al., 2005). This program employed social marketing strategies similar to those that specifically target Latino gay and bisexual clients, and has been successful in recruiting participants from a wider geographic range than that achieved prior to the social marketing campaign.

Cultural conflicts similar to those experienced by Latino MSM may also be encountered by older gay men who developed their sexual identities in an age when it was more prudent to keep one's sexual orientation hidden. This group may be at particular disadvantage in dealing with the effects of societal heterosexualism. For example, in the United Kingdom, surviving partners of homosexual relationships cannot claim property, register the partner's death, or claim other social benefits available to heterosexual spouses. In addition, disability and lack of avenues for care may necessitate disclosure of previously unknown sexual orientation, leaving clients open to discrimination on the basis of both age and sexual orientation (Price, 2005).

Societal attitudes toward what many consider deviant behavior may lead to prejudice, discrimination, harassment, and victimization. For example, more than 50% of gay men reported experiencing discrimination in their lives, compared to only 34% of heterosexual men (Mays & Cochran, 2001), and associations have been found among psychosocial distress, perceptions of discrimination, and experiences of victimization in MSM. In some studies, 28% of gay men reported violence or criminal activity directed at them because of their sexual orientation. Gay, lesbian, and bisexual youth are more likely to be involved in physical fighting in school than other youth (25% to 38% of gay youth versus 7% to 19% of others) (Huebner, Rebchook, & Kegeles, 2004). Similarly, half of older gay men and lesbians report being physically abused, and three fourths report verbal abuse (Heath, 2002). In 2002, Federal Bureau of Investigation statistics indicated 1,464 hate crimes in the United States based on sexual orientation, 68% of which were directed at homosexual men (U.S. Census Bureau, 2005). Gay men have also been found to be disproportionately victimized by heterosexual men in prison settings. Most male-to-male sexual assaults involve unprotected anal intercourse, with the attendant risks of trauma and STD (Dean & Bradford, 2000).

Family interaction is another element of the sociocultural dimension that affects the health of gay, bisexual, and transgender men. Disclosure of homosexuality or transgenderism to family members and their response, homosexual relationships, and homosexual parenting are the three primary aspects of family interaction to be assessed by the community health nurse.

Two different themes occur in families' responses to disclosure of a family member's homosexuality: loving acceptance or conventionality, which results in rejection of the homosexual family member. All families who come to know of homosexual or transgender members need to deal with feelings of grief, guilt, and fear for their child or sibling.

For those families that are able to accept homosexuality or transgenderism in one of their members, acceptance appears to come about in stages similar to the stages of grief experienced with the loss of a loved one. The first stage is one of grief, followed by a period of denial during which parents may see their child's professed sexual identity as a "phase" that he or she will grow out of. This stage is followed successively by stages characterized by guilt and anger and, finally, acceptance (Barret & Robinson, 2000). Unfortunately, some families never achieve the stage of acceptance of their loved one's sexual orientation.

Parental response to the disclosure of homosexuality is strongly influenced by a variety of factors: the strength of traditional gender role conceptions, perceptions of the probable attitudes of significant others in the family's social network, and parental age and education level (younger and better educated parents tend to be more accepting). Affiliation with conservative religious ideologies and intolerance of other stigmatized groups are other factors that suggest a negative response to disclosure.

Gay males may face decisions about disclosure to wives as well as parents and siblings. Contrary to popular belief, many homosexual men are or have been married, and about half of these men have children. Some gay men do not become aware of their homosexuality until after marriage. Others marry in an attempt to deny or hide their sexual orientation. Responses of wives to the disclosure of homosexuality vary considerably and may include feelings of living with a "stranger," guilt, development of an asexual friendship or a semi-open relationship in which both husband and wife are free to take outside lovers, or a desire for divorce. Transgender identity changes can be particularly devastating to marital relationships, as the spouse questions not only the husband's sexual identity but her own as well (Sember, 2000). Community health nurses should assess the extent of clients' disclosure of their sexual identities and the effects of the responses received. Nurses should also assess the needs of family members for assistance in dealing with the disclosure.

Disclosure to family members is usually not a one-time event. As families grow and change, both the homosexual family member and others face decisions regarding disclosure to extended family members, to in-laws as siblings marry, and possibly to children and grandchildren (Barret & Robinson, 2000).

Parenting by gay, bisexual, and transgender men brings its own stresses, many of them similar to those experienced by lesbian parents. Gay or bisexual men may become fathers in a number of ways: in heterosexual relationships prior to coming out, as foster parents or through adoption, or in cooperation with a lesbian woman or surrogate mother. Gay fathers may be marginalized by both the heterosexual and homosexual communities, and partners may resent the intrusion of children into the relationship (Barret & Robinson, 2000). Gay fathers may also be forced to be less open about their sexual identities than they might otherwise be in order to prevent court actions and potential loss of custody. This often means that they cannot openly live with a same-sex partner and may be denied the companionship and support afforded to heterosexual and even lesbian couples (Lambert, 2005).

The mistaken societal view that homosexuality can be transmitted to children has motivated a great deal of research on the effects of homosexual parenting on children. Heteronormative family forms require such research to be defensive in nature, effectively proving that living in a homosexual household is not detrimental to children (Hicks, 2005). In actuality, gay fathers have been found to show greater warmth and responsiveness to children and to provide more limits to children's behavior than heterosexual fathers. Gay fathers are also more likely than lesbian mothers to encourage play with gender-specific toys. In general, parental sexual orientation has not been found to affect children's gender identity or sexual orientation. Children of gay and lesbian parents may be more open to early experimentation with same-sex behaviors than those of heterosexual parents, but no relationship has been shown to final gender identification or sexual orientation. Similarly, no effects have been noted for children's personal development, although younger children of homosexual parents may be somewhat more likely than others to be teased. This effect seems to dissipate as children get older, and children of homosexual parents develop normal peer relationships (Lambert, 2005).

Disclosure of one's sexual identity to children is another dilemma faced by gay, bisexual, and transgender men. Depending on when and how disclosure occurs, children may exhibit the same range of responses shown by other family members. Some considerations in disclosure of sexual identity to children are provided below.

SPECIAL CONSIDERATIONS

DISCLOSURE OF SEXUAL ORIENTATION OR IDENTITY TO CHILDREN

- Come to grips with your own sexual identity before trying to explain it to children.
- Children are never too young to be told, but explanations must be couched in terms the child can understand.
- Disclose to children before they suspect or are informed by others.
- Plan the disclosure; do not let it occur in an impromptu fashion.
- Make the disclosure in a private setting where interruptions are unlikely.
- Inform the child in an objective and straightforward manner; do not "confess."
- Stress that your relationship with the child will not change.
- Be prepared for questions and respond to them honestly.

Data from: Barret, R. L., & Robinson, B. E. (2000). Gay fathers: Encouraging the hearts of gay dads and their families. San Francisco: Jossey-Bass.

BUILDING OUR KNOWLEDGE BASE

Savin-Williams and Esterberg (as cited in Lambert, 2005) suggested several areas for research regarding parenting by gay and lesbian clients. These areas include:

- How is gay or lesbian parenthood viewed in the context of the current legal and social system in the United States?
- How do gay and lesbian parents construct identities as parents as well as homosexuals? How do their identities differ with their circumstances?
- How do gay and lesbian parents interact with social institutions related to parenting (e.g., schools)? What are the effects of this interaction on parents and social systems?
- How is the transition to parenthood for gay and lesbian parents similar to and different from that of their heterosexual counterparts?
- How does parenthood affect the character of gay and lesbian relationships?
- What support is available to gay and lesbian parents from their social networks (both traditional and within the gay and lesbian community)?

How might you design a study to address one or more of these questions? How might you include ethnic minority groups whose participation in research on homosexuality has been limited?

Gay men frequently establish long-term partnerships with same-sex partners, although cohabitation by same-sex couples is less socially acceptable than among heterosexual couples (Casper & Bianchi, 2002). Gay couples' relationships are subjected to the same kinds of stress as heterosexual relationships, but this stress may be exacerbated by the absence of social support for the marital role. Therapists who work with gay and lesbian couples have identified several additional issues that threaten the stability of their relationships. These issues include differences in the stages of coming out between partners, differences with respect to extended family involvement, inequalities of power, and financial conflict and disparity in income (Barret & Robinson, 2000). With the exception of the stage of coming out, these same issues may also affect the stability of relationships among heterosexual couples.

Gay, bisexual, and transgender men may experience violence and abuse in intimate relationships, just as partners in heterosexual relationships do. In one study of four U.S. cities, for example, 34% of MSM reported psychological or symbolic battering, 22% reported physical battering, and 5% reported sexual battering by their partners in the last 5 years. Battering was more likely to occur if the victim was younger, had a low educational level, or was HIV-infected (Greenwood et al., 2002).

The occupational risks and concerns experienced by gay men, another consideration in the social environment, relate primarily to avoiding discrimination and rejection in the workplace. For example, 22.5% of gay men report not being hired for a position versus 18.5% of heterosexual men. Similarly, gay men are more likely than heterosexual men to report being passed over for promotion (17% versus 13%) (Mays & Cochran, 2001). No clearly established occupational health risks pertain to gay or bisexual lifestyles. It should, however, be noted that in occupational settings where masculine roles are stereotypical and exaggerated (e.g., construction), there may be an increased incidence of acting out of homophobic thinking, resulting in an increased risk of assault. Nursing assessment should focus on such potential safety risks and should consider the possibility that gay men who are unable to accept their sexual orientation may themselves enact exaggerated masculine roles and experience the related safety risks these behaviors may entail.

Societal attitudes toward nonheterosexual orientations have changed somewhat in some segments of the American population and elsewhere in the world. For example, a 1999 survey indicated that only 13% of the U.S. population thought that gay men and lesbians should not have equal rights regarding employment, compared to 33% in 1977. Although many people continue to see homosexuality as a moral issue, others are more tolerant than was previously the case, and people who are personally acquainted with gay and lesbian individuals are more accepting of this population than those who are not (Casper & Bianchi, 2002). In spite of these changes, there is continuing evidence of discrimination and violence against gay, bisexual, and transgender men.

Gay, bisexual, and transgender men may participate in the "gay culture," although transgender men may be less likely to do so than others. Some authors have noted, however, that some elements of gay and lesbian networks (e.g., gay bars) are not supportive and may promote alcohol and drug use in MSM (Ridge et al., 2003; Thiede et al., 2003; Webster et al., 2005).

Behavioral Considerations

Behavioral factors are also important influences on the health of gay, bisexual, and transgender men. One study conducted in seven U.S. cities indicated drug use prevalence in 66% of gay men, and 28% of MSM reported using three or more drugs. In addition, 29% of study respondents used drugs frequently, and 4% were injection drug users. Drug use was found to be more common in bisexual men, those who self-identified as heterosexual, runaway youth, and those subjected to forced sexual intimacy (Thiede et al, 2003). Drug use may be higher among MSM in some parts of the country than others. For example, 37% of MSM in South Beach, Florida, reported using three or more recreational drugs in the previous year, compared to 18% in New York City, Chicago, San Francisco, and Los Angeles (Webster et al., 2005). Increased risk of HIV infection has been linked to methamphetamine and other "club" drug use among

EVIDENCE-BASED PRACTICE

Webster et al. (2005) described the use of a population-based survey of men who have sex with men (MSM) in the South Beach, Florida, area to tailor interventions to this subpopulation in preventing HIV infection. Community members responded to survey findings by creating a community-wide education effort to address the intertwined problems of recreational drug use, unprotected intercourse, and HIV infection. The survey highlighted differences in the extent of HIV infection in the local population of MSM and contributing factors from other high-incidence areas throughout the country. These differences permitted development of tailored interventions specific to the population at greatest risk. How might a similar approach be used to identify key factors and intervention strategies in your own area?

MSM. Methamphetamine use is also associated with higher-risk sexual behaviors (Boddiger, 2005). Bisexual men, in particular, have been shown to engage in a variety of high-risk behaviors (Russell, Driscoll, & Truong, 2002).

MSM are also more likely to smoke and to initiate smoking at an earlier age than their heterosexual counterparts; gay, lesbian, bisexual, and transgender youth have been particularly targeted by tobacco company marketing campaigns (Washington, 2002). In one study, 31.4% of MSM were smokers, compared to 24.7% of men in the general population (Greenwood et al., 2005). General figures for smoking prevalence lie at 46% for gay men. In addition to smoking more, gay men tend to find smoking cessation more difficult than their heterosexual counterparts, and gay youth who smoke are more likely than others to engage in other high-risk behaviors. Besides being damaging to health in terms of increased risk for lung and other cancers and heart disease, smoking triggers immune system changes that affect prognosis of hepatitis C and other STDs common among MSM (Washington, 2002).

In addition to smoking and drug use, many MSM engage in high-risk sexual behaviors such as "bare backing." *Bare backing* is the term for intentional unprotected anal intercourse (UAI) (Craft et al., 2005). In part, the move away from condom use to UAI is motivated by perceptions among gay, bisexual, and transgender men that HIV/AIDS is now "curable" with the advent of newer, more effective drugs (Hawke, 2002). Other reasons for UAI reported in the literature include general tendencies toward risk taking, identifying HIV infection with being gay or as a rite of passage, guilt about personal survival when others have died of the disease, a desire to be metaphorically "impregnated," and attempts to get attention due to illness (Ridge et al., 2003). Additional reasons for failing to use condoms include perceptions of their ineffectiveness in preventing HIV infection and associations with erectile dysfunction (Webster et al., 2005).

Unprotected receptive anal intercourse in the previous 6 months was reported by 48% of MSM in a study conducted in six U.S. cities, and 55% reported unprotected insertive anal intercourse (Koblin et al., 2003). Some MSM also engage in oral-anal sexual encounters that put them at increased risk of hepatitis A infection (Allard et al., 2001) and transmission of syphilis, particularly during the secondary stage of the disease. Oral lesions also increase the potential for HIV transmission (Division of STD Prevention, 2004b). In fact, MSM accounted for 40% of all cases of primary and secondary syphilis diagnosed in 2002, and diagnosis was strongly associated with HIV coinfection (Division of STD Prevention, 2003). From 1999 to 2002, MSM accounted for 60% of new diagnoses of HIV infection (Division of HIV/AIDS Prevention, 2003b). Hepatitis C, on the other hand, has not been shown to be transmitted by sexual activity among MSM except in the context of intravenous drug use (Alary et al., 2005).

Sexual motivation, quality of relationships, disclosure of sexual orientation and HIV status, and sex trading are some of the factors that influence UAI among MSM. Craft and associates (2005) found four types of needs that were satisfied by sexual encounters among MSM. Pleasure-focused motivations reflected perceptions of sexual intimacy as meeting personal physical, emotional, and sexual needs. Partner-focused motivations reflected sexual activity to meet the needs of the partner. MSM motivated by substitution needs used sexual intimacy to meet other personal needs, such as relief of depression, and so on. Sexual activity based on relationship needs was motivated by attempts to strengthen relationships with the sexual partner. MSM motivated by pleasure-focused and substitution needs were more likely than other MSM to engage in casual sexual interactions. Those motivated by relationship-focused needs were more likely to have a steady partner.

Relationships with steady or casual partners have also been shown to influence UAI, although the direction of influence is not consistent. In some studies, UAI is more likely to occur with steady than casual partners. For example, in Craft et al.'s (2005) study, 70% of UAI occurred among steady partners. In another study, 29% of those in steady partnerships with someone whose HIV status was negative or unknown engaged in UAI (Denning & Campsmith, 2005), and 25% of men with nonsteady partners who reported insertive anal intercourse engaged in UAI (Division of HIV/AIDS Prevention, 2004).

Many MSM do not disclose their sexual orientation and may self-identify as heterosexual. **Disclosure** is the term used to describe the explicit revealing of one's sexual orientation to others. Nondisclosure is prevalent among MSM who self-identify as heterosexual (Denning & Campsmith, 2005). These men are at particular risk for HIV infection (Division of HIV/AIDS Prevention, 2003a). Other gay, bisexual, and transgender men may

choose to disclose their sexual orientation to certain people and not to others. MSM may also fail to disclose HIV status. MSM with steady partners are more likely to disclose their HIV status to their "main partner." For example, only 19% of MSM in one study had not disclosed HIV status to their regular partner, but 43% failed to disclose their status to casual partners. HIV-positive MSM have been found to be more likely to disclose their status if the partner is known to also be HIV-positive and least likely to disclose if the partner's HIV status is unknown, possibly for fear of rejection (Poppen, Reisen, Zea, Bianchi, & Echeverry, 2005). Disclosure of HIV status influences condom use, with condoms more likely to be used when partners are "seroconcordant," either both positive or both negative.

Sex trading, or engaging in sexual activity in return for money, drugs, shelter, or food, also occurs among MSM, particularly those who do not self-identify as gay. In one study, sex trading occurred among 62.5% of MSM, and MSM who engaged in sex trading were more likely than other MSM to engage in unprotected sexual activity. Sex trading places the individual MSM at risk for STDs as well as endangering his non-sex-trade male and female sexual partners. Sex trading was associated with crack cocaine and injection drug use, childhood abuse, and homelessness (Newman, Rhodes, & Weiss, 2004). A higher percentage of transgender men than other MSM may engage in sex trading to pay for sexual reassignment surgery. Because transgender prostitutes are stigmatized by both heterosexual and gay and lesbian prostitutes, they are often forced to take the least desirable customers who are least likely to agree to condom use. In addition, transgender individuals may resort to self-injecting hormones and engage in needle sharing, which increases their risk of HIV infection and hepatitis B (Sember, 2000).

Health System Considerations

The final category to be addressed in the epidemiology of gay, bisexual, and transgender men's health is the health system dimension. Gay, bisexual, and transgender men may encounter homophobia and heterosexism among health care workers and care delivery systems. In addition, the perception of homophobia represents a significant barrier to health care. For example, gay men and lesbians have been found to be somewhat more likely to perceive that heterosexual individuals are made more uncomfortable by them than is actually the case (Casper & Bianchi, 2002).

Despite possible exaggerations of perceptions of discrimination, however, gay, bisexual, and transgender men are subjected to discrimination in some health care settings (Perkins, 2004). In a survey of members of the Gay and Lesbian Medical Association, 67% indicated seeing gay and lesbian clients receive substandard care based on their sexual orientation (White, Bradford, Silenzio, & Wolfe, 2000). In another study, 3.1% of gay and bisexual men reported being denied care or given inferior care (Mays & Cochran, 2001). Even when the health care provider, whether an individual or an institution, is devoid of homophobia, various circumstances may threaten the gay client and act as health barriers. For example, assessment questions about birth control practices, if answered truthfully, might have the effect of requiring that a client disclose his sexual identity. For the client who fears loss of health care benefits (due to assumed higher risk of AIDS for all gay men), this is a situation to be avoided. Confidentiality issues may also prevent gay and bisexual men at risk for HIV infection from being tested. An estimated half of gay men in the United Kingdom do not disclose their sexual orientation to their primary providers, and one third of them would be unhappy for their providers to have this information. Reasons given for nondisclosure include perceptions that the information is not relevant, fear of stigma or discrimination, and fear of release of information to insurance companies and others (Durham, 2004).

Another problem in the current health care system is the lack of providers who are knowledgeable regarding the health care needs of gay, bisexual, and transgender clients. This lack exists among providers of mental health and other services as well. Inability to communicate effectively with gay, bisexual, and transgender clients may lead to inaccurate diagnoses and inappropriate treatment plans as well as impaired compliance with health-related recommendations (White, Bradford, & Silenzio, 2000). In some reports as many as 50% of gay men and lesbians who seek counseling report dissatisfaction with the services received (Savage et al., 2005).

The effects of the health care system on transgender men in the United States may be even more profound than for gay and bisexual men. Sexual reassignment surgery is covered under national health insurance in the Netherlands, Great Britain, and Australia. In the United States, requests for coverage under Medicaid are addressed on an individual basis and are frequently not decided in favor of the client. Availability of surgery is often dependent on the individual client's ability to pay for services out of pocket. The long-term effects of surgery have not been adequately studied, although immediate responses to surgery have been almost uniformly favorable. Hormone therapy does, however, have some adverse side effects, including a twentyfold increase in thromboembolism for men receiving estrogen, some reports of breast cancer, liver disease, increased risk for heart disease, increased blood pressure, sterility, mood changes, and a decreased sex drive, among others. For women receiving testosterone, side effects may include increased cholesterol and lipid levels, heart disease, mood changes, male pattern baldness, acne, and cessation of menses (Sember, 2000).

ASSESSING THE HEALTH OF THE MALE POPULATION

The first requisite for effectively meeting the health needs of men is an accurate assessment of their health status and health needs. Here we will focus on assessing the health of men as a segment of the population. A tool that can be adapted for use in assessing the health status and needs of individual male clients is included in Appendix I on the Companion Website. A tool specifically designed to assess men's health is included in the *Community Assessment Reference Guide* designed as a companion volume to this text.

In conducting an assessment of this population, the community health nurse would gather data related to factors in each of the six dimensions of health discussed earlier. Information related to the biophysical dimension would be primarily derived from local morbidity and mortality data. Mortality data and a great deal of morbidity information will be available from the local health department. Other morbidity data (e.g., the extent of hospitalizations for specific conditions such as diabetes, cardiovascular disease, or asthma among men) may be available from local hospitals. Other health care agencies (e.g., clinics, disease registries, or voluntary organizations) may also have relevant morbidity and mortality data for male clients. For example, local emergency departments may be able to provide statistics on accidental injuries among men. Similarly, local police departments may have data on accident-related calls and the injuries suffered. For other conditions, such as erectile dysfunction and immunization levels among men, there are often no statistical data available and information may be best obtained by means of community surveys. Community surveys or rehabilitation service data might address the extent of activity limitation in the male population. The focused assessment provided below can assist the community health nurse in determining biophysical factors that influence the health of the male population.

With respect to psychological dimension factors, local psychiatric units should be able to provide

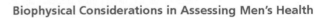

FOCUSED ASSESSMENT

Biophysical Considerations in Assessing Men's Health

- What is the age composition of the male population?
- What is the racial/ethnic composition of the male population?
- What are the main causes of mortality in the male population?
- What acute and chronic illnesses are prevalent in the male population? What factors contribute to the prevalence of these conditions?
- What is the prevalence of sexual dysfunction in the male population?
- What is the level of immunity to specific communicable diseases among the male population?

information regarding hospitalizations for mental health problems. Again, police departments may have figures on arrests made for aberrant behavior, or clients taken to psychiatric facilities. Psychiatric service providers can also be interviewed to get an estimate of the numbers of men who seek care for mental health issues such as depression and PTSD. Data on the extent of suicide among men will be available from local mortality figures. Community surveys may be used to gain information regarding the levels of stress experienced by the male population, coping strategies used, and their effectiveness. Cultural immersion or interviews with persons knowledgeable regarding local cultures are effective means for determining male gender socialization and its effects on health status and health-related behaviors. Questions to guide the assessment of psychological factors affecting the health of men in the population are included in the focused assessment provided below.

General information related to the physical environment and its effects on the health of men would be similar to that gathered for a comprehensive community assessment. In addition, the nurse would obtain information regarding occupational and recreational exposures to hazardous conditions. The local Chamber of Commerce or Business Association will probably have data on the types of business and industry present in the community. The telephone book may be a good source of information on recreational opportunities available to men in the community. In addition, direct observation by means of a "windshield survey" could provide information related to physical environmental conditions and their effects on men's health. Police departments may also have data on dangerous intersections or other road hazards that contribute to motor vehicle accidents. Assessment questions related to physical environmental factors influencing men's health are provided above right.

Community health nurses assessing the health of the male population would also obtain information

related to sociocultural dimension factors. Much of this data will be available from community census figures. For example, information regarding income, employment, educational levels, and single parenthood among men in the population is available through the census. Local government may also have figures on the extent of homelessness among men in the community. Interviews with local informants will provide information on typical family roles played by men and their gender socialization to these roles. Local authorities will also have some information on the extent to which men are perpetrators or victims of violence. General employment and unemployment figures are available from census data,

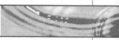

FOCUSED ASSESSMENT

Physical Environmental Considerations in Assessing Men's Health

- To what environmental health hazards are men in the population exposed?
- What environmental hazards are posed by occupational settings? By recreational pursuits among men?
- To what extent does the physical environment promote or impede healthy behaviors by men (e.g., physical activity)?

FOCUSED ASSESSMENT

Sociocultural Considerations in Assessing Men's Health

- What are the social roles expected of men? What effects do these role expectations have on men's health?
- What opportunities for social interaction are available to men in the population? How do men in the population typically interact with others?
- To what extent are men perpetrators or victims of violence? What are the health effects of exposure to violence?
- What is the extent of social support available to men in the population?
- What is the percentage of single-parent families headed by men in the population?
- What is the typical educational level of men in the population?
- What is the economic status of men in the population? What is the average income of men in the population?
- What effects do economic, educational, and employment levels have on men's health?
- What transportation opportunities are available to men in the population?
- To what extent do men in the population function as caretakers for other family members? To what extent do these men experience caretaker burden?
- What percentage of men in the population is employed? What are the typical occupations for men in the population? What effects do occupation and employment setting have on men's health? What support do employers provide for men's other roles and responsibilities?
- What childcare services are available to working single male parents? What is the cost of these services?

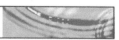

FOCUSED ASSESSMENT

Psychological Considerations in Assessing Men's Health

- What are the sources of stress to which men in the population are exposed?
- What are the incidence and prevalence of mental illness in the male population? What specific mental health problems are prevalent in the population?
- What is the rate of suicide in the male population?
- How are men socialized in the population? Does socialization contribute to health problems among men? How does male socialization affect coping abilities?
- What is the extent of nonheterosexual orientation in the population? How does this affect the level of stress experienced by men in the population?

and current levels of employment can be obtained from local employment offices. Information on the types of employment available in the community can be obtained from local newspapers as well as the Chamber of Commerce or Business Association discussed earlier. Information on marriage and divorce among the male population is available from vital statistics collected by local government agencies. The focused assessment provided on the previous page includes questions for assessing the effects of sociocultural dimension factors on the health of the male population.

Most information regarding consumption patterns, exercise and leisure, sexual activity, and other behavioral dimension factors that influence health will be obtained primarily from community surveys. In some instances, indirect measures of behavior are available. For example, information regarding sales of tobacco and alcohol or arrests for illicit drug use would give some idea of the extent of these behaviors. Similarly, the prevalence of STDs in the population would suggest lack of condom use. Some information related to exercise and leisure activities can be obtained from observation or from interviews with owners of businesses that support these activities. For example, the nurse can observe the number of men who walk or jog in the park in the evening or speak with proprietors of exercise facilities regarding the extent of their use by men in the community. Assessment of behavioral considerations in men's health can be guided by the focused assessment questions included below.

Finally, the community health nurse would assess factors related to the health system dimension such as the extent to which men in the population use available health services. Such data can be obtained from the providers of health care services or from insurers who pay for them. In addition, the nurse would obtain information on the extent of health insurance coverage in the male population. In part, this information can be extrapolated from unemployment figures since the unemployed are unlikely to have health insurance. Local agencies may also have information regarding the extent of health insurance in the population. For example, a

FOCUSED ASSESSMENT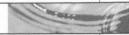

Health System Considerations in Assessing Men's Health

- What percentage of the male population has a regular source of health care?
- What are the attitudes of men to health and health care services? How do they define health and illness?
- What percentage of the male population has health insurance coverage?
- What health services are available to men in the population? Are health care services needed by men available to all segments of the population?
- What barriers to obtaining health care do men encounter?
- What are the attitudes of health care providers to care of men? To care of nonheterosexual men? How do these attitudes affect health care utilization by men?

local hospital would have data on the number of male clients served who did not have health insurance coverage. Similarly, local businesses could provide data on the number of employees who receive employment-based health insurance benefits. Information on health insurance status can also be obtained through community surveys.

Similar types of information related to factors in each dimension of health would be obtained with respect to the gay, bisexual, and transgender population. Unfortunately, information may be more difficult to obtain for this population than for the general population of men, but a few data sources may exist. For example, mortality data for suicide may provide some indication of the number of suicidal men who were members of the gay, bisexual, or transgender community. For the most part, however, community surveys, interviews, and observation will be the most profitable means of obtaining information for these subgroups of men. The focused assessment included above can assist the community health nurse in gathering data related to health system factors affecting the health of men in the population.

DIAGNOSTIC REASONING IN THE CARE OF MEN

Community health nurses use data from their assessment of the male population to identify health needs and determine appropriate nursing diagnoses. Nursing diagnoses may reflect positive or negative health states or increased risk for disease. A positive diagnosis might be "High prevalence of adequate physical activity due to presence of multiple low-cost opportunities for exercise." An example of a negative diagnosis might be "increased risk of sexually transmitted diseases among young adult men due to unprotected sexual activity." Based on the diagnoses derived from the assessment of men's health status and health needs, the community health nurse would

FOCUSED ASSESSMENT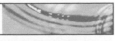

Behavioral Considerations in Assessing Men's Health

- What are the dietary consumption patterns typical of men in the population?
- What is the prevalence of smoking among men in the population?
- What is the extent of alcohol and other drug use in the population?
- To what extent do men in the population engage in safety practices (e.g., seat belt use)?
- To what extent do men who are sexually active engage in safe sexual practices?
- To what extent do men engage in health screening practices such as testicular self-exam?

collaborate with other segments of the community to plan, implement, and evaluate health care delivery programs to meet the needs of this population.

PLANNING AND IMPLEMENTING HEALTH CARE FOR MEN

Interventions to improve the health status of men in the population may occur at primary, secondary, or tertiary levels of prevention. The level of prevention chosen for community health nursing interventions depends on the status of health problems to be addressed.

Primary Prevention

Although it is difficult to generalize about male clients' attitudes toward health promotion activities, there are some commonly encountered patterns of health behavior among men. One such behavior is a tendency to view exercise as sufficient to compensate for unhealthy behaviors such as a high intake of fats in the diet. Men also tend to attribute greater significance to health changes they can sense than to those they cannot (e.g., they can sense pain but not elevated blood pressure). Because men tend to rate their health as very good or excellent more often than women, they may feel they do not need to be actively involved in health promotion activities. They may also err in their health appraisal efforts, stemming from a tendency to believe that their past athletic or current work activities may provide for their present health needs ("When I was a teenager I would run all day." "I work hard all day in the fresh air. What could be healthier than that?"). Community health nurses may need to advocate among men for changing attitudes to health and health-related behaviors through health education initiatives and reframing approaches.

Reframing, which focuses on helping men to see the same situation in a different light, is one technique that can be used to promote positive behavioral change. A second technique for promoting change involves emphasizing alternate ways of coping with anxiety or fearfulness. Education, of course, is a crucial aspect of any primary prevention strategy. Education is perhaps most effective when teaching is initiated with school-age male youngsters, as this is the stage when lifelong health values and habits are forming. Health promotion by family members is known to be a significant motivator and predictor of client compliance and outcomes, and involvement of family members in educational efforts and treatment planning is usually of significant benefit.

General approaches to promoting health among men are included in the HEALTH program, a six-point program intended to facilitate creation of health care services that better meet the health promotion needs of men. HEALTH is an acronym that stands for **H**umanize, **E**ducate, **A**ssume, **L**ocate, **T**ailor, and **H**ighlight. Health services for men should humanize the experience of illness by emphasizing the normality of experiencing and acknowledging pain, weakness, fear, and similar emotions to defuse the "macho" gender socialization to which men are subjected. Community health nurses can advocate for realistic health-related messages that emphasize the normality of these experiences and assist men to see them in the light of catalysts for health-related behaviors. Community health nurses working with men should educate them regarding the need for screening, primary prevention, and risk reduction. It may also be helpful in working with men to assume the worst and to overexaggerate risks to make the point of the need for change in health-related behaviors. Community health nurses and other health care providers should also locate support for men's health through follow-up telephone calls and return visits for health promotion purposes after acute care needs have been met. Health care services for men should also be tailored to their specific needs with input from those involved. Community health nurses, in particular, are in a position to advocate for the inclusion of men in planning health services relevant to their needs. For example, a community health nurse might identify men who are single parents and encourage them to be involved in the development of support services for men who are parenting alone. Finally, effective health care services for men highlight strengths and lay out the costs and benefits of health-promoting behaviors such as smoking cessation, hypertension control, and so on, in terms that are relevant to men (Monts & Smith, 2002). Community health nurses can help to draft health-related messages in language that is meaningful to men, addressing consequences and benefits in meaningful terms. For example, a community health nurse might approach the need for health promotion and illness prevention among men in terms of their continued ability to work or support their families, both elements of male gender socialization.

Primary prevention for health concerns specific to men focuses on increasing their use of health-promoting behaviors in the areas of chronic disease prevention, coping, immunization, safety practices, and elimination of high-risk behaviors. Chronic diseases in men can be prevented through adequate nutrition, physical activity, and weight control and elimination of behaviors such as smoking. Education for the prevention and control of other underlying diseases can also help to prevent chronic disease. For example, compliance with hypertension treatment can minimize the risk of developing cardiovascular disease.

Environmental modification can also help to prevent chronic diseases and injuries. For example, community health nurses can be advocates for environments that promote physical activity among men and for the elimination of hazardous exposures in work and other settings that put men at risk for environmentally caused diseases.

Promoting coping strategies among men would focus primarily on moving men from a reliance on avoidant coping mechanisms to more confrontive types of coping. This may necessitate specific education for coping as early as grade school and continuing on throughout the educational process. Coping education can also be employed in settings where men experience considerable stress such as the workplace. Community health nurses can advocate for and develop coping skills training programs tailored to men in both school and work settings.

Immunizations for men should focus on prevention of diseases such as tetanus, hepatitis A and B, influenza, and pneumonia for those at highest risk of disease due to occupational exposure (e.g., working outdoors or around animals) or high-risk behaviors such as oral-anal intercourse or injection drug use. Gay, bisexual, and transgender men are at particular risk for hepatitis A in the context of oral-genital and oral-anal sexual encounters and should be immunized. Concerted immunization efforts in this population are particularly warranted in the event of outbreaks of hepatitis A (Allard et al., 2001). Men with chronic conditions, particularly chronic respiratory conditions, or who work with susceptible populations should routinely receive immunizations for influenza and pneumonia. Because most adult men are part of the workforce, community health nurses may need to advocate for immunization services at times and locations that fit busy schedules. In addition, they can advocate for workplace policies that promote immunization, particularly in settings where risk of infectious disease is high. For example, a community health nurse might promote development and enforcement of a policy mandating regular tetanus boosters among construction workers. The nurse working in this setting might also monitor immunization status among employees and provide tetanus immunizations as needed.

Health promotion related to safety issues for men would focus on both injury prevention and safe sexual practices. Because of men's socialization to accept personal risk and their tendency to engage in high-risk behaviors, injury prevention often depends on legislation and regulation. Community health nurses can advocate for the passage and enforcement of legislation related to use of seat belts and other protective devices. Community health nurses can also monitor and report occupational safety hazards that put men at risk for injury or toxic exposures. Legislative advocacy may also be required in this area. Groups of men can also be educated regarding the need for effective injury prevention and the possible long-term consequences of injury.

Education may also need to focus on safe sexual practices. The Alan Guttmacher Institute (2005a) has recommended an ABC approach for sexual health promotion for men: Abstinence, Being faithful to one partner, and Condom use. Specific services are needed for men's reproductive health needs as well as women's. For example, one hospital instituted a program for addressing the sexual needs of young men that resulted in 83% of young men participating reporting that they would be able to resist peer pressure for sexual activity and 94%

Think Advocacy

Howard, Davis, Evans-Ray, Mitchell, and Apomah (2004) described the establishment of a "teen-friendly" clinic for both male and female adolescents to meet the need for sexual clinical and education services for this age group. The clinic was established based on the evaluation of an educational program in which adolescent boys achieved gains in knowledge about and changes in attitudes toward sexual activity and indicated that they would use protection during sexual intercourse if available. Provision of such services is often resisted in many communities in the belief that it promotes sexual activity among adolescents. How would such a service be viewed in your community? Where might resistance to the program originate? How would you go about advocating for such a program?

reporting intentions to use STD protection during intercourse (Howard, Davis, Evans-Ray, Mitchell, & Apomah, 2004). Again, community health nursing advocacy may be required before such programs for men are developed.

The ABC approach would also be effective for promoting safe sexual activity among MSM. Additional preventive practices may also be warranted in this population. For example, the Division of Bacterial and Mycotic Diseases (2005) of the Centers for Disease Control and Prevention recommends that MSM who have diarrhea refrain from oral-genital or anal-genital activity, and that MSM wash their hands and genital areas with soap and water before and after sexual intercourse. Additional recommendations include the use of gloves during digital-anal contact, condoms for oral-genital or anal-genital sexual activity, and dental dams for oral-anal contact to prevent transmission of enteric pathogens. Programs to prevent UAI among men who have sex with men have yielded mixed results, however. In one study, for example, the prevalence of UAI among MSM exposed to an educational intervention decreased from 37% to 27%, whereas that for the control group increased. Unfortunately, although UAI reportedly decreased in the experimental group, 31% of the participants compared to only 21% of the controls developed at least one new STD during the study period (Imrie et al., 2001). The SOLAAR program discussed earlier has been somewhat more successful in promoting monogamous relationships and decreased risk of STD exposure in Latino MSM (Conner et al., 2005). Community health nurses can be actively involved in educating MSM for safer sexual practices and in advocating these practices in venues that reach MSM. For example, a community health nurse might advocate for a condom dispenser in a prominent location in a gay bar or convince gay publications to include articles advocating safer sexual practices. Nurses might even volunteer to write health-related articles for these publications.

Another approach to primary prevention in men is the elimination of high-risk behaviors. Elimination of high-risk sexual behaviors has already been addressed, but attention should also be given to smoking cessation and prevention or cessation of illicit drug use. Community health nurses can educate men about the need for smoking cessation and make referrals to smoking cessation services. They can also advocate for smoke-free workplace legislation to limit places where smoking is permitted or for coverage of smoking cessation assistance under health insurance plans. They can engage in similar interventions related to drug use. Community health nurses may also need to advocate for the availability of such services and for their coverage under health insurance.

One additional primary preventive intervention for gay, bisexual, and transgender men is that of empowerment. There is a need for this population to "reconstruct their interpersonal and intrapersonal spheres to yield positive self-concepts and to diminish heterosexism" (Savage et al., 2005). Empowerment for this subset of men involves both psychological and community empowerment. Psychological empowerment occurs within the individual at three levels: intrapersonal, interactional, and behavioral. Intrapersonal empowerment entails constructing positive perceptions of self in the context of one's sexual orientation. Interactional empowerment reflects the individual's perceptions of the social environment, and behavioral empowerment involves action to influence one's social and political environments. Community empowerment occurs at the group level and entails efforts by the gay and lesbian community to address issues through political activity (Savage et al., 2005).

Community health nurses can work with individual gay, bisexual, and transgender men to promote psychological empowerment. They can also work at the societal level to promote community empowerment for this population. In part, they can accomplish community empowerment by working to eliminate heterosexism, particularly in health care settings, and by assisting groups of gay, bisexual, and transgender men to form coalitions with other marginalized groups and represent their position in a variety of social venues (Savage et al., 2005). Table 3◆ presents a summary of the major foci in primary prevention for men as well as examples of community health nursing interventions related to each focus.

Secondary Prevention

Secondary prevention involves the earliest possible detection of health needs through effective screening. It also encompasses the actual treatment of the health needs or disorders themselves.

Community health nurses may participate in health screening activities by providing or encouraging the client's use of such health measures as blood pressure screening and cardiovascular risk-assessment programs in public, educational, or occupational settings. Men are more likely than women to have multiple risk factors for heart disease and stroke (Division of Adult and Community Health, 2005b), and community health

TABLE 3	Primary Prevention Foci and Sample Interventions in the Care of Men
Focus	Sample Interventions
Reframing	• Creating health care systems tailored to address men's needs and health-related perceptions
Preventing chronic illnesses	• Promoting healthy diet • Promoting physical activity • Advocating for environmental modifications to promote health • Referring for treatment of underlying conditions that contribute to chronic illness (e.g., hypertension) • Advocating for available and accessible health preventive services
Enhancing coping	• Teaching confrontive coping strategies
Providing immunization	• Educating men on the need for immunizations • Providing immunization services • Advocating for availability and insurance coverage of adult immunization services
Promoting safety	• Educating men regarding the need to use safety devices • Educating men regarding safe sexual practices • Monitoring and eliminating environmental safety hazards • Advocating for safety legislation
Eliminating risk behaviors	• Educating men regarding smoking and drug use • Referring men for smoking and drug use cessation programs • Advocating for insurance coverage for smoking and drug use cessation services
Advocating empowerment	• Promoting personal psychological empowerment at all levels • Assisting the gay, bisexual, and transgender community with community empowerment activities

nurses can design, implement, and promote participation in risk assessments for the male population. Blood cholesterol screening is one example of such services. In 2003, nearly three fourths of U.S. men (71.8%) had received blood cholesterol screening services in the previous 5 years, slightly less than among women (74.4%). At that time, only two states had achieved the *Healthy People 2010*◆ objective of cholesterol screening in 80% of the U.S. adult population (Division for Heart Disease and Stroke Prevention, 2005). Men with elevated cholesterol levels, however, are twice as likely as women to have them controlled (Division of Adult and Community Health, 2005a).

Nurses can also facilitate the offering and use of screening examinations by other health care professionals within the community, such as rectal examinations and blood testing for prostate cancer and chest x-rays for lung cancer. Early detection of testicular cancer is an important area for secondary prevention by community health nurses.

One intervention that facilitates detection of testicular cancer is teaching the testicular self-examination

(TSE) technique. In one study, as many as 64% of men rarely or never engaged in TSE (Wynd, 2002). Because testicular cancer occurs primarily in young men, the community health nurse can often educate and motivate clients efficiently (and minimize individual embarrassment in the process) by working with groups of males in school or work settings.

Prostate cancer screening can employ a digital rectal examination or testing for prostate-specific antigen (PSA), although both are limited in their effectiveness in identifying disease. Because prostate cancer may not have adverse effects in many men, widespread screening programs are controversial. It is also unknown whether or not treatment increases survival rates, since the prognosis for 5-year survival is high even without treatment. In addition, treatment of prostate cancer may have a variety of adverse effects, including erectile dysfunction, urinary incontinence, depression, and hot flashes. The suggested approach to determining the need for screening and treatment for prostate cancer includes informing the client regarding the consequences of the disease and the potential benefits and disadvantages of available screening and treatment options, dealing with questions and concerns, discussing rationale for different choices, and coming to a joint decision with the client regarding the advisability of screening and/or treatment (Pinkelman, 2002b).

Routine screening procedures for men include tobacco use and alcohol misuse, colorectal cancer, hypertension, lipid disorders, and obesity. Other screening tests are recommended for men at particular risk for certain conditions. Recommendations of the U.S. Preventive Services Task Force (2005) for screening in men are presented in Table 4◆. Community health nurses may need to advocate for access to routine screening services, particularly among low-income men and those without health insurance.

Community health nurses may refer men with existing health problems for medical evaluation and treatment. They may also participate in the treatment of illnesses experienced by male clients. In the case of ischemic and certain other cardiac disorders, for example, stress has been shown to impact negatively on treatment outcomes, in some cases leading to a threefold increase in mortality (e.g., in post–myocardial infarction clients). Treatment programs that identify high-stress clients during hospitalization, that track and reduce their stress levels after discharge, and that provide prompt assistance from nurses in the community when episodes of increased stress occur can result in significant reduction of the stress-related mortality experienced by post–myocardial infarction clients. Again, advocacy may be required to assure access to diagnostic and treatment services for men. For example, a community health nurse might assist in the development of stress reduction programs in the workplace or in the development of coping skills training programs in school and work settings.

TABLE 4	Routine Screening Recommendations for Men
Type of Screening	**Recommendation**
Alcohol misuse	All adult men
Colorectal cancer	Men over 50 years of age (fecal occult blood &/or sigmoidoscopy); no evidence of effectiveness of screening colonoscopy
Depression	Adult men in practice settings where follow-up is available
Diabetes	Adult men with hypertension or hyperlipidemia
Hypertension	All men 18 years of age and older
HIV infection	All men at risk of infection
Lipid disorders (total cholesterol and HDL-C)	All men over 35 years of age; men under 35 years of age with risk factors
Obesity	All adult men
Syphilis	All men at risk
Tobacco use	All adult men

Data from: U.S. Preventive Services Task Force. (2005). The guide to clinical preventive services, 2005. Retrieved August 13, 2005, from http://www.ahrq.gov/clinic/pocketgd.pdf

A special treatment issue for transgender men involves counseling regarding their options. Not all transgender men (or women) are happy with the results of sexual reassignment surgery (SRS), and clients should be assisted to examine the benefits of treatment options. These options include hormone therapy, surgical intervention, and assistance with legal, emotional, and financial issues. There is also a need for social advocacy to promote options other than SRS as legitimate grounds for changing one's gender legally (Fee, Brown, & Laylor, 2003).

Tertiary Prevention

Tertiary prevention for men is directed at those disorders that influence men's health in some ongoing manner or that have a likelihood of recurrence. The goals of tertiary prevention are to assist men in coping with the continuing manifestations of illness and to reduce the likelihood of future episodes of an illness. To this end, it is useful to group tertiary prevention measures into care directed toward those disorders that affect men's sexual functioning or sexual identity or as they present a threat to notions about male strength. Tertiary prevention measures also would be directed at supporting compliance with long-term therapy.

One area for tertiary prevention measures by the community health nurse involves those disorders that affect the male client's sexual functioning or sexual identity, such as testicular cancer and erectile dysfunction. Male clients with testicular cancer may face significant emotional distress owing to the effects of treatment on their sexuality. Treatment for testicular cancer is surgical removal of the affected testes followed by hormonal therapy. These treatments, along with their side effects

Advocacy in Action

A Hypertensive Emergency

Every once in a while, a community health nurse finds him- or herself advocating for something with a client rather than on the client's behalf. This is what occurred when community health nurses working in an information and referral center encountered a client with a soaring blood pressure. The client, an African American gentleman in his late forties to early fifties, had a blood pressure of 210/170. This was his first visit to the nursing center, so the nurses had no previous blood pressure readings for him. He did not have a history of hypertension and was symptom free.

After allowing him to rest, we took several more blood pressure readings. They remained extremely high, and the nurses strongly suggested that he go immediately to the emergency department. Because the client did not feel ill and did not have health insurance or a regular provider, he was extremely reluctant to do so. The nurses finally talked him into going to the ED. Once there, he was admitted, and an emergency angioplasty was performed. When he subsequently returned to the center, his blood pressure had approximated normal levels, and he was recovering well from the angioplasty.

(loss of fertility, emasculation), can have a profound impact on the client's self-image and psychosocial functioning (Gurevich et al., 2003). Community health nurses may need to advocate for development of and access to services dealing with sexual dysfunction. They may also be instrumental in changing men's attitudes to sexual dysfunction and their willingness to seek help.

An important area of tertiary prevention in this regard involves encouraging men to join support groups. Interaction with other men who have experienced the same problems can be very effective in facilitating adjustment to treatments that so tangibly affect men's sense of masculinity. On a one-to-one basis, the nurse can be accepting, supportive, and facilitative of the male client's expression of his feeling of loss. Community health nurses may also be instrumental in initiating supportive groups for these men or in advocating their availability in the community.

Some disorders may affect men's sense of strength; this is particularly true of cardiovascular disorders. The heart is a symbol of masculine strength for some men. Consequently, cardiovascular disorders not only can leave residual symptoms and physiological impairment, but can also threaten a man's self-image. Men with cardiovascular disease often benefit from interventions that support their self-image as masculine and from discussing their feelings about their illness. As noted elsewhere, stress management training also can have a significant positive effect on outcomes for men who have cardiovascular disease. These interventions are essential to promote adjustment and compliance with treatment.

Of course, community health nurses should also support and reinforce men's positive responses to cardiac rehabilitation efforts initiated in other treatment settings. Foremost among these would be weight control, limited intake of saturated fats, regular exercise, compliance with follow-up examinations and medications, and control of other disorders that exacerbate cardiovascular disease (hypertension, diabetes).

In the case of some chronic disorders, especially those producing no overt symptoms, men tend to be lax about complying with long-term treatment recommendations. This is especially true for male clients with hypertension. Interventions that help men understand the importance of controlling this disorder and that build on their perceptions of masculinity are very helpful. Maintaining a regimen of antihypertensive medications may be especially difficult for men when side effects interfere with necessary masculine roles. Examples of such side effects could include impotence, dizziness, and decreased tolerance for physical activity. Nurses can assist the men by teaching ways to compensate for these side effects, thereby helping them to maintain a sense of control over circumstances. In cases in which the side effects are not manageable and are affecting clients' masculinity (impotence), collaborating with the client's physician or assisting the client to discuss the problem with the physician can lead to acceptance of the treatment for hypertension.

Preventing recidivism, or rehospitalization, in instances of substance abuse is a major tertiary intervention in working with men. Interventions that decrease the likelihood of recidivism include encouraging the use of therapeutic support groups (Alcoholics Anonymous) and education regarding factors that predispose one to continued substance abuse (poor coping skills, co-dependent relationships, maintaining social contacts with abusers). It is also important for the community health nurse to consider the client's family and significant others when caring for substance-abusing men. Families and significant others can be either enablers of substance abuse or corrective forces leading to its elimination. Education of family and support persons regarding behaviors that produce improvement and those that permit further substance abuse is essential, and referrals to family treatment and support services are also of value.

Two special considerations in tertiary prevention for men include assisting transgender men to adjust to the effects of sexual reassignment surgery and use of the Internet for disease self-management information. SRS may result in loss of sexual feeling and appetite. In addition, the continuation of male facial features may make male-to-female transgender persons less satisfied with the outcome of surgery than might otherwise be expected. Facial feminization surgery is possible, but usually at an additional cost of up to $30,000 (Fee et al., 2003). In addition, community health nurses must help monitor transgender individuals for effects related to hormone therapy such as increased risk of heart disease, stroke, and breast cancer.

The Internet may be a particularly valuable tool for educating men regarding tertiary prevention and self-management of chronic illnesses as well as for motivating primary prevention activities by men (Division of STD Prevention, 2003). More and more, the U.S. population is turning to the Internet as a source of information. Community health nurses can help to create Web sites to provide such information as well as monitor existing sites for their accuracy and credibility.

EVALUATING HEALTH CARE FOR MEN

As in working with other population groups, community health nursing plans and interventions are evaluated by determining the degree to which population health goals have been met. It is also important to determine whether interventions were efficient. Could the same results have been accomplished with less expense of time or other resources?

The effects of interventions for men at the aggregate level can be assessed in terms of the accomplishment of national health objectives. The current status of selected objectives related to men's health is presented below. Information about objectives related to men's health is available on the *Healthy People 2010*◆ Web site at http://wonder.cdc.gov/data 2010. As we can see in the table, many of the objectives are actually moving away from their 2010 targets, and only three objectives have actually been met. Even for most of the objectives that are actually progressing toward the established targets, progress is so slight as to suggest that target goals will not be met by 2010 without additional concerted efforts.

Men have a variety of health care needs that they may or may not acknowledge. Community health nurses can be actively involved in encouraging men to seek health care as needed. They may also provide direct services to male clients, particularly with respect to education for primary prevention. In addition, community health nurses may be involved in advocacy activities to assure the availability and accessibility of needed services to improve men's health status.

HEALTHY PEOPLE 2010
Goals for Population Health◆

OBJECTIVE	BASELINE	MOST RECENT DATA	TARGET
1-1. Increase the proportion of men with health insurance	81%	82%	100%
1-4. Increase the proportion of men with a source of ongoing care	84%	85%	96%
2-3. Reduce the proportion of men with chronic joint symptoms	1.6%	ND	1.2%
2-11. Reduce activity limitation due to chronic back pain (per 1,000 men)	31	29	25
3-1. Reduce cancer deaths (per 100,000 men)	251.9	238.9	159.9
3-2. Reduce lung cancer deaths (per 100,000 men)	76.9	73.2	44.9
3-7. Reduce prostate cancer deaths (per 100,000 men)	33.3	27.9	28.8*
3-8. Reduce melanoma cancer deaths (per 100,000 men)	2.6	2.6	2.5
5-2. Prevent new cases of diabetes (per 1,000 men)	5.5	6.7	2.5#
5-5. Reduce the diabetes death rate (per 100,000 men)	89	91	45#
12-1. Reduce coronary heart disease deaths (per 100,000 men)	260	180	166
12-7. Reduce stroke deaths (per 100,000 men)	63	57	48
12-9. Reduce the proportion of men with high blood pressure	30%	ND	16%
12-14. Reduce the proportion of men with high blood cholesterol levels	19%	ND	17%
12-15. Increase the proportion of men who have had their blood cholesterol checked in the last 5 years	64%	ND	80%
13-2. Reduce the number of AIDS cases among MSM	17,847	15,917	13,385
14-3f. Reduce the number of cases of hepatitis B in MSM	7,135	8,063	1,808#
14-6. Reduce new cases of hepatitis A (per 100,000 men)	12.7	3.7	4.5*
14-28b. Increase hepatitis B vaccine coverage among MSM	9%	ND	60%

Continued on next page

HEALTHY PEOPLE 2010 *continued*

■ 15-2. Reduce hospitalization for nonfatal spinal cord injuries (per 100,000 men)	7.6	5.4	2.4
■ 15-3. Reduce firearm-related deaths (per 100,000 men)	18.4	18.6	4.1#
■ 15-12. Reduce emergency department visits due to injury (per 1,000 men)	146	154	126#
■ 15-13. Reduce unintentional injury deaths (per 100,000 men)	49.8	51.5	17.5#
■ 15-15. Reduce motor vehicle accident deaths (per 100,000 men)	20.4	21.3	0.2#
■ 15-32. Reduce homicides (per 100,000 men)	9.1	9.4	3.0#
■ 15-34. Reduce physical assault by intimate partners (per 100,000 men)	1.3	0.08	3.3*
■ 15-37. Reduce physical assaults (per 1,000 men)	37.4	23.9	13.6
■ 18-1. Reduce suicide deaths (per 100,000 men)	17.4	18.4	5#
■ 19-2. Reduce the proportion of men who are obese	20%	28%	15%#
■ 20-1. Reduce occupational injury deaths (per 100,000 men)	7.7	6.9	3.2
■ 22-1. Reduce the proportion of men who engage in no leisure-time physical activity	36%	35%	20%
■ 25-2. Reduce new cases of gonorrhea (per 100,000 men)	125	124	19
■ 25-3. Reduce cases of primary and secondary syphilis	3.6	3.8	0.2#
■ 26-1. Reduce deaths and injuries due to alcohol and drug-related motor vehicle accidents (per 100,000 men)	9.2	ND	4.0
■ 26-3. Reduce drug-induced deaths (per 100,000 men)	9.4	11.7	1.0#
■ 27-1. Reduce tobacco use by men	26%	25%	12%
■ 27-5. Increase smoking cessation attempts by men who smoke	39%	42%	75%

NDA—No data available

* Objective has been met

 # Objective moving away from target

Data from: Centers for Disease Control and Prevention. (2005). Healthy people data. Retrieved September 5, 2005, from http://wonder.cdc.gov/data2010

Case Study

Promoting Sexual Health in Men

There is a high rate of sexually transmitted diseases among men in the community where you are employed as a community health nurse. Particularly high incidence rates are noted for *Chlamydia trachomatis* and gonorrhea. Significant disparities are noted in incidence rates among Caucasian, African American, and Latino men, with incidence higher among young African American and Latino men than among Caucasians, although incidence among all three groups is high. STD incidence does not seem to be associated with sexual orientation since high rates are noted for both exclusively heterosexual men and those who have sex with other men.

1. How might you address the problem of STD incidence at the population level?
2. What additional information might you need to determine appropriate interventions for the problem?
3. What other segments of the community would you involve in developing your interventions?

Test Your Understanding

1. What are the major factors in the biophysical, psychological, physical environmental, sociocultural, behavioral, and health system dimensions influencing men's health?

2. What are some of the factors that contribute to adverse health effects for gay, bisexual, and transgender men?

3. Identify at least four areas for primary prevention with men. How might the community health nurse be involved in each?

4. What are the major secondary prevention considerations for men? Give an example of at least one community health nursing intervention related to each consideration.

5. Identify areas of emphasis in tertiary prevention for men. How might the community health nurse be involved in each? In what kinds of situations might tertiary prevention be required?

EXPLORE MediaLink

http://www.prenhall.com/clark
Resources for this chapter can be found on the Companion Website.

Audio Glossary
Appendix I: Adult Health Assessment and
    Intervention Guide
Exam Review Questions

Case Study: Promoting Men's Health
MediaLink Application: Prostate Cancer (video)
Media Links
Challenge Your Knowledge

Update *Healthy People 2010*
Advocacy Interviews

References

Alam, S., Niederberger, C. S., & Meacham, R. B. (2004). Evaluation and treatment of male infertility. In R. S. Kirby, C. C. Carson, M. G. Kirby, & R. N. Farah (Eds.), *Men's health* (2nd ed., pp. 261–266). London: Taylor & Francis.

Alan Guttmacher Institute. (2002). *Sexual and reproductive health: Women and men.* Retrieved September 18, 2005, from http://www.guttmacher.org/pubs/fb_10-02.html

Alan Guttmacher Institute. (2004). *In their own right: Addressing the sexual and reproductive health of American men.* Retrieved September 18, 2005, from http://www.guttmacher.org/pubs/summaries/exs_men.html

Alan Guttmacher Institute. (2005a). *In their own right: Addressing the sexual and reproductive health of men worldwide.* Retrieved September 18, 2005, from http://www.guttmacher.org/pubs/summaries/exs_itorintl.pdf

Alan Guttmacher Institute. (2005b). *Sexual and reproductive health information and services for men dangerously lacking.* Retrieved September 18, 2005, from http://www.guttmacher.org/media/presskits/2005/03/15/index.html

Alary, M., Joly, J. R., Vincelette, J., Lavoie, R., Turmel, B., & Remis, R. S. (2005). Lack of evidence of sexual transmission of hepatitis C virus in a prospective cohort of men who have sex with men. *American Journal of Public Health, 95,* 502–505.

Allard, R., Beauchemin, J., Bedard, L., Dion, R., Tremblay, M., & Carsley, J. (2001). Hepatitis A vaccination during an outbreak among gay men in Montreal, Canada, 1995–1997. *Journal of Epidemiology and Community Health, 55,* 251–256.

Anderson, W. R., & Holmes, S. A. (2004). Genital piercing. In R. S. Kirby, C. C. Carson, M. G. Kirby, & R. N. Farah (Eds.), *Men's health* (2nd ed., pp. 407–414). London: Taylor & Francis.

Archambault, D. (2002). The health needs of homeless men. *Community Health Forum, 3*(5), 37–39.

Artazcoz, L., Benach, J., Borrell, C., & Cortes, I. (2004). Unemployment and mental health: Understanding the interactions among gender, family roles, and social class. *American Journal of Public Health, 94,* 82–88.

Banks, M. (2002). Richard Roundtree's road to recovery from male breast cancer. *Community Health Forum, 3*(5), 22–25.

Barret, R. L., & Robinson, B. E. (2000). *Gay fathers: Encouraging the hearts of gay dads and their families.* San Francisco: Jossey-Bass.

Boddiger, D. (2005). Methamphetamine use linked to rising HIV transmission. *The Lancet, 365,* 1217–1218.

Bufalini, M. (2002). Barriers to state coverage for single males. *Community Health Forum, 3*(5), 46–48.

Calandra, J. (2004). Transition—Not "male menopause"—The norm for middle-aged men. *Nurseweek, 17*(26), 27–28.

Campbell, I. W. (2004). Obesity and men's health. In R. S. Kirby, C. C. Carson, M. G. Kirby, & R. N. Farah (Eds.), *Men's health* (2nd ed., pp. 55–62). London: Taylor & Francis.

Carson, C. (2004). Erectile dysfunction: Diagnosis and treatment. In R. S. Kirby, C. C. Carson, M. G. Kirby, & R. N. Farah (Eds.), *Men's health* (2nd ed., pp. 343–357). London: Taylor & Francis.

Casper, L. M., & Bianchi, S. M. (2002). *Continuity and change in the American family.* Thousand Oaks, CA: Sage.

Centers for Disease Control and Prevention. (2004a). *Health, United States, 2004.* Retrieved August 9, 2005, from http://www.cdc.gov/nchs/data/hus/hus04.pdf

Centers for Disease Control and Prevention. (2004b). Indicators for chronic disease surveillance. *Morbidity and Mortality Weekly Report, 53*(RR-11), 1–114.

Centers for Disease Control and Prevention. (2005). *Healthy people data.* Retrieved September 6, 2005, from http://wonder.cdc.gov/data2010

Chua, D., & Bakris, G. (2004). Hypertension. In R. S. Kirby, C. C. Carson, M. G. Kirby, & R. N. Farah (Eds.), *Men's health* (2nd ed., pp. 89–100). London: Taylor & Francis.

Conner, R. F., Takahashi, L., Ortiz, E., Archuleta, E., Muniz, J., & Rodriguez, J. (2005). The SOLAAR HIV prevention program for gay and bisexual Latino men: Using social marketing to build capacity for service provision and evaluation. *AIDS Education and Prevention, 17,* 361–374.

Cooke, C. L. (2004). Joblessness and homelessness as precursors of health problems in formerly incarcerated African American men. *Journal of Nursing Scholarship, 36,* 155–160.

Craft, S. M., Smith, S. A., Serovich, J. M., & Bautista, D. T. (2005). Need fulfillment in the sexual relationships of HIV-infected men who have sex with men. *AIDS Education and Prevention, 17,* 217–226.

Culpepper, K. S., & McKee, P. H. (2004). Cutaneous melanoma. In R. S. Kirby, C. C. Carson, M. G. Kirby, & R. N. Farah (Eds.), *Men's health* (2nd ed., pp. 171–183). London: Taylor & Francis.

Curry, L. C., & Hogstel, M. O. (2002). Osteoporosis. *American Journal of Nursing, 102*(1), 26–31.

Dean, L., & Bradford, J. (2000). Violence and sexual assault. In Gay and Lesbian Medical Association & Center for Lesbian, Gay, Bisexual, and Transgender Health (Eds.), *Lesbian, gay, bisexual, and transgender health: Findings and concerns* (pp. 29–32). New York: Author.

Denning, P. H., & Campsmith, M. L. (2005). Unprotected anal intercourse among HIV-positive men who have a steady male sex partner with negative or unknown HIV serostatus. *American Journal of Public Health, 95,* 152–158.

Denton, M., Prus, S., & Walters, V. (2004). Gender differences in health: A Canadian study of the psychosocial, structural, and behavioral determinants of health. *Social Science & Medicine, 58,* 2585–2600.

Division for Heart Disease and Stroke Prevention. (2005). Trends in cholesterol screening and awareness of high blood cholesterol—United States, 1991–2003. *Morbidity and Mortality Weekly Report, 54,* 865–870.

Division of Adult and Community Health. (2005a). Disparities in screening for and awareness of high blood cholesterol—United States, 1999–2002. *Morbidity and Mortality Weekly Report, 54,* 117–119.

Division of Adult and Community Health. (2005b). Racial/ethnic and socioeconomic disparities in multiple risk factors for heart disease and stroke—United States, 2003. *Morbidity and Mortality Weekly Report, 54,* 113–117.

Division of Adult and Community Health. (2005c). Racial/ethnic disparities in the prevalence and impact of doctor-diagnosed arthritis—United States, 2002. *Morbidity and Mortality Weekly Report, 54,* 119–123.

Division of Bacterial and Mycotic Diseases. (2005). *Shigella flexneri* type 3 infections among men who have sex with men—Chicago, Illinois, 2003–2004. *Morbidity and Mortality Weekly Report, 54,* 820–822.

Division of Cancer Prevention and Control, National Center for Chronic Disease Prevention and Health Promotion. (2004). Cancer survivorship—United States, 1971–2001. *Morbidity and Mortality Weekly Report, 53,* 526, 528–529.

Division of HIV/AIDS Prevention—Intervention, Research, and Support. (2002). Unrecognized HIV infection, risk behaviors, and perceptions of risk among young black men who have sex with men—Six U.S. cities, 1994–1998. *Morbidity and Mortality Weekly Report, 51,* 734–736.

Division of HIV/AIDS Prevention, National Center for HIV, STD, and TB Prevention. (2003a). HIV/STD risks in young men who have sex with men who do not disclose their sexual orientation—Six U.S. cities, 1994–2000. *Morbidity and Mortality Weekly Report, 52,* 81–68.

Division of HIV/AIDS Prevention, National Center for HIV, STD, and TB Prevention. (2003b). Increases in HIV diagnoses—29 states, 1999–2002. *Morbidity and Mortality Weekly Report, 52,* 1145–1148.

Division of HIV/AIDS Prevention. (2004). High-risk sexual behavior by HIV-positive men who have sex with men—16 sites, United States, 2000–2002. *Morbidity and Mortality Weekly Report, 53,* 891–894.

Division of STD Prevention, National Center for HIV, STD, and TB Prevention. (2003). Internet use and early syphilis infection among men who have sex with men—San Francisco, California, 1999–2003. *Morbidity and Mortality Weekly Report, 52,* 1229–1232.

Division of STD Prevention, National Center for HIV, STD, and TB Prevention. (2004a). Lymphogranuloma venereum among men who have sex with men—Netherlands, 2003–2004. *Morbidity and Mortality Weekly Report, 53,* 985–987.

Division of STD Prevention, National Center for HIV, STD, and TB Prevention. (2004b). Transmission of primary and secondary syphilis by oral sex—Chicago, Illinois, 1998–2002. *Morbidity and Mortality Weekly Report, 53,* 966–968.

Donaldson, S. L. (2004). Inequalities and men's health. In R. S. Kirby, C. C. Carson, M. G. Kirby, & R. N. Farah (Eds.), *Men's health* (2nd ed., pp. 8–14). London: Taylor & Francis.

Durham, N. (2004, August 30). Over half of gay men not out to GPs. *General Practitioner,* 17–18.

Fee, E., Brown, T. M., & Laylor, J. (2003). One size does not fit all in the transgender community. *American Journal of Public Health, 93,* 899–900.

Gotsch, K. E., Annest, J. L., Mercy, J. A., & Ryan, G. W. (2001). Surveillance for fatal and nonfatal firearm-related injuries—United States, 1993–1998. *Morbidity and Mortality Weekly Report, 50*(SS-2), 1–34.

Greenwood, G. L., Paul, J. P., Pollack, L. M., Binson, D., Catania, J. A., Chang, J., et al. (2005). Tobacco use and cessation among a household-based sample of US urban men who have sex with men. *American Journal of Public Health, 95,* 145–151.

Greenwood, G. L., Relf, M. V., Huang, B., Pollack, L. M., Canchola, J. A., & Catania, J. A. (2002). Battering victimization among a probability-based sample of men who have sex with men. *American Journal of Public Health, 92,* 1964–1969.

Griffiths, S. (2004). Men as risk takers. In R. S. Kirby, C. C. Carson, M. G. Kirby, & R. N. Farah (Eds.), *Men's health* (2nd ed., pp. 243–250). London: Taylor & Francis.

Gurevich, M., Bishop, S., Bower, J., Malka, M., & Nyhof-Young, J. (2003). (Dis)embodying gender and sexuality in testicular cancer. *Social Science & Medicine, 58,* 1597–1607.

Hawke, M. (2002). Just like everyone else. *Nursing Spectrum, Western Edition, 3*(12), 20–21.

Heath, H. (2002). Opening doors: Working with older lesbians and gay men. *Nursing Standard, 16*(48), 18–19.

Hendry, W. F., & Christmas, T. J. (2004). Testicular cancer. In R. S. Kirby, C. C. Carson, M. G. Kirby, & R. N. Farah (Eds.), *Men's health* (2nd ed., pp. 359–366). London: Taylor & Francis.

Hicks, S. (2005). Is gay parenting bad for kids? Responding to the "very idea of difference" in research on lesbian and gay parents. *Sexualities, 8,* 153–168.

Hjelm, K. G., Bard, K., Nyberg, P., & Apelqvist, J. (2005). Beliefs about health and diabetes in men of different ethnic origin. *Journal of Advanced Nursing, 50,* 47–59.

Howard, M., Davis, J., Evans-Ray, D., Mitchell, M., & Apomah, M. (2004). Young men's sexual education and health services. *American Journal of Public Health, 94,* 1332–1335.

Huebner, D. M., Rebchook, G. M., & Kegeles, S. M. (2004). Experiences of harassment, discrimination, and physical violence among young gay and bisexual men. *American Journal of Public Health, 94,* 1200–1203.

Huey, F. L. (2001). Global impact of innovations on chronic disease in the genomics era. *The Pfizer Journal, 11*(2), 13.

Imrie, J., Stephenson, J. M., Cowan, F. M., Wanigaratne, S., Billington, A. J. P., Copas, A. J., et al. (2001). A cognitive behavioral intervention to reduce sexually transmitted infections among gay men: Randomised trial. *British Medical Journal, 322,* 1451–1456.

Johnson, B. K. (2004). Prostate cancer and sexuality: Implications for nursing. *Geriatric Nursing, 25,* 341–347.

Kirby, M. (2004). Erectile dysfunction: Cardiovascular risk and the role of the primary care physician. In R. S. Kirby, C. C. Carson, M. G. Kirby, & R. N. Farah (Eds.), *Men's health* (2nd ed., pp. 145–157). London: Taylor & Francis.

Kirby, R. S., & Kirby, M. (2004). Benign and malignant diseases of the prostate. In R. S. Kirby, C. C. Carson, M. G. Kirby, & R. N. Farah (Eds.), *Men's health* (2nd ed., pp. 285–298). London: Taylor & Francis.

Koblin, B. A., Chesney, M. A., Husnik, M. J., Bozeman, S., Celum, C. L., Buchbinder, S., et al. (2003). High risk sexual behaviors among men who have sex with men in 6 US cities: Baseline data from the EXPLORE study. *American Journal of Public Health, 93,* 926–932.

Lambert, S. (2005). Gay and lesbian families: What we know and where to go from here. *The Family Journal: Counseling and Therapy for Couples and Families, 13*(1), 43–51.

Lim, L. S., & Fitzpatrick, L. A. (2004). Osteoporosis in men. In R. S. Kirby, C. C. Carson, M. G. Kirby, & R. N. Farah (Eds.), *Men's health* (2nd ed., pp. 203–221). London: Taylor & Francis.

Mannino, D. M., Homa, D. M., Akinbami, L. J., Ford, E. S., & Redd, S. C. (2002). Chronic obstructive pulmonary disease surveillance—United States, 1971–2000. *Morbidity and Mortality Weekly Report, 53*(SS-6), 1–16.

Marston, C. (2004). Gendered communication among young people in Mexico: Implications for sexual health interventions. *Social Science & Medicine, 59,* 445–456.

Mays, V. M., & Cochran, S. D. (2001). Mental health correlates of perceived discrimination among lesbian, gay, and bisexual adults in the United States. *American Journal of Public Health, 91,* 1869–1876.

McLeer, S. V. (2004). Mental health services. In H. S. Sultz & K. M. Young, *Health care USA: Understanding its organization and delivery* (4th ed., pp. 335–366). Sudbury, MA: Jones and Bartlett.

Meyer, I., & Bowen, D. (2000). Lesbian, gay and bisexual health concerns: Cancer. In Gay and Lesbian Medical Association & Center for Lesbian, Gay, Bisexual, and Transgender Health (Eds.), *Lesbian, gay, bisexual, and transgender health: Findings and concerns* (pp. 15–17). New York: Author.

Meyer, I., Rothblum, E., & Bradford, J. (2000). Mental health and mental disorders. In Gay and Lesbian Medical Association & Center for Lesbian, Gay, Bisexual, and Transgender Health (Eds.), *Lesbian, gay, bisexual, and transgender health: Findings and concerns* (pp. 21–26). New York: Author.

Meyer, I., Silenzio, V., Wolfe, D., & Dunn, P. (2000). Introduction/background. In Gay and Lesbian Medical Association & Center for Lesbian, Gay, Bisexual, and Transgender Health (Eds.), *Lesbian, gay, bisexual, and transgender health: Findings and concerns* (pp. 4–9). New York: Author.

Monts, R. (2002a). Depression among migrant farm workers. *Community Health Forum, 3*(5), 52–54.

Monts, R. (2002b). Men don't seek treatment for depression. *Community Health Forum, 3*(5), 54.

Monts, R., & Smith, S. (2002). Why don't men obtain preventive care? *Community Health Forum, 3*(5), 8–13.

Murray, S. O. (2000). *Homosexualities.* Chicago: University of Chicago Press.

Murty, S. A., Peek-Asa, C., Zwerling, C., Stromquist, A. M., Burmeister, L. F., & Merchant, J. A. (2003). Physical and emotional abuse reported by men and women in a rural community. *American Journal of Public Health, 93,* 1073–1075.

Mussolino, M. E., Looker, A. C., & Orwoll, E. S. (2001). Jogging and bone mineral density in men: Results from NHANES III. *American Journal of Public Health, 91,* 1056–1059.

Natinsky, P. (2002). The return of syphilis. *Community Health Forum, 3*(5), 30–31.

National Center for Chronic Disease Prevention and Health Promotion. (2004). Self-reported frequent mental distress among adults—United States, 1993–2001. *Morbidity and Mortality Weekly Report, 53,* 963–966.

Newman, P. A., Rhodes, F., & Weiss, R. (2004). Correlates of sex trading among drug-using men who have sex with men. *American Journal of Public Health, 94,* 1998–2003.

Nickel, J. C. (2004). Prostatitis. In R. S. Kirby, C. C. Carson, M. G. Kirby, & R. N. Farah (Eds.), *Men's health* (2nd ed., pp. 315–327). London: Taylor & Francis.

Nnko, S., Boerma, J. T., Urassa, M., Mwaluko, G., & Zaba, B. (2003). Secretive females or swaggering males? An assessment of the quality of sexual partnership reporting in rural Tanzania. *Social Science & Medicine, 59,* 299–310.

Paul, J. P., Catania, J., Pollack, L., Moskowitz, J., Canchola, J., Mills, T., et al. (2002). Suicide attempts among gay and bisexual men: Lifetime prevalence and antecedents. *American Journal of Public Health, 92,* 1338–1345.

Perkins, R. (2004). Diversity in Health Care Delivery. *Pfizer Journal, VIII*(2), 4–14.

Pinhey, T. K., & Millman, S. R. (2004). Asian/Pacific Islander adolescent sexual orientation and suicide risk in Guam. *American Journal of Public Health, 94,* 1204–1206.

Pinkelman, M. A. (2002a). In their own right: Men's sexual and reproductive health issues on the line. *Community Health Forum, 3*(5), 20.

Pinkelman, M. A. (2002b). Search for consensus: Prostate. *Community Health Forum, 3*(5), 17–19.

Poppen, P. J., Reisen, C. A., Zea, M. C., Bianchi, F. T., & Echeverry, J. J. (2005). Serostatus disclosure, seroconcordance, and unprotected anal intercourse among HIV-positive Latino men who have sex with men. *AIDS Education and Prevention, 17,* 227–237.

Price, E. (2005). All but invisible: Older gay men and lesbians. *Nursing Older People, 17*(4), 16–18.

Prigerson, H. G., Maciejewski, P. K., & Rosenheck, R. A. (2002). Population attributable fractions of psychiatric disorders and behavioral outcomes associated with combat exposure among US men. *American Journal of Public Health, 92,* 59–63.

Purcell, H., Daly, C., & Petersen, S. (2004). Coronary heart disease in men (reversing the "descent of man"). In R. S. Kirby, C. C. Carson, M. G. Kirby, & R. N. Farah (Eds.), *Men's health* (2nd ed., pp. 101–109). London: Taylor & Francis.

Ridge, D., Hulme, A., & Peasley, D. (2003). Queering health: The health of young same-sex-attracted men and women. In P. Liamputtong & H. Gardner (Eds.), *Health, social change and communities* (pp. 283–305). Oxford: Oxford University Press.

Russell, S. T., Driscoll, A. K., & Truong, N. (2002). Adolescent same-sex romantic attractions and relationships: Implications for substance use and abuse. *American Journal of Public Health, 92,* 198–202.

Russell, S. T., & Joyner, K. (2001). Adolescent sexual orientation and suicide risk: Evidence from a national study. *American Journal of Public Health, 91,* 1276–1281.

Savage, T. A., Harley, D. A., & Nowak, T. M. (2005). Applying social empowerment strategies as tools for self-advocacy in counseling lesbian and gay male clients. *Journal of Counseling & Development, 83,* 131–137.

Scout, & Robinson, K. (2000). HIV/AIDS. In Gay and Lesbian Medical Association & Center for Lesbian, Gay, Bisexual, and Transgender Health (Eds.), *Lesbian, gay, bisexual, and transgender health: Findings and concerns* (pp. 18–20). New York: Author.

Sell, R. (2000). Methodological challenges to studying lesbian, gay, bisexual, and transgender health. In Gay and Lesbian Medical Association & Center for Lesbian, Gay, Bisexual, and Transgender Health (Eds.), *Lesbian, gay, bisexual, and transgender health: Findings and concerns* (pp. 43–47). New York: Author.

Sember, R. (2000). Transgender health concerns. In Gay and Lesbian Medical Association & Center for Lesbian, Gay, Bisexual, and Transgender Health (Eds.), *Lesbian, gay, bisexual, and transgender health: Findings and concerns* (pp. 32–43). New York: Author.

Shepherd, A. J. (2004). An overview of osteoporosis. *Alternative Therapies, 10*(2), 26–33.

Silenzio, I. (2000). Immunization and infectious diseases. In Gay and Lesbian Medical Association & Center for Lesbian, Gay, Bisexual, and Transgender Health (Eds.), *Lesbian, gay, bisexual, and transgender health: Findings and concerns* (p. 21). New York: Author.

Singleton, J. A., Greby, S. M., Wooten, K. G., Walker, F. J., & Strikas, R. (2000). Influenza, pneumococcal, and tetanus toxoid vaccination of adults—United States, 1993–1997. *Morbidity and Mortality Weekly Report, 49*(SS-9), 39–62.

Solomon, H., & Jackson, G. (2004). Risk factors in men with erectile dysfunction. In R. S. Kirby, C. C. Carson, M. G. Kirby, & R. N. Farah (Eds.), *Men's health* (2nd ed., pp. 159–170). London: Taylor & Francis.

Stall, R., Mills, T. C., Williamson, J., Hart, T., Greenwood, G., Paul, J., et al. (2003). Association of co-occurring psychosocial health problems and increased vulnerability to HIV/AIDS among urban men who have sex with men. *American Journal of Public Health, 93,* 939–942.

Taylor, B. (1999). "Coming out" as a life transition: Homosexual identity formation and its implications for health care practice. *Journal of Advanced Nursing, 30,* 520–525.

Thiede, H., Valleroy, L. A., MacKellar, D. A., Celentano, D. D., Ford, W. L., Hagan, H., et al. (2003). Regional patterns and correlates of substance abuse among young men who have sex with men in 7 urban areas. *American Journal of Public Health, 93,* 1915–1921.

U.S. Census Bureau. (2004a). *Historical health insurance tables.* Retrieved October 1, 2004, from http://www.census.gov

U.S. Census Bureau. (2004b). *Poverty: 2003 highlights.* Retrieved September 30, 2004, from http://www.census.gov

U.S. Census Bureau. (2005). *Statistical abstract of the United States: 2004–2005.* Retrieved August 16, 2005, from http://www.census.gov/prod/2004pubs/04statab

U.S. Department of Health and Human Services. (2000). *Healthy people 2010* (Conference edition, in two volumes). Washington, DC: Author.

U.S. Preventive Services Task Force. (2005). *The guide to clinical preventive services, 2005.* Retrieved August 13, 2005, from http://www.ahrq.gov/clinic/pocketgd.pdf

Washington, H. (2002). Burning love: Big tobacco takes aim at LGBT youths. *American Journal of Public Health, 92,* 1086–1095.

Webster, R. D., Darrow, W. W., Paul, J. P., Roark, R. A., Taylor, R. A., & Stempel, R. R. (2005). Community planning, HIV prevention, and a needs assessment for men who have sex with men: The South Beach health survey. *Sexually Transmitted Diseases, 32,* 321–327.

Weidner, G., & Cain, V. S. (2003). The gender gap in heart disease: Lessons from Eastern Europe. *American Journal of Public Health, 93,* 768–770.

Weitoft, G. R., Burstrom, B., & Rosen, M. (2004). Premature mortality among lone fathers and childless men. *Social Science & Medicine, 59,* 1449–1459.

White, A. K., & Banks, I. (2004). Help seeking in men and the problems of late diagnosis. In R. S. Kirby, C. C. Carson, M. G. Kirby, & R. N. Farah (Eds.), *Men's health* (2nd ed., pp. 1–7). London: Taylor & Francis.

White, J., Bradford, J., & Silenzio, V. (2000). Health communication. In Gay and Lesbian Medical Association & Center for Lesbian, Gay, Bisexual, and Transgender Health (Eds.), *Lesbian, gay, bisexual, and transgender health: Findings and concerns* (pp. 11–13). New York: Author.

White, J., Bradford, J., Silenzio, V., & Wolfe, D. (2000). Access to quality health services. In Gay and Lesbian Medical Association & Center for Lesbian, Gay, Bisexual, and Transgender Health (Eds.), *Lesbian, gay, bisexual, and transgender health: Findings and concerns* (pp. 10–12). New York: Author.

Williams, D. R. (2003). The health of men: Structured inequalities and opportunities. *American Journal of Public Health, 93,* 724–731.

World Health Organization. (2005). *World health statistics 2005.* Retrieved September 21, 2005, from http://www.who.int/healthinfo/statistics/whostat2005en1.pdf

Wynd, C. A. (2002). Testicular self-examination in young adult men. *Journal of Nursing Scholarship, 34,* 251–255.

Meeting the Health Needs of Older Clients

Advocacy in Action

The Credit Card

Mrs. A. is an 83-year-old widow who lives alone in a small four-plex that she owns. She has a son who lives in the area and stops by frequently to check on her. He has a learning disability and does not read, so he is not involved in her financial affairs, nor does she want him to be.

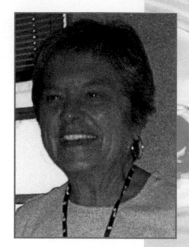

Because of problems with her teeth, including pain and not being able to chew, Mrs. A. went to a local dentist. While she was at the dentist's office having x-rays taken, a clerk came in and asked her to sign a paper without any explanation. Mrs. A. signed the paper but did not know why or ask any questions. Later she said she thought it was permission for them to do the dental work.

Six weeks later Mrs. A. received a bill from a credit card company for over $2,000, including finance charges. The bill was a prepayment for dental work that would be done over several office visits. This was the first she knew that she had signed for a credit card while at the dentist's office. Mrs. A. does not have any credit cards at present, and her only experience with a credit card was a bad one years ago. She had planned to pay for the dental work herself, as it was done, and had no desire to put the bill on credit. She called the credit card company but was unable to get a satisfactory answer. She also called the dentist's office, but they would only say that she signed for the card.

The community health nurse working with Mrs. A. called the credit card company and explained the situation. They were sympathetic and asked for a written synopsis of the details, but did not offer much hope. The next step was to contact the elder abuse division of the district attorney's office. Mrs. A. was advised to send a registered letter to the dentist. She received no response. The next week, Mrs. A. and the community health nurse met with the dentist. Mrs. A. indicated that she no longer wanted him as her dentist and that she would never have signed the credit card if she had known what it was. After a lengthy discussion and threats to report the dentist to the Better Business Bureau, he agreed to waive all credit card charges, including interest. The dentist wrote a check to the credit card company, and an agreement was signed.

Without the intervention of the community health nurse, Mrs. A. would have been faced with an extensive bill and finance charges for dental work that had not yet even been done.

Connie Curran, MSN, RN, PHN

Community Health Nurse

Bayside Community Center

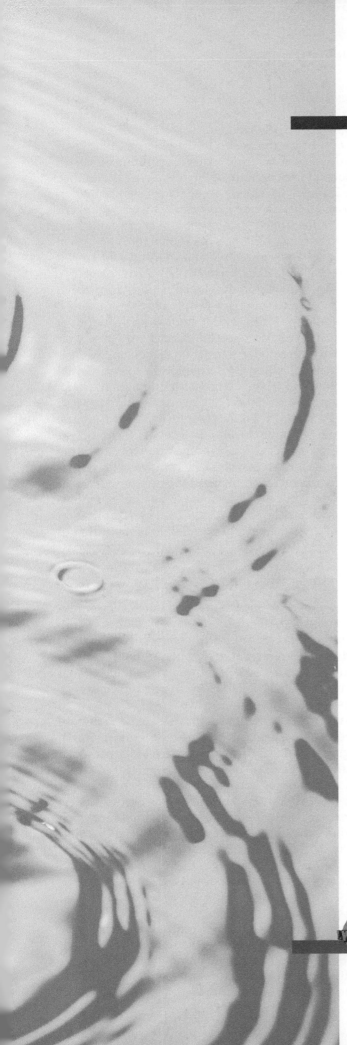

Meeting the Health Needs of Older Clients

CHAPTER OBJECTIVES

After reading this chapter, you should be able to:

1. Describe three categories of theories of aging.
2. Describe biophysical, psychological, physical environmental, sociocultural, behavioral, and health system factors influencing the health of the elderly population.
3. Identify major considerations in primary prevention in the care of older adults and analyze community health nursing roles related to each.
4. Describe secondary preventive measures for at least four health problems common among older clients.
5. Identify at least three foci for tertiary prevention with older clients and give examples of related community health nursing interventions.
6. Identify considerations that may influence the community health nurse's approach to health education for older clients.
7. Analyze the influence of factors unique to older clients on evaluation of nursing care.

KEY TERMS

advanced activities of daily living (AADLs)
ageism
aging
basic activities of daily living (BADLs)
comorbidity
dementia
elderly support ratio
functional status
instrumental activities of daily living (IADLs)
life-sustaining treatment
old-age dependency ratio
palliative care
respite
senescence
social network
transnationalism
validation therapy

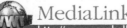

MediaLink
http://www.prenhall.com/clark

Additional interactive resources for this chapter can be found on the Companion Website. Click on Chapter 19 and "Begin" to select the activities for this chapter.

According to the Federal Interagency Forum on Aging-related Statistics (2004), the older population of the United States increased tenfold during the 20th century and is expected to increase to 87 million by 2050. Increased longevity and decreasing fertility are continuing to change the proportion of elderly people in relation to other age groups in the population. Life expectancy has increased by 2 years each decade over the last 50 years and is expected to increase by another 10 years worldwide by 2050 (Plese, 2005b). In the United States, although overall life expectancy at birth was 77.2 years, additional life expectancy for a person who was 65 years of age in 2001 was another 18.1 years (Centers for Disease Control and Prevention [CDC], 2004b). Worldwide, Japan has the highest life expectancy at birth at 82 years (World Health Organization [WHO], 2005).

By 2030, the elderly population throughout the world is expected to increase to 973 million people, and the number of older adults will more than triple in developing countries, which will account for 71% of the world's elderly population. In 2004, elderly persons already constituted more than 20% of the total population of 22 countries. Italy had the highest proportion of elderly residents at nearly a quarter of the population (24.5%) (World Health Organization, 2004), but China has the largest elderly population in the world in terms of actual numbers (You, Deans, Liu, Zhang, & Zhang, 2004). The number of centenarians (people over 100 years of age) is expected to increase fifteenfold by 2050 to 2.2 million persons worldwide, and in 2005 there were already 300 to 450 "super centenarians" (those more than 110 years of age) in the world (Plese, 2005b).

In the United States, the proportion of the population over 65 years of age is expected to increase from 12.4% in 2000 to 19.6% in 2030, and the actual number of elderly people will more than double from 35 million to 71 million. In addition, the number of people over 80 years of age in the United States is expected to increase from 9.3 million in 2000 to 19.5 million in 2030 (Division of Adult and Community Health, 2003c). Much of this increase will come in ethnic minority populations, with a decrease in the proportion of non-Hispanic White residents from 87% to 67% of the elderly population, an elevenfold increase in the Hispanic elderly population, and small increases in the proportion of elderly residents of other minority groups (Manly & Mayeux, 2004).

As the world's population ages, there will be a growing demand for health care services that improve the quality of life as well as longevity. This emphasis on quality of life can be seen in the national health objectives for 2010 addressing the health needs of the elderly. A major thread throughout these objectives is to reduce activity limitations that impair the quality of life for older persons (U.S. Department of Health and Human Services [USDHHS], 2000). These objectives can be viewed on the *Healthy People 2010*◆ Web site, which can be accessed at http://wonder.cdc.gov/data2010.

Concern for the health of the older population of the world also stems from a desire to minimize health care expenditures. Because of the prevalence of multiple chronic illnesses, the elderly account for a significant percentage of all health care expenditures worldwide. For example, in the United States, people over 65 years of age accounted for 45% of all days of hospital care and 38% of hospital discharges in 2003 (National Center for Health Statistics [NCHS], 2005d). Health care costs for people age 65 years and over in developed nations are three to five times those for younger people (Division of Adult and Community Health, 2003c). Improving the health of this population can decrease the societal burden of their care as well as promoting a better quality of life.

Nurses have long provided care to individual older clients and to the elderly as a population group. The American Association of Colleges of Nursing and the John A. Hartford Foundation Institute for Geriatric Nursing (2000) have developed a set of 30 competencies required of baccalaureate preparation for care of the elderly in the United States. These competencies primarily address knowledge required for care of individual elderly clients, but can be adapted to the care of the elderly as a vulnerable population. This latter application to the health of the elderly population is the thrust of this chapter.

THEORIES OF AGING

Aging is defined as "maturation and senescence of biological systems" (Albert, Im, & Raveis, 2002, p. 1214). Some authors prefer the term **senescence**, which is defined as "progressive deterioration of body systems that can increase the risk of mortality as an individual gets older" (Tabloski, 2006, p. 15). Aging or senescence involves a gradual and progressive loss of function over time that is not synonymous with an increase in disease (Malavolta, Mocchegiani, & Bertoni-Freddari, 2004), although the effects of aging may place older people at higher risk for disease.

A number of different theories have been advanced to explain how and why aging occurs. Generally speaking, these theories can be divided into three categories: biological theories, psychological theories, and sociological theories. Biological theories attempt to explain the biophysical changes that occur in aging and are of two basic types, programmed theories and error theories. Programmed aging theories propose that genetic codes regulate cell reproduction and death and that organ deterioration and eventual death are programmed in one's genetic makeup (Saxon & Etten, 2002). Specific programmed aging theories address longevity, declining endocrine function, and declining immune function. In error theories, hypothesized

TABLE 1	Stages and Foci of Erikson's and Peck's Developmental Theories	
Life Stage	Erikson's Stages	Focus
Infancy	Stage 1: Trust vs. mistrust	Erikson: Development of a sense of trust in self and others
Childhood	Stage 2: Autonomy vs. shame and doubt	Erikson: Development of the ability to express oneself and cooperate with others
Childhood	Stage 3: Initiative vs. guilt	Erikson: Development of purposeful behavior and the ability to evaluate one's own behavior
Childhood	Stage 4: Industry vs. inferiority	Erikson: Development of belief in one's own abilities
Adolescence	Stage 5: Identity vs. role confusion	Erikson: Development of a sense of self and plans to actualize one's potential
Adolescence/early adulthood	Stage 6: Intimacy vs. isolation	Erikson: Development of one's capacity for reciprocal relationships
Middle age	Stage 7: Generativity vs. stagnation	Erikson: Promotion of creativity and productivity and development of the capacity to care for others Peck: Development of the ability to value wisdom over physical competence Shifting relationships to emphasize friendship and companionship over sexual satisfaction Development of flexibility in roles and relationships Development of mental and intellectual flexibility
Late adulthood	Stage 8: Ego identity vs. despair	Erikson: Acceptance of one's life as unique and worthwhile Peck: Development of the ability to value one's self outside of work roles Development of abilities to adapt to physical changes and effects of aging Maintenance of an active interest in the external world

cumulative environmental assaults stretch the body's ability to respond and cause accumulation of metabolic toxins that impair normal function (Tabloski, 2006).

Psychological theories of aging focus on psychological changes that occur with age and propose that effective aging requires development of effective coping strategies over time. Major theories in this area include Jung's theory of individualism, in which the individual's mental focus changes from the external to the internal world, and the developmental theories (Tabloski, 2006). Erik Erikson's stage theory of development proposed eight stages of life in which the individual needed to accomplish specific developmental tasks that would facilitate task accomplishment in later stages. Peck took Erikson's last two stages, which encompass the last 40 to 50 years of life, and subdivided them into seven more discrete stages that cover middle age and older adult life (Saxon & Etten, 2002). In Peck's final stage, the individual engages in life review in preparation for death. Table 1◆ presents an overview of developmental theories and associated foci for task accomplishment.

Sociological theories of aging focus on changes in roles and relationships that occur with advancing age. Theories in this group tend to be mutually exclusive. For example, disengagement theory proposes that individuals disengage from life as a means of making way for a younger generation in preparation for death. The process may actually work in reverse, however, with society disengaging from and isolating older individuals as a result of **ageism**, which is prejudice or discrimination based on chronological age or appearance of age. In activity and continuity theories, however, older persons maintain their interest in life, but their specific interests change (Tabloski, 2006).

THE EPIDEMIOLOGY OF HEALTH FOR OLDER CLIENTS

Factors in each of the six dimensions of health influence the health of the older population, often with greater effects than on the health of people in younger age groups. Here we will examine some of the major

CULTURAL COMPETENCE

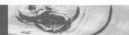

*D*ifferent cultural groups have differing attitudes toward the elderly and the conditions that often affect them. For example, in many cultures, the elderly are revered and respected for their wisdom, yet in these same cultures, stigma attached to certain conditions may make caring for older clients with these conditions difficult. Zhan (2004) described the additional burden on caregivers of family members with Alzheimer's disease (AD) due to perceived stigma among Chinese clients. In a qualitative study of Chinese caregivers for older clients with AD, she noted that diagnosis was often delayed because, even though family members recognized problems, they were ashamed to admit them to others, including health care providers. There were also differences in perceptions of the disease between caretakers, who saw AD as a brain dysfunction, and family members and others in the community, who ascribed AD to fate, wrongdoing, getting old and forgetful, worrying too much, being crazy, and bad *feng shui*. Some also thought AD was communicable and so shunned both client and family members to avoid contagion. Cultural factors, such as inability to speak English, also prevented clients and families from obtaining access to some services for persons with AD.

Cultural values did have one positive aspect, however. Because of the strong cultural value given to care of the elderly, caregivers felt satisfaction in their caregiving that allowed them to cope with the stresses of caregiving as well as the stigma in the community.

What are the responses of other cultural groups to diagnoses such as AD in the elderly? How do cultural factors influence the care of these older persons? How might community health nurses intervene in cultural groups that attach stigma to AD and similar diseases?

influences on the health of the older population in each dimension.

Biophysical Considerations

Major considerations related to the biophysical dimension of health include those related to maturation and aging and physiologic function, including immunization status.

Maturation and Aging

Whatever the ultimate causes of aging, aging has certain rather universal effects that result in a number of changes in both form and function. These changes may be the result of senescence or of cumulative exposures to risk factors over long periods of time (Albert et al., 2002). The major change involved in aging is loss of physical reserve capacity, which results in both cognitive and physical slowing, increased response to stress, a more easily disrupted equilibrium, and a need to pace oneself (Saxon & Etten, 2002). These effects are seen in slowed reaction times, decreased psychomotor and walking speed, loss of verbal memory, declining strength, decreased urine flow, and loss of skeletal muscle. The physiologic changes that occur with aging occur at different rates for different people and are normal effects. They may, however, increase the older client's

risk of developing illness and disability. Physical changes related to aging and their possible implications for health are summarized in Table 2◆.

Aging also results in changes in patterns of disease that may make diagnosis or treatment of illness more difficult. These changing disease patterns include comorbidity, differences in symptom experience, and perceptions of many symptoms of disease as a normal part of aging (Williams, 2005). **Comorbidity**, the coexistence of many chronic physical and/or mental illnesses in the same person at the same time, complicates both diagnosis and treatment of illness in older adults. For example, drug therapies for one condition may interact with treatment of another condition, interfering with therapeutic effects or causing adverse effects. In addition, older people may not present with classic symptoms of a given condition, making diagnosis more difficult. For example, many older people do not experience the chest pain typical of myocardial infarction. Finally, older clients, family members, and health care providers may inaccurately interpret abnormal symptoms as facets of normal aging (e.g., many people believe that pain and stiffness are normal concomitants of age).

The goal of community health nursing with respect to aging is to foster healthy aging and to promote active aging, defined by WHO as "the process of optimizing opportunities for health, participation, and security in order to enhance quality of life as people age" (quoted in Plese, 2005b, p. 5). Three requisites have been proposed for healthy aging: (a) accepting the limitations posed by bodily changes, (b) modifying one's lifestyle as needed to accommodate these changes, and (c) developing new personal standards of achievement and life goals consistent with the constraints imposed by the effects of aging (Saxon & Etten, 2002). The role of the community health nurse is to assist the elderly population to mitigate the adverse effects, prevent unnecessary deterioration in function, and promote quality of life for older clients.

Physiologic Function

Older populations experience increased mortality and morbidity rates relative to younger groups of people. They also experience higher rates of many other problems that affect their quality of life, such as pain and incontinence. A few of these physiologic effects will be discussed here. With respect to mortality, age-specific death rates increase with age for most diseases. For example, the mortality rate for heart disease in 2002 was 241.5 per 100,000 persons aged 55 to 64 years, but more than doubled for the next age group (615.9 per 100,000), then nearly tripled for those aged 75 to 84 years (1,677 per 100,000), then more than tripled again for those over age 85 (5,466 per 100,000). Similar escalation with age is noted in mortality rates for cerebrovascular disease, malignancies, chronic lower respiratory diseases, and other chronic illnesses (CDC, 2004a).

TABLE 2	Common Physical Changes of Aging and Their Implications for Health	
System	Changes Noted	Possible Health Implications
Integumentary		
Skin	Decreased turgor, sclerosis, and loss of subcutaneous fat, leading to wrinkles	Lowered self-esteem
	Increased pigmentation, cherry angiomas	
	Cool to touch, dry	Itching, risk of injury, insomnia
	Decreased perspiration	Hyperthermia, heatstroke
Hair	Thin, decreased pigmentation	Lowered self-esteem
Nails	Thickened, ridges, decreased rate of growth	Difficulty trimming nails, potential for injury
Cardiovascular	Less efficient pump action and lower cardiac reserves	Decreased physical ability, fatigue with exertion
	Thickening of vessel walls, replacement of muscle fiber with collagen	Elevated blood pressure, varicosities, venous stasis, pressure sores
	Pulse pressure up to 100	
	Arrhythmias and murmurs	
	Dilated abdominal aorta	
Respiratory	Decreased elasticity of alveolar sacs, skeletal changes of chest	Decreased gas exchange, decreased physical ability
	Slower mucus transport, decreased cough strength, dysphagia	Increased potential for infection or aspiration
	Postnasal drip	
Gastrointestinal	Wearing down of teeth	Difficulty chewing
	Decreased saliva production	Dry mouth, difficulty digesting starches
	Loss of taste buds	Decreased appetite, malnutrition
	Muscle atrophy of cheeks, tongue, etc.	Difficulty chewing, slower to eat
	Thinned esophageal wall	Feeling of fullness, heartburn after meals
	Decreased peristalsis	Constipation
	Decreased hydrochloric acid and stomach enzyme production	Pernicious anemia, frequent eructation
	Decreased lip size, sagging abdomen	Change in self-concept
	Atrophied gums	Poorly fitting dentures, difficulty chewing, potential for mouth ulcers, loss of remaining teeth
	Decreased bowel sounds	Potential for misdiagnosis
	Fissures in tongue	
	Increased or decreased liver size (2–3 cm below costal border)	Potential for misdiagnosis
Urinary	Decreased number of nephrons and decreased ability to concentrate urine	Nocturia, increased potential for falls
Reproductive		
Female	Atrophied ovaries, uterus	Ovarian cysts
	Atrophy of external genitalia, pendulous breasts, small flat nipple, decreased pubic hair	Lower self-esteem
	Scant vaginal secretions	Dyspareunia
	Vaginal mucosa thinned and friable	
Male	Decreased size of penis and testes, decreased pubic hair, pendulous scrotum	Lowered self-esteem
	Enlarged prostate	Difficulty urinating, incontinence

Continued on next page

TABLE 2	Common Physical Changes of Aging and Their Implications for Health *(continued)*	
Musculoskeletal	Decreased muscle size and tone	Decreased physical ability
	Decreased range of motion in joints, affecting gait, posture, balance, and flexibility	Increased risk of falls, decreased mobility
	Kyphosis	Lowered self-esteem
	Joint instability	Increased risk of falls, injury
	Straight thoracic spine	
	Breakdown of chondrocytes in joint cartilage	Osteoarthritis, joint pain, reduced abilities for activities of daily living
	Osteoporosis	Increased risk of fracture
Neurological	Diminished hearing, vision, touch, and increased reaction time	Increased risk for injury, social isolation
	Diminished pupil size, peripheral vision, adaptation, accommodation	
	Diminished sense of smell, taste	Decreased appetite, malnutrition
	Decreased balance	Increased risk of injury
	Decreased pain sensation	Increased risk of injury
	Decreased ability to problem-solve	Difficulty adjusting to new situations
	Diminished deep tendon reflexes	
	Decreased sphincter tone	Incontinence (fecal or urinary)
	Diminished short-term memory	Forgetfulness
Endocrine		
Thyroid	Irregular, fibrous changes	
Female	Decreased estrogen and progesterone production	Osteoporosis, menopause
Male	Decreased testosterone production	Fatigue, weight loss, decreased libido, impotence, lowered self-esteem, depression

Older populations are even more prone to morbidity from acute and chronic illness than to death, and the bulk of the burden of many of these conditions is borne by the older segments of the population.

ACUTE HEALTH CONDITIONS Because of decreased organ function and immune function that accompanies aging, older people are often at greater risk for acute illnesses and injuries as well as for developing serious complications of disease. Accidental injuries are acute conditions that significantly affect the health of the elderly. For example, in 2002, the rate of injury-related emergency department visits for older clients was 1,192.5 per 10,000 men and 1,369.4 per 10,000 women (CDC, 2004a). Accidental injuries are the seventh leading cause of death over age 65 years and the fifth leading cause for people over age 85 (Hurley et al., 2004). Most of these injuries are related to falls, with one third of older adults in the United States each year experiencing a fall (Huang & Acton, 2004). Mortality is 12% to 20% higher among older people experiencing a hip fracture as a result of a fall than among non-fallers. Annual costs for hip fractures resulting from falls in the United States amount to $6 billion (Yuan et al.,

2001). Injuries are addressed in more detail in the section on safety later in this chapter.

Influenza and pneumonia are two other acute health conditions that disproportionately affect the elderly. Influenza causes more than 36,000 deaths each year (Harper, Fukuda, Uyeki, Cox, & Bridges, 2005). From 1990 to 1999, more than 32,000 influenza-related deaths occurred each year among people over 65 years of age (Epidemiology and Surveillance Division, 2004). Similar patterns are evident for pneumococcal pneumonia, with hospitalizations among the elderly increasing by 93.5% from 1991 to 1998 (Baine, Yu, & Summe, 2001) and more than 3,000 deaths in people over 65 years of age in 1999 alone (CDC, 2004b). In 2001, influenza and pneumonia together constituted the fifth leading cause of death in people over 85 years of age (U.S. Census Bureau, 2005).

Although a smaller proportion of the population is affected than in other age groups, 10% of AIDS cases occur in people over 50 years of age in the United States. In addition, from 1991 to 1996, the incidence of AIDS increased more in the population over 50 years of age than in the 13- to 49-year-old group (Rose, 2004). In 2002, an estimated 8,900 people over 65 years of age in the United States were living with AIDS (U.S. Census

Bureau, 2005). In 2003, incidence rates for AIDS in people over 60 years of age were 6.3 per 100,000 men and 1.5 per 100,000 women (CDC, 2004a). Although these rates are less than a quarter of those for people aged 13 to 59 years, they are significant because many providers do not think of AIDS in the older population and because of the added complication posed by AIDS in the control of other health problems among the elderly. Community health nurses may need to advocate for treatment facilities that meet the specific needs of older clients with AIDS or for health education programs particularly targeted to this population.

CHRONIC DISEASE AND DISABILITY Both the incidence and prevalence of chronic illnesses increase with age. An estimated 84% of people over 65 years of age have at least one chronic illness, and 62% have two or more chronic conditions (Tanner, 2004). By age 80, three fourths of women have two or more chronic conditions, the major contributors to disease burden being arthritis, hypertension, heart disease, and hearing and vision problems (Yoon & Horne, 2004). Chronic illness contributes to an increasing number of days in bed. For example, in 2003, the average number of days in bed due to chronic disease was only 3.5 for people aged 18 to 44 years and 6 days for those aged 45 to 64 years, but increased with age to 6.6 days for those 65 to 74 years old and 9.4 days for those over 75 years of age (NCHS, 2005a).

Arthritis affects 60% of people over 65 years of age in the United States. The percentage of people affected by this disease is expected to remain relatively stable through 2030 (58% of the elderly population), but the actual number of people with arthritis or chronic joint symptoms is expected to double to 41.1 million (Division of Adult and Community Health, 2003b). Arthritis is the most frequent cause of disability in the United States. Arthritis pain limits movement, which leads to deconditioning of joints and muscles and greater pain with movement. Without treatment, arthritis leads to a continuous pain-movement cycle that limits function and increases the potential for disability (Davis, Hiemenz, & White, 2002).

Hypertension and consequent cardiovascular disease are other common chronic illnesses in older populations. From 1999 to 2002, for example, hypertension affected 59% of men aged 65 to 74 years and 68% of those over 75 years of age. The percentage of women in each age group is even higher, at 72.5% of those 65 to 74 years of age and 83% of those over age 75 (CDC, 2004a). Heart disease and stroke incidence also increase with increasing age. In 2001, for example, 50% to 74% of hospitalizations for cardiovascular disease, coronary heart disease, angina, or stroke occurred among people over 65 years of age, and people over 85 years of age constitute 84% of cardiovascular and coronary heart disease deaths (Johnson, 2004). The risk of cardiovascular disease increases substantially in women after menopause (Lewis, 2004).

The rate of hospitalization for stroke also increases with age. In 2001, for example, the rate of stroke hospitalization nearly doubled each decade after age 65 years, from 10.3 per 100,000 people aged 65 to 74 years to 20.5 per 100,000 of those 75 to 84 years of age, to 29.9 per 100,000 of those over age 85 years (Division of Adult and Community Health, 2003a).

Cardiovascular disease often leads to congestive heart failure (CHF), and 7% to 10% of people over age 80 have some degree of CHF. The incidence of CHF increases ninefold for men and elevenfold for women with every decade from age 50 to 80 years (Resnick, 2005).

Malignant neoplasms are the leading cause of death in people 65 to 74 years of age in the United States, at which point they are replaced by heart disease as the leading cause of death (U.S. Census Bureau, 2005). Approximately 60% of all new cancer diagnoses each year occur in people over 65 years of age, and people in this age group account for 61% of all cancer survivors (Division of Cancer Prevention and Control, 2004). Prostate cancer incidence in men increases with age; men aged 60 to 79 years have a twelvefold higher risk than younger men (Calabrese, 2004). An estimated 8% of men over age 80 have prostate cancer (Pinkelman, 2002). Breast cancer mortality in women also increases with age. For example, in 2002, mortality rates increased from 56.2 per 100,000 women aged 55 to 64 years to 191.5 per 100,000 women 85 years of age and over (CDC, 2004a).

Diabetes is another chronic illness that affects the health status of the elderly. From 1999 to 2000, for example, approximately 19% of people over 60 years of age had diabetes (CDC, 2004a). About 4.5 million women over age 60 years have diabetes, and nearly one fourth of them remain undiagnosed (National Center for Chronic Disease Prevention and Health Promotion, 2002a).

Chronic obstructive pulmonary disease (COPD) is a group of diseases that affect pulmonary function and includes chronic bronchitis, chronic obstructive bronchitis or emphysema, and combinations of these diseases. COPD is the fourth leading cause of death in the United States and is expected to become the third leading cause by 2020 (National Heart, Lung, and Blood Institute, 2003). In 2002, the latest year for which statistics are available, the overall age-adjusted U.S. mortality rate for lower respiratory diseases including COPD was 43.5 per 100,000 population. COPD death rates are far higher among the elderly, however, climbing to 163 per 100,000 among people age 65 to 74 and 637.6 among those 85 years of age and older (NCHS, 2005b). COPD may make even minimal exertion difficult for those affected and is a significant cause of disability among the elderly.

Even for chronic diseases that do not have a higher incidence among older adults, the effects of disease may be more pronounced with age. For example, only 45% of people with multiple sclerosis (MS) are over 55 years of age, but older persons with MS must deal with continuing deterioration as well as the usual effects of aging. In addition, older people with MS tend to display a more rapid rate of decline in function than those diagnosed at younger ages (Finlayson, Van Denend, & Hudson, 2004).

Chronic disease in the elderly often leads to functional limitations and disability. **Functional status** is the ability to perform tasks and fulfill expected social roles. Assessment of functional status includes exploration of abilities at three levels of task complexity: basic, intermediate or instrumental, and advanced activities of daily living. **Basic activities of daily living (BADLs)** are personal-care activities and include the ability to feed, bathe, and dress oneself, and toileting and transfer skills (getting in or out of a chair or bed). Intermediate or **instrumental activities of daily living (IADLs)** are tasks of moderate complexity, including household tasks such as shopping, laundry, cooking, and housekeeping, as well as abilities to take medications correctly, manage money, and use the telephone or public transportation. **Advanced activities of daily living (AADLs)** involve complex abilities to engage in voluntary social, occupational, or recreational activities.

Disability in the older population is defined as "difficulty with household and personal self-maintenance activities severe enough to threaten independent living" (Albert et al., 2002, p. 1215). Some authors propose three distinct pathways leading to disability in the elderly (Albert et al., 2002). In the first pathway, senescence, or the normal effects of aging, lead to frailty, which is seen as a preclinical stage to disability. Frailty is characterized by increasing weakness, slowness, and poor endurance, which make it difficult for the older person to engage in activities of daily living (ADLs). When these effects reach a threshold of "physical and cognitive capacity required for completion of daily tasks" (p. 1215), disability results.

The second pathway to disability reflects the direct effects of chronic diseases on stamina, strength, sensibility, dexterity, and the effect of pain and balance difficulties that decrease the capacity to perform ADLs. Albert

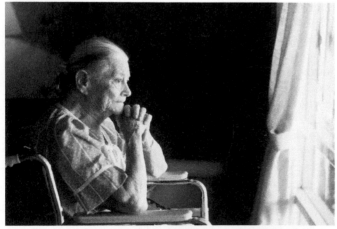

Disability may result in social isolation for many older clients. (Mark Richards)

and associates (2002) noted that senescence and disease can interact to contribute to disability. In the third pathway, environmental factors contribute to disability when difficulties in performing ADLs are compounded by lack of access to assistive and prosthetic devices or absent social and psychological resources to offset these difficulties. In one study, approximately 54% of disability in the elderly was attributed to the direct effects of chronic disease, 28% to frailty alone, and 18% was potentially related to environmental conditions (Albert et al., 2002). Other authors noted that more than 3 million people in Britain experienced locomotor disability, the inability to walk, climb stairs, or maintain balance. They found that personal difficulties arose primarily from the gap between the disability and environmental conditions that would allow people to function effectively in the face of the disability (Ebrahim, Papacosta, Wannamethee, & Adamson, 2004).

The extent of disability in the elderly population declined from 25% in 1984 to 20% in 1999. Despite the decrease in the percentage of the population affected, the actual number of older people experiencing disability increased due to the increasing size of this population (Federal Interagency Forum on Aging-related Statistics, 2004).

In 2002, an estimated 42% of people over 65 years of age in the United States experienced one or more disability. For 29% the disability was physical in nature; 14% experienced sensory limitations; 11% had mental disabilities of some kind; 9.5% experienced self-care limitations; and 20% were unable to go outside their homes without assistance. Just over 6% of people over age 65 experienced limitations in ADLs, and twice as many (12%) had difficulties with IADLs (U.S. Census Bureau, 2005).

Activity limitations vary with age and gender. In 2002, 25% of people aged 65 to 74 years experienced activity limitations, compared to 45% of those over age 75 (U.S. Census Bureau, 2005). The percentage of people aged 65 to 74 years with BADL limitations was 2.7%, whereas 9.6% of those over age 75 had BADL limitations. With respect to IADLs, the respective percentages were 6% and 18.9% (CDC, 2004a). The cause of disability may also vary with age. Between 65 and 84 years of age, disability is most often due to chronic physical conditions such as arthritis, hypertension, and heart disease. After age 85, disability due to cognitive and sensory problems, such as Alzheimer's and vision and hearing impairment, are more common (Huey, 2001). For example, memory impairment is found in approximately 5% of people aged 65 to 69 years, but 32% of those over 80 years of age (Federal Interagency Forum on Aging-related Statistics, 2004). Nearly 4% of women and 10% of men aged 65 to 74 years have hearing problems, and these figures increase to 13% of women and 18% of men who are 75 years of age or older (NCHS, 2005c). Approximately 18% of people over 70 years of age in the United States have visual difficulties, and 8.6% have both hearing and vision problems. People with both hearing and vision impairment were nearly three times more likely to consider themselves in poor health and were half as likely as those with neither impairment to report their health as excellent. Similarly, those with impairments in both senses were almost three times as likely as those with neither impairment to be depressed or confused and to have difficulty walking and were nearly four times more likely to have difficulty preparing meals. Those with vision problems were three times more likely to have difficulty going places and were more than twice as likely to have problems taking medications as people with neither hearing nor vision problems (Crews & Campbell, 2004).

The prevalence of disability in the older population also varies by gender. Although women have lower mortality rates than men and lower incidence and prevalence rates for some chronic illnesses, they tend to report lower quality of life and more disability and physical limitations than men. In general, about half of women over 65 years of age have some sort of functional disability (National Center on Birth Defects and Developmental Disabilities, 2005). In studies, 52% of older women report functional limitations compared to 37% of men. Women also report more limitations and greater disability than men do. Mobility limitations were reported by women one and a half times more often than men, and women were also more likely than men to report use of assistance in ADLs. In addition, women reported more pain and stiffness and greater fatigue related to chronic illness than men (Murtaugh & Hubert, 2004).

In addition to impaired quality of life for older people, disability presents significant costs to society. For example, in 1995 the estimated cost of older people transitioning from an independent to a dependent status due to disability amounted to a total of $26.1 billion. Average annual costs for people who developed a disability in a given year but remained in their home were $3,400. For those living at home who began and ended the year with a disability, average costs were doubled to $6,800. When disability resulted in nursing home placement, annual costs escalated to $21,000 per person (Guralnik, Alecxih, Branch, & Wiener, 2002).

PAIN Pain is a symptom that accompanies a wide variety of acute and chronic illnesses and is a common problem experienced by the older population. It is estimated that at least 70% of older adults experience chronic pain, most often as a result of arthritis and neuralgias (Davis et al., 2002). Unrelieved pain can diminish quality of life for the elderly through its functional, cognitive, emotional, and social effects. The normal effects of aging may lead to a slightly higher pain threshold for the elderly, such that older clients may not experience the pain typical of some conditions, making diagnosis more difficult. Pain is, however, prevalent and is often undertreated in older persons. The incidence of pain has been found to double

after the age of 60 years and increases each decade thereafter (Hanks-Bell, Halvey, & Paice, 2004).

Poor pain management in the elderly centers around client and provider decisions related to pain management. One study identified several barriers to arthritis pain management that are relevant to other causes of pain. These barriers included lack of access to care or treatment, an accelerating pain-movement cycle, lack of use of adaptive resources, emotional distress and its effects on pain and pain management, knowledge deficits regarding pain management, age-related perceptions by clients and providers that pain is normal in old age, and poor communication with providers (Davis et al., 2002).

INCONTINENCE Incontinence is another manageable physiologic condition that affects the quality of life of the elderly. Urinary incontinence has both psychological and social effects for older individuals, as well as economic consequences. For example, it is estimated that the 2002 cost of urinary incontinence was $2.2 billion (Phillips, 2004). Approximately 17 million people in the United States experience urinary incontinence or overactive bladder, but only about 15% of them seek help with the condition. Estimated prevalence in U.S. community-dwelling elders is 37% to 41%, with European studies suggesting that 20% of men and 24% of women are affected (Cooper & Kaplan, 2004; Heidrick & Wells, 2004).

Urinary incontinence may be of four general types: stress incontinence, overflow incontinence, urge incontinence, and functional incontinence (Dash, Foster, Smith, & Phillips, 2004). Stress incontinence occurs with movements that stress the urethral sphincter, such as coughing or sneezing. Overflow incontinence is due to residual urine remaining in the bladder from incomplete emptying. Urge incontinence is characterized by a sudden uncontrollable need to urinate, and functional incontinence is due to impaired mobility to reach the toilet in

ETHICAL AWARENESS

You are caring for an elderly gentleman with terminal lung cancer. He is experiencing considerable pain and has been given a prognosis of about 6 months' survival time. He tells you that he and his wife have been exploring the idea of assisted suicide and have found a physician who may be willing to help them. His wife experiences severe pain due to her arthritis and is never pain free, although pain medications decrease the level of pain to some extent. He had been doing most of the work in the home (cooking, washing, etc.) until recently. They have no family in the area and his wife's older brother lives in another state and is caring for his wife, who has Alzheimer's disease. Your client is afraid that when he dies, his wife will have no one to care for her and will suffer even more. He says they would "like to be together in death" just as they have been in life for over 50 years. Assisted suicide is illegal in your state. What will you do in this situation?

time or decreased manual dexterity in undressing. Incontinence in any given individual may combine several types (Teunissen, de Jonge, van Weel, & Lagro-Janssen, 2004). Incontinence may also be related to medications, such as anticholinergics, psychotropics, antidepressants, diuretics, sedatives, alpha-adrenergic blockers and agonists, calcium channel blockers, and muscle relaxants, or to alcohol or caffeine use (Dash et al., 2004).

Older clients may also experience fecal incontinence related to limited mobility and difficulty getting to the toilet and removing their clothing. Other causes of fecal incontinence include diarrhea caused by a variety of factors, constipation resulting in overflow incontinence, irritable bowel syndrome, incomplete evacuation, rectal neoplasms, neurological problems (e.g., stroke, multiple sclerosis, dementia), congenital malformations, accidental or surgical trauma, and pelvic floor denervation due to vaginal delivery, rectal prolapse, or chronic straining at stool (International Foundation for Functional Gastrointestinal Disorders, 2006a). Approximately 2.2% to 6.9% of the general population experiences fecal incontinence, but prevalence may be as high as 47% of elderly nursing home residents (International Foundation for Gastrointestinal Disorders, 2003). Although fecal incontinence is more common in older clients than in younger ones, it is not a normal part of aging (National Digestive Diseases Information Clearinghouse, 2004).

Both fecal and urinary incontinence are distressing to older clients because of the loss of control and feelings of reversion back to babyhood. Clients with incontinence may isolate themselves from others and become virtually housebound due to feelings of embarrassment and incompetence. They may also be reluctant to share problems of incontinence with health care providers. Community health nurses may need to advocate with older clients themselves to encourage them to seek treatment. They may also need to educate the public regarding incontinence and the potential for treatment.

Psychological Considerations

Psychological considerations that particularly influence the health of the older population include cognitive impairment, stress, and depression. Although cognitive impairment has a number of biophysical causes, it is addressed here because the majority of its effects are mental, with physiological effects arising from the mental deficits caused. Some other psychiatric illnesses will be noted in the elderly population, some of which may be superimposed on other physical illnesses or may result from physical illness. By 2030, 15 million older adults in the United States are expected to have some form of psychiatric illness, the most common of which will be dementia, depression, and anxiety disorders. Symptoms of schizophrenia seem to diminish with age, but older clients are at greater risk for extrapyramidal side effects of psychotropic medications than younger people. In addition, hearing and vision impairments that often accompany aging may increase the potential for confusion and delusions (Calandra, 2003).

Cognitive Impairment

Elements of cognitive function that may be impaired in the elderly include attention span, concentration, judgment, learning ability, memory, orientation, perception, problem solving, psychomotor ability, reaction time, and social intactness. Although slight decline in some of these areas (e.g., memory) or increased slowness in others (e.g., learning or reaction time) may be expected with age, marked changes are not consistent with the normal aging process. **Dementia** is a loss of intellectual function in multiple domains including memory, problem-solving ability, judgment, and others (Garand, Buckwalter, & Hall, 2000). *Dementia* is a general term used to encompass cognitive deficits that include progressive memory loss and at least one other symptom such as aphasia (difficulty with written or verbal communication), apraxia (inability to correctly use objects), or agnosia (loss of comprehension of auditory, visual, or tactile sensations) (Vogel, 2003). Dementia is found in 2% of people aged 65 to 70 years and 11% to 40% of those over 80 years of age (Chang, Nitta, Carter, & Markham, 2004).

Alzheimer's disease (AD) is the most common cause of dementia, affecting 3% of people over 65 years of age in the United States, and 20% of those over 85 years of age (Vogel, 2003). In the future as many as 47% of people over age 85 are expected to develop the disease. Similarly, the estimated prevalence of dementia in the United Kingdom is 4% to 6% (Minardi & Blanchard, 2004). During the 1990s, as many as 360,000 new cases were diagnosed each year in the United States, and this number is expected to climb to 959,000 per year by 2050 (Hurley et al., 2004; National Institute on Aging, 2002). There are currently 4 million Americans with Alzheimer's disease (Kolanowski, Fick, Waller, & Shea, 2004), and the number who will require care due to the effects of dementia is expected to increase by 350% before 2050 (Brown & Alligood, 2004). These figures may be even higher for ethnic minority groups who tend to have higher rates of cognitive impairment, dementia, and Alzheimer's disease than the non-Hispanic White population (Manly & Mayeux, 2004). Although Alzheimer's disease is the primary cause of dementia, it may also be caused by other conditions. For example, 20% to 60% of people with Parkinson's disease, especially severe disease, develop dementia. Other potential causes of dementia include Pick's disease (a rare degenerative neurological disease), Korsakov's syndrome (due to prolonged alcohol abuse), HIV infection, head trauma, and classic Creutzfeldt-Jakob disease (CDC, 2005a; Vogel, 2003). Circulatory deficiencies in chronic heart failure may also lead to cognitive deficits in memory, learning ability, executive function, and psychomotor speed. In fact, cognitive deficits may occur in as many as 30% to 80% of clients with congestive heart failure (Bennett, Suave, & Shaw, 2005).

Alzheimer's dementia usually progresses in stages characterized by progressive impairment. In the early stage, the client experiences mild cognitive impairment, increased difficulty learning and retaining new material, and difficulty with complex tasks that require reasoning, spatial orientation, and language. Additional characteristics of this stage include increasing difficulty with problem solving, managing finances, accomplishing routine tasks, and remembering specific words. People in middle-stage Alzheimer's disease exhibit inability to recognize family and friends not seen regularly, difficulty in completing simple tasks, wandering and becoming lost, mood changes, irritability, agitation, and sleep disturbance. Late Alzheimer's disease is

characterized by a substantial decline in verbal, recognition, and comprehension skills; inability to comprehend language; gait disturbances and loss of the ability to walk; urinary incontinence; and loss of the ability to feed oneself and swallow, with consequent poor nutrition (Vogel, 2003).

The confusion experienced in Alzheimer's disease may be exacerbated by changes in one's surroundings, and maintenance of familiar surroundings may help clients remain comfortable and retain some functional abilities. This is due to the fact that priming or conditioning memory (habit) tends to be retained in many people with AD, in contrast to explicit memory (conscious, directed effort to recall information) and procedural memory related to learned skills such as feeding oneself (Son, Therrien, & Whall, 2002). The focused assessment below contains questions to guide assessment of cognitive function in older clients.

FOCUSED ASSESSMENT

Assessing Cognitive Function in Older Clients

Attention Span

- Does the client focus on a single activity to completion?
- Does the client move from activity to activity without completing any?

Concentration

- Is the client able to answer questions without wandering from the topic?
- Does the client ignore irrelevant stimuli while focusing on a task?
- Is the client easily distracted from a subject or task by external stimuli?

Intelligence

- Does the client understand directions and explanations given in everyday language?
- Is the client able to perform basic mathematical calculations?

Judgment

- Does the client engage in action appropriate to the situation?
- Are client behaviors based on an awareness of environmental conditions and possible consequences of action?
- Are the client's plans and goals realistic?
- Can the client effectively budget income?
- Is the client safe driving a car?

Learning Ability

- Is the client able to retain instructions for a new activity?
- Can the client recall information provided?
- Is the client able to correctly demonstrate new skills?

Memory

- Is the client able to remember and describe recent events in some detail?
- Is the client able to describe events from the past in some detail?

Orientation

- Can the client identify him- or herself by name?
- Is the client aware of where he or she is?
- Does the client recognize the identity and function of those around him or her?
- Does the client know what day and time it is?
- Is the client able to separate past, present, and future?

Perception

- Are the client's responses appropriate to the situation?
- Does the client exhibit evidence of hallucinations or illusions?
- Are explanations of events consistent with the events themselves?
- Can the client reproduce simple figures?

Problem Solving

- Is the client able to recognize problems that need resolution?
- Can the client envision alternative solutions to a given problem?
- Can the client weigh alternative solutions and select one appropriate to the situation?
- Can the client describe activities needed to implement the solution?

Psychomotor Ability

- Does the client exhibit repetitive movements that interfere with function?

Reaction Time

- Does the client take an unusually long time to respond to questions or perform motor activities?
- Does the client respond to questions before the question is completed?

Social Intactness

- Are the client's interactions with others appropriate to the situation?
- Is the client able to describe behaviors appropriate and inappropriate to a given situation?

Stress, Coping, and Depression

Like people in other age groups, older clients experience stress and have a broad range of abilities to cope with stress. Unlike others, however, older people may have fewer resources to allow them to cope effectively with stress. During 2001–2002, for example, 2.4% of the U.S. population over 65 years of age reported serious psychological distress (CDC, 2004a). Coping with the helplessness and loss of power often associated with chronic illness may be particularly difficult for older persons, who often need to achieve a balance between assistance and independence (Tanner, 2004). Studies of older people suggest that they prefer to manage stress themselves whenever possible. This has been found to be true in Asian populations, perhaps because of the cultural imperative to "save face" or in response to the absence of effective social support. Approaches to stress management found among older Asian clients include participation in enjoyable activities, having positive thoughts, and expressing thoughts and feelings to family and friends. Study subjects were less likely to seek professional help due to fear of stigma, cost, not wanting to worry others, difficulty communicating with providers, not knowing where to go, or perceptions that help would not be effective (Kwong & Kwan, 2004).

When older people cannot cope with the stress encountered in their lives, they may become depressed. Estimates of the overall prevalence of depression in the elderly vary from 2% (with 15% to 30% experiencing mild or "subsyndromal depression") (Antai-Otong, 2004) to 15% to 20% of the general elderly population (Loughlin, 2004; Weeks, McGann, Michaels, & Penninx, 2003) to 26% to 44% of the homebound elderly (Loughlin, 2004). According to the Federal Interagency Forum on Aging-related Statistics (2004), 11% of older men and 18% of women are clinically depressed. These figures may increase as "baby boomers" begin to age, because this group has higher rates of depression, suicide, anxiety, and substance abuse disorders than previous cohorts (McLeer, 2004).

Many older clients with depression have a previous personal history of depressive disorders; others develop depression for the first time late in life. Risk factors for late-onset depression include family history of depression, cognitive impairment, loss of interest in life, low socioeconomic status, inadequate support systems,

negative life events such as retirement or loss, physical or mental comorbidity, and divorce, separation, or widowhood (Antai-Otong, 2004). Depression has also been linked to loneliness and decreased life satisfaction (Minardi & Blanchard, 2004).

In addition to diminished quality of life, depression in the elderly has been associated with diminished immunity and increased risk of substance abuse as a means of coping with depression (Calandra, 2003). Depression has also been linked to falls in the elderly, perhaps as a result of postural and gait changes that often occur in the context of depression. Conversely, antidepressant therapy may also predispose the elderly to falls (Turcu et al., 2004). Depression increases health care use and costs and may lead to functional decline and dependence (Weeks et al., 2003).

Depression may be difficult to diagnose in the elderly for several reasons. Comorbid depression is often missed in the presence of critical illness or undertreated when it is recognized (Weeks et al., 2003). Providers and family members may miss symptoms of depression, attributing them to aging. At the same time, older clients may feel shame related to their perceived inability to cope and not voice their feelings of depression, or may fail to recognize them for what they are (Calandra, 2003). Many medications used to treat chronic illness in the elderly may also contribute to feelings of depression. Some authors have voiced a need for standardized tools for screening for depression in the elderly that account for the many confounding factors (Weeks et al., 2003).

At its extreme, depression may lead to suicide, which is a significant problem among the elderly, particularly among older men. From 2000 to 2003, the average annual suicide rate for people over 65 years of age in the United States was 27.34 per 100,000 men and 4.43 per 100,000 women (National Center for Injury Prevention and Control, 2005a). Suicide rates increase with age for older men, but decrease slightly among women. In 2002, for example, suicide mortality affected 13.5 per 100,000 men aged 65 to 74 years, rose to 17.7 per 100,000 for 75- to 84-year-olds, and was highest among men 85 years of age or older. Comparable figures for women in these age groups were 4.1, 4.2, and 3.8 per 100,000 women (CDC, 2004a). White men over 85 years of age have the highest suicide rate of any age or racial group (American Association of Retired Persons [AARP], 2002).

BUILDING OUR KNOWLEDGE BASE

Turcu et al. (2004) found that among patients who were admitted to a geriatric unit as a result of a fall, those who were depressed had lower motor ability scores than those who were not depressed. They noted, however, that their data did not suggest whether depression was a contributing factor in the falls or was a consequence of injury sustained in a fall. How might you design a study to address this issue?

Physical Environmental Considerations

Conditions in the physical environment also affect the health of older populations. For example, living in neighborhoods with problems of traffic, noise, crime, trash and litter, poor lighting, and inadequate public transportation has been associated with increased risk of functional loss among elderly residents. As the number of problems in the neighborhood increased, greater loss of physical function occurred. Neighborhood factors have also been linked to problems of social isolation, hearing impairment, cognitive impairment, and depression in the elderly (Balfour & Kaplan, 2002). Similar findings have been noted for functional deterioration in unsafe neighborhoods (Blazer, Sachs-Ericsson, & Hybels, 2005).

Physical environmental conditions may also have a direct effect on physical health status. For example, in 2002, 45% of older persons in the United States lived in counties with ozone levels above federal standards. This figure represented an increase from 26% in 2000. Another 19% lived in areas with excessive particulate matter (Federal Interagency Forum on Aging-related Statistics, 2004). Both ozone and particulate matter have an adverse effect on respiratory function, particularly in people with chronic respiratory diseases. In fact, a 4-year national study found that older people had higher rates of cardiovascular and respiratory diseases than younger people when exposed to fine particle pollution, and that disease rates increased with age even among the elderly (National Institute of Environmental Health Sciences, 2006).

Safety hazards are another major consideration with respect to the physical environment of the elderly. Older clients may live in older housing with multiple safety hazards. Or, given recent energy prices, older persons on fixed incomes may have significantly more difficulty heating or cooling their homes than in the past. Both heat and cold have more profound effects on elderly persons than on younger ones due to changes in heat-regulating mechanisms that occur with aging. For example, heat wave mortality has been associated with increasing age, particularly in the presence of lower socioeconomic status, poor housing quality, and lack of air conditioning (Center for Climatic Research, 2004). The companion *Community Assessment Reference Guide* 📄 designed to accompany this text provides a tool for assessing home safety for older clients.

Conversely, older people may live in settings that promote health and independence. Residential areas that provide opportunities for safe exercise by the elderly or assist with accomplishment of routine tasks can delay functional deterioration. Unfortunately, in 2002, only 2% of the Medicare population lived in settings with at least one such service available (Federal Interagency Forum on Aging-related Statistics, 2004).

Sociocultural Considerations

Sociocultural considerations that have a major impact on the health of the elderly population include family roles and responsibilities, social support, and economic and employment factors. Abuse and violence are other sociocultural factors that have a profound influence on the health of this vulnerable population.

Family Roles and Responsibilities

Family configurations and the resulting roles and responsibilities change over time. Children grow up and marry or move away; spouses divorce or die. Older clients may need to adjust to a variety of changes in family roles and responsibilities, some of which are looked forward to and some of which are not. In 2003, 3% of people over 65 years of age in the United States had never married, 56.5% were married, 31.6% were widowed, and 8% were divorced (U.S. Census Bureau, 2005).

Living arrangements for older clients are many and varied. In 2003, people over 65 years of age constituted 36% of those living alone in the United States and constituted 26% of heads of households. Thirty one percent of people lived alone, 54% with spouses, and 15% with others (usually grown children) (U.S. Census Bureau, 2005). Women constitute 80% of older persons living alone, and older women are three times more likely than older men to be widowed (Callen, 2004). In fact, approximately 40% of all older women live alone, compared to 73% of older men who live with spouses (Leenerts, Teel, & Pendleton, 2002). Baby boomers are particularly likely to live alone as they age (Plese, 2002).

Older people are accepting greater responsibility for raising grandchildren than in the past. In 2000, for example, an estimated 42% of people over 65 years of age assumed at least partial responsibility for caring for their grandchildren (U.S. Census Bureau, 2005). In 2003, 14.5% of U.S. grandmothers had been caring for their grandchildren for 6 months or longer. These responsibilities

GLOBAL PERSPECTIVES

*I*n many cultural groups, care of aging parents is expected to be performed by children. Lee and Law (2004) noted that in Hong Kong, this traditional pattern of intergenerational care is rapidly changing due to societal changes. Some of these changes include the increasing economic pressure on women to be employed, career plans, smaller families with fewer children to share the burden of elder care, and weakening family bonds. Although the pattern of care is changing, most elderly residents in Hong Kong have engaged in little or no planning with respect to retirement. The authors make the case that advance planning with respect to financial, health, residential, and psychological issues is associated with better adjustment and quality of life among retirees. In their study, however, they found that most Hong Kong residents moving toward retirement age had engaged in only 3 of 19 retirement planning activities, if any retirement planning was done at all. More than half of the respondents (52%) had initiated financial savings for retirement, and 57% had begun to quit unhealthful behaviors such as smoking to enhance health status. An additional 51.5% had begun to exercise regularly to promote their health. Far fewer people had engaged in such activities as buying life or accident insurance, arranging for regular health care services, planning living arrangements, considering how to spend time after retirement, obtaining information about retirement from a variety of sources, or discussing retirement with family, friends, and others.

To what extent do you think these findings are typical of the U.S. pre-retirement population? Of people in other parts of the world? How might you go about obtaining information on retirement attitudes and planning practices in other cultural settings?

often devolved on grandparents when their adult children died, were divorced, were mentally ill, or were incarcerated. Caring for grandchildren has been linked to depression, insomnia, hypertension, diabetes, functional limitations, and poor self-reported health in caregivers. In fact, in one study, caring for grandchildren 21 hours a week or more increased coronary heart disease risk by 150% (Lee, Colditz, Berkman, & Kawachi, 2003).

Caregiving responsibilities may also be undertaken by older persons in the care of aging spouses. Societal policies to promote "aging in place," or allowing people to remain in their own homes as they grow older, will increase the requirements for assistance and caregiving by family members (Magnusson & Hanson, 2005). More than one fifth of U.S. households include someone who requires caregiving, and in 81% of these households the recipient of care is someone over 50 years of age (Plese, 2005a). More than half of the adult population in the United States (54%) have provided care to a family member in a given year; 44% of these caregivers are men. A surprising number of caregivers are young people, many of them young men. Studies indicate that anywhere from 12% to 18% of adult caregivers in the United States are between the ages of 18 and 25 years (Levine et al., 2005). A caregiver is defined as "an individual aged 16 or over who provides or intends to provide a substantial amount of care on a regular basis for another individual who is 18 or over" (Merrell, Kinsella, Murphy, Philpin, & Ali, 2005, p. 550).

Family caregivers have been described as an "unpaid extension of the health care system" (Hunt, quoted in Plese, 2005a, p. 5). The average family caregiver, for instance, provides nearly 18 hours of care per week, and 17% of caregivers provide more than 40 hours of care a week (Plese, 2005a). For women, in particular, caring may become their "life's work" by the time they have spent several years caring for children, then for aging parents, and later for aging spouses (Plese, 2002). Caregiver responsibilities range from personal physical care and assistance with activities of daily living to supervision to financial management and guardianship to complete care (Davis, Burgio, Buckwalter, & Weaver, 2004). Roughly one fourth of family caregivers provide assistance with three or more ADLs, and 80% assist with IADLs. Both men and women provide assistance with IADLs, but women are more likely than men to assist with personal care. The broad range of responsibilities required of caregivers necessitates expertise in many areas that some older clients do not have (Plese, 2005a).

Research has suggested that when caregiving is based on mutually agreed-upon rules for the relationship, there is less strain for both caregiver and recipient (Coeling, Biordi, & Theis, 2003). Unfortunately, such mutual decision making often cannot occur in the face of Alzheimer's disease and other forms of dementia. Studies of caregivers of older people with AD indicate a

number of concerns and challenges. These include dealing with change, managing competing responsibilities, providing the broad spectrum of care discussed above, finding and using community resources, and dealing with physical and emotional responses to caregiving (Farran, Loukissa, Perraud, & Paun, 2004). More than half (57%) of those caring for elderly family members are employed, and an estimated 12% of the U.S. workforce provide care for elderly relatives, yet only 42% of large employers have programs in place to assist family caregivers, leaving caregivers to juggle work and caregiving responsibilities on their own (Plese, 2005a). Some states provide for family medical leave for care of ill family members. Unfortunately, although family medical leaves permit caretakers to keep their jobs, most such leaves are unpaid, and caretakers may not be able to afford to take advantage of them.

Frequently, even when resources are available from employers or others in the community, older caregivers are not aware of them or do not perceive themselves as caregivers eligible for assistance. Older caregivers have been found to be less likely to request assistance from either formal or informal support networks, since they may perceive their care as part of an ongoing relationship, rather than as caregiving per se (McGarry & Arthur, 2001). Changes in social structure related to smaller families, more women working, higher divorce rates, and an increasingly mobile population have diminished the social networks of many older people, often leaving them to deal with caregiving tasks in relative isolation (Hoskins, Coleman, & McNeely, 2005).

Most caregivers for people with Alzheimer's disease are aging spouses who have their own health problems that are compounded by the physical and psychological burdens of caregiving. The ability to initiate or continue caregiving activities is predicated on maintenance of the same level of health in both caregiver and recipient (McGarry & Arthur, 2001). Unfortunately, the stress of caregiving often leads to diminished health for caregivers. For example, spouses caring for persons with dementia have been found to have more anxiety disorders, falls, rheumatologic disease, and diabetes. Caregiver strain has also been associated with increased cardiovascular disease risk (Kolanowski et al., 2004). Women caregivers of aging spouses have been referred to as "hidden patients" because of the lack of attention to the physical and emotional effects of caregiving (Jansson, Nordberg, & Grafstrom, 2001). Older

Think Advocacy

What groups might be approached to form a coalition to advocate for support services for caretakers of older clients with Alzheimer's disease? Why would you include these specific groups in your coalition?

caregivers, in general, have poorer self-reported health status than their non-caregiving counterparts, and caregivers may not attend to their own health care needs. For example, 85% of older caregivers in one study reported previously engaging in a variety of health-promotive activities, but only 63% still performed these activities at the time of the study (Matthews, Dunbar-Jacob, Sereika, Schulz, & McDowell, 2004).

Caregiver strain is also heightened by changes in relationships, particularly in the face of dementia. Relationship changes occur with both the care recipient and other family members (Vellone, Sansoni, & Cohen, 2002). Loss of companionship of the care recipient and social isolation are two of the relationship changes that Alzheimer's caregivers have noted as creating strain (Hoskins et al., 2005). Caregivers may also experience loneliness, which has been found to be less frequent when caregiver and recipient live together. Cohabitation, however, may lead to greater social isolation when activities with others are constrained by caregiving responsibilities (Ekwall, Sivberg, & Hallberg, 2005). In some cultural groups, caregiving may also be accompanied by the stress of stigma. For example, Chinese caregivers for people with Alzheimer's disease face stigma related to cultural perceptions of AD as a result of fate, wrongdoing, worrying too much, craziness, bad feng shui, or contagion (Zhan, 2004).

Caregiving by older people also has financial burdens for both caregivers and for society. For example, approximately 60% of care costs for persons with dementia are paid out-of-pocket by caregivers (Kolanowski et al., 2004). Average monthly costs for caregiving for those with the highest care needs amount to $200 to $325 (Plese, 2005a).

Social Support

Social support is another major sociocultural influence on the health of the elderly population. Social support occurs at societal, neighborhood, and individual levels. At the societal level, social support is a function of the sense of solidarity felt by subsegments of the population with other segments. In many European countries, for example, there is greater solidarity in which younger people feel a greater responsibility for the welfare of older generations than is usually the case in the United States (Edwards, 2004). In stable neighborhoods, opportunities for social interaction increase social support available from neighbors who can be called upon at short notice because of their propinquity (McGarry & Arthur, 2001).

Social support may arise from either informal or formal social networks. A **social network** is the web of social relationships within which one interacts with other people and from which one receives social support. Social support includes emotional, instrumental, or financial assistance from the social network. The informal social network consists of friends, family members, and neighbors, whereas the formal network comprises health and social service providers. Religious affiliation may provide a form of social support that often bridges the formal and informal networks. For example, many congregations provide material and emotional support to their members. In addition, religious affiliation has been associated with greater use of preventive services (Benjamins & Brown, 2004).

Some authors have noted that examination of the health of elderly populations should include consideration both of the social support available and perceptions of its adequacy among recipients (Tanner, 2004). Most older persons seek social support most often from family members, particularly spouses. In one Japanese study, for example, for married older adults with spouses, the spouse was the most important source of social support, followed by adult children and others. For elders without spouses, adult children were the most important source of support (Okabayashi, Liang, Krause, Akiyama, & Sugisawa, 2004). The quality of support provided, however, is affected by several factors, including residential propinquity, co-residence, and past relationships (Davey, Janke, & Savla, 2005). Residential propinquity is associated with household assistance, but not financial assistance, and prior financial support from parents has been linked to later financial support of parents by their children. Co-residence may involve mutual support between generations or couples. For example, adult children may provide housing for their parents, who, in turn, provide assistance with childcare.

For immigrant families, intergenerational support may be transnational in nature, where some family members live in one country and some in another. **Transnationalism** is defined as "the process by which immigrants forge and sustain multistranded social relations that link together their societies of origin and resettlement" (Basch, Glick, Schiller, & Szanton Blanc, as quoted in Burholt & Wenger, 2005, p. 154). Transnational social support may be made more difficult by monetary exchanges, immigration laws, and other forces that regulate movement of people and objects across international borders. Some refugee immigrant families may not even have transnational support available. Many refugee families have been separated or have had family members killed. In addition, family members left in the country of origin may not have the freedom to contact immigrant members or may have little in the way of support to offer. Community health nurses can be actively involved in linking these clients to other sources of support (e.g., churches or other organizations). They may also advocate for the availability of necessary support services for these older clients.

Economic and Employment Factors

Although older people in the United States are somewhat better off financially as a total group than some other age groups, economic forces still have a significant impact on the health of the elderly. In 2002, for example, the median household income for people over 65 years of age was $23,152, up from $16,882 in 1974 (Federal Interagency Forum on Aging-related Statistics, 2004), compared to a median income of $42,409 for all U.S. households (U.S. Census Bureau, 2005). From 1984 to 2001, the median net worth of older households increased by 82% (Federal Interagency Forum on Aging-related Statistics, 2004), and older adults control 70% of U.S. wealth and 75% of the wealth of the United Kingdom (Plese, 2005b). Poverty among U.S. elderly declined from 25% in 1970 to 11% in 1996 (Imamura, 2002), and from 1965 to 1986 social welfare spending for the elderly in the United States increased from 21% of national expenditures to 33% (Newacheck & Benjamin, 2004). Despite these figures, approximately 10% of the U.S. elderly population in 2003 had an annual income below poverty level (U.S. Census Bureau, 2004b). Nearly a third (31%) of households headed by persons over 65 years of age had annual incomes below $15,000 in 2002, and the elderly comprised nearly 9% of food stamp recipients (U.S. Census Bureau, 2005). More than 20% of U.S. elderly fall into the lowest quartile for income, compared to only 6% in the Netherlands (Edwards, 2004), and older women are twice as likely as men to be poor (National Center for Chronic Disease Prevention and Health Promotion, 2002a).

Most of the income for this age group (39%) derives from Social Security payments, 25% from continued earnings, 19% from retirement pensions, and 14% from other asset income. For the lowest fifth of the population, 83% of annual income is derived from Social Security. Although many older people own their own homes, 40% of those in the lowest quintile for annual income spend 40% of their income on housing alone (Federal Interagency Forum on Aging-related Statistics, 2004).

Income levels influence access to health care as well as to other necessary goods and services. For example, in 2003, less than 54% of older adults with incomes below poverty level received influenza vaccinations, compared to 58% of the total Medicare population and 71% of those who could afford supplemental insurance in addition to Medicare (Immunization Services Division, 2005). Similarly, in 1999 1.2 million Medicare beneficiaries did not have a prescription filled, half of them due to the cost of the medication (AARP, 2002). In addition, in one study, socioeconomic status as measured by home and car ownership was associated with decreased risk of disability in older men (Ebrahim et al., 2004).

Employment and retirement are other factors that affect the health of older people indirectly through their effects on economic status as well as more directly. In 2003, 3.3% of the U.S. population over 65 years of age were employed, with approximately equal percentages among men and women (U.S. Census Bureau, 2005). Older workers are just as productive as younger ones,

but they do have increased health risks in some areas. For example, occupational injury rates in 2002 were nearly twice as high among those over age 65 as among other age groups (CDC, 2004a), and disability risk is higher in occupations involving manual labor than in other occupational groups (Ebrahim et al., 2004). As noted earlier, older workers are also at greater risk of disease and complications related to influenza, which is rapidly transmitted in workplace environments.

There is a great deal of concern lately about retirement funding. Much has been written in the United States about the Social Security and Medicare systems in particular. At present, most countries have set 65 years of age as the minimum age for drawing public pension benefits, and many employers have mandatory retirement at a specific age. Only Australia and the United States prohibit mandatory retirement except in certain age-dependent occupations (Edwards, 2004). Retirees throughout the world have been promised benefits of 37% to 70% of their earnings per year, with the United States about in the middle of this range at 45% (Plese, 2005b). Because of increased longevity,

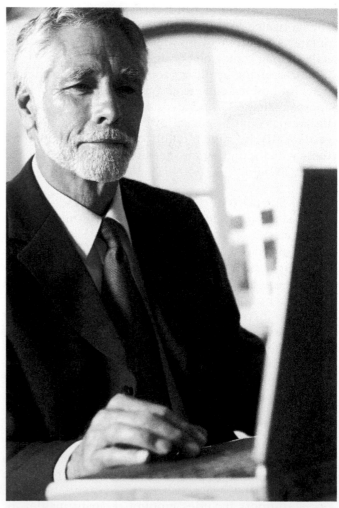

Older individuals may continue to be successfully employed beyond the typical retirement age. (Image Source)

many people can expect to spend a quarter of their lives in retirement (Lee & Law, 2004). The **old-age dependency ratio**, or the number of nonworking elders to workers, is expected to double in the developed world and triple in less developed nations from current figures of one elder per nine workers to one to four, or even one to two. Another related concept is the **elderly support ratio**, or the number of people over 65 years of age per 100 people aged 20 to 64 years (Division of Adult and Community Health, 2003c). Increases in these two ratios result in a declining tax base from which to fund services to the elderly as well as other segments of the population.

With the increasing numbers of elderly, the cost of public pension and health care benefits is expected to increase from 12% to 24% of the gross domestic product (GDP) by 2040. To stabilize expenditures at the current percentage of GDP, benefits would need to be cut by 30% to 60% (Plese, 2005b). With respect to health care services, however, reducing benefits would be a short-term solution at best. Reducing access to and payment for health care will only add to later societal costs for conditions that could have been prevented or treated in much less expensive fashion earlier.

In addition to the increased expenditures for elderly services, there will be a stagnation of markets with less money available for other forms of personal and government spending. More caregiving will be required of fewer young family members, resulting in what has been labeled the "4-2-1 phenomenon"—four aging grandparents and two aging parents to be cared for by one working adult (Plese, 2005b). Some countries such as China and Japan have already begun to experience this phenomenon.

Another result of the aging of the population is an aged workforce and employers losing skilled and experienced employees to retirement. Because of the smaller number of younger people in the workforce, employers will have difficulty replacing these people at all, much less with people of comparable levels of expertise. One solution proposed to address all of these concerns is that of "reinventing the last third of life as a time of continued productivity rather than retired leisure" (Plese, 2005, p. 8). Retaining older employees in the workforce would have benefits for employers as well as for the employees. Employers will continue to retain highly competent employees who will continue to be productive rather than a drain on society. Continued employment, whether paid or volunteer, full-time or part-time, has been found to have health benefits for older persons. Not working, on the other hand, has been linked to increased incidence of suicide and other health effects. In one study, for example, not working reduced longevity by as much as 14 years (Plese, 2005b). Retaining employees in the workforce might have the added benefit of improving the health of family members as well. For instance, news media recently addressed a new phenomenon in Japan called "retired husband syndrome." This syndrome is experienced by wives of men who retire and expect their wives to meet their demands for service (N. A., 2005).

For older clients to continue to be productively employed, a number of changes will be required in the workplace and in society at large. Increased emphasis on health promotion in the workplace will be required to keep employees healthy and productive. Societal changes will be required to promote a move to an "age-neutral" society in which older workers are not seen as less creative or productive. Employers will also need to develop more flexible work patterns and schedules to accommodate employees who prefer part-time work and retraining programs to help older employees keep up with new skill needs. Finally, both local and societal action will be required to end age discrimination in and out of the workplace (Plese, 2005b).

Abuse and Violence

One final sociocultural consideration that affects the health of the older population is that of violence and abuse. The increase in the older population has been accompanied by a disproportionate increase in elder abuse or maltreatment. Between 1986 and 1996, reports of elder abuse increased by 150%, compared to only a 10% increase in the population. In part, this increase may be due to better reporting, but also probably stems from an actual increase in abusive events. Elder abuse is defined as "the mistreatment, neglect, or exploitation of an elderly person" (Orhon, 2002, p. 22).

From 3% to 6% of people over 65 years of age in the United States experience abuse or neglect each year (Meeks-Sjostrom, 2004). This amounts to 700,000 to 1.2 million cases of abuse per year (Fulmer, 2002). In 2001, more than 33,000 older adults were treated for assault-related injuries in U.S. emergency departments (National Center for Injury Prevention and Control, 2003). Elder abuse occurs throughout the world, with 27.5% of elders in Hong Kong reporting at least one incident of abuse by a caretaker in the past year and overall prevalence of abuse at 4.6% of elders in Australia and 15.5% in Greece. In Canada, the prevalence of abuse ranges from 1.1% for verbal abuse in some studies to 20% for financial abuse. In other studies in the United Kingdom, 45% of caregivers admitted to at least one form of abuse of an older person (Yan & Tang, 2004). The average U.S. homicide rate for people over 65 years of age from 2000 to 2003 was 2.3 per 100,000 population overall (CDC, 2004a), 2.8 per 100,000 men, and 1.38 per 100,000 women (National Center for Injury Prevention and Control, 2005a). Elder abuse may be physical, verbal or emotional, sexual, or financial, or involve neglect, abandonment, or self-neglect (Fulmer, 2002; Meeks-Sjostrom, 2004; Mouton et al., 2004), and its effects may be physical or psychological.

Behavioral Considerations

Research has indicated that sociocultural and behavioral lifestyle factors have greater effects on biological systems in the older population than aging itself (Williams, 2005). Behavioral factors, such as diet and other consumption patterns, physical activity, sexuality, and medication use, have important influences on the health of the older population. Factors in each of these areas will be briefly addressed.

Diet

Diet figures significantly in many health problems experienced by older clients. Conversely, health problems such as loss of teeth may affect dietary intake. Nearly 8% of the total U.S. population is edentulous (without any teeth), but this percentage increases to nearly 25% of those over 60 years of age (Beltran-Aguilar et al., 2005). Presence or absence of teeth, diminished gastric secretion and motility, and diminished sense of taste or smell may affect older clients' ability or desire to eat a nutritious diet.

Some of the nutrition-related problems experienced by the older population include malnutrition, obesity, elevated cholesterol levels, dehydration, and deficiencies in certain specific nutrients. Between 2% and 16% of the elderly population in the United States is malnourished. Annual hospitalization costs for malnourished elders are twice those of older people who are not malnourished, with an average length of stay 5.6 days longer. In one study of older clients admitted to an acute care setting, none of those assessed as malnourished perceived themselves to be so (Callen, 2004).

Another 30% of the elderly population is obese, and during the period of 1999 to 2002, 69% of all those over 65 years of age in the United States were overweight (Federal Interagency Forum on Aging-related Statistics, 2004). Older individuals with disabilities are even more likely to be obese. For example, a 1998–1999 survey in eight states and the District of Columbia found that, although obesity affected 14% of all those over 65 years of age, 24% of disabled elderly were obese (Division of Human Development and Disability, 2002). In addition, nearly 14% of men and 33% of women aged 65 to 74 years had elevated cholesterol levels. These figures decreased slightly in the population over 75 years of age to 10% and 26.5%, respectively (CDC, 2004a).

Interestingly, obesity in women over 70 years of age has been associated with the absence of health promotion measures. For example, obese older women were less likely than women of normal weight to receive influenza immunizations in one study (Østbye, Taylor, Yancy, & Krause, 2005). These women may choose not to seek care for routine health promotion due to embarrassment regarding their weight or fears that providers will chastise them for their obesity.

Chronic dehydration is another dietary problem that occurs frequently in older populations. In one study, as many as 48% of elderly clients seen in emergency departments suffered from chronic dehydration. Dehydration leads to loss of muscle function, depression, altered states of consciousness, and renal failure and contributes to increased potential for medication toxicity, hypo- or hyperthermia, and infection. Dehydration is often unrecognized in the elderly, and mortality may be as much as seven times higher in dehydrated elders than in the general elderly population. Annual costs of dehydration in the older population are estimated at more than $1 billion, but this may be an underestimate because of the tendency for this diagnosis to be missed in older clients (Bennett, Thomas, & Riegel, 2004).

Finally, older clients may be lacking in specific nutrients such as iron, protein, and calcium. Calcium, in particular, is needed to prevent or ameliorate the effects of osteoporosis. Many older women, however, do not know that they should continue calcium intake into their older years. In one study, even after an educational intervention related to the need for dietary calcium, many women most at risk for osteoporosis had not increased their calcium intake (Sandison, Gray, & Reid, 2004). Many older clients also take a variety of vitamins and food supplements. In fact, it is estimated that two thirds of people aged 60 to 100 years take vitamins and food supplements, and limit caffeine, sugar, and fat intake (Matthews et al., 2004).

Other Consumption Patterns

Other consumption patterns that affect the health status of the older adult population include alcohol and tobacco use. According to the Federal Interagency Forum on Aging-related Statistics (2004), 10% of older men and 9% of women smoked in 2002. Elderly smokers are more likely than their younger counterparts to have health-related effects due to diminished respiratory function as a result of aging. An estimated 70% of smokers want to quit the habit, and 46% of them make the attempt (Andrews, Heath, & Graham-Garcia, 2004).

Many older clients believe that smoking cessation will not make much difference with respect to their health. Smoking cessation at any age, however, can have beneficial effects. For example, smoking cessation at age 65 years has been found to add 1.4 to 2 years of life for men and 2.7 to 3.7 years for women (Taylor, Hasselblad, Henley, Thun, & Sloan, 2002).

Alcohol consumption may also affect the health of the older adult population. In one study, half of the men and women 55 to 65 years of age consumed alcohol three or more times a week, and 38% of women and 48% of men reported seven or more drinks per week (Moos, Brennan, Schutte, & Moos, 2004). Misuse of alcohol and other drugs (e.g., benzodiazepines) is relatively common, particularly among older women. An estimated 1.8 million women (7%) over 59 years of age abuse alcohol, and 2.8 million (11%) abuse psychotropic drugs. Approximately one third of women who misuse drugs and alcohol begin to do so after 60 years of age.

Aging diminishes the ability of the body to metabolize alcohol and other drugs. Increased body fat also results in slower excretion of alcohol, which is a water-soluble substance. These factors contribute to higher alcohol-related mortality among older women than men (50% to 100% higher) (Finfgeld-Connett, 2004). In addition to its direct effects on the body, alcohol-related disease increases the risk of hip fracture by more than twofold (Yuan et al., 2001).

Physical Activity

As with their perceptions of the need for continued calcium intake, many older people do not believe they need to engage in much physical activity. Exercise by older adults, however, has been shown to prevent disability and hospital admission, improve lipid profiles, reduce body fat, and prevent osteoporosis (Schneider, Mercer, Herning, Smith, & Prysak, 2004). In addition, exercise in the presence of congestive heart failure increases exercise capacity, decreases symptoms, and improves quality of life (Resnick, 2004).

Exercise provides both physical and psychological benefits for older clients. In the physical realm, exercise contributes to improved cardiovascular function, better control of hypertension and hyperlipidemia, cancer prevention, and prevention of gallstones as well as osteoporosis. Additional physical benefits include reduction in diabetes risk; increased muscle, bone, and joint strength; and decreased risk of falls (National Center for Chronic Disease Prevention and Health Promotion, 2002b). Psychologically, physical activity contributes to emotional well-being and improved self-assurance and self-concept and may be linked to improvements in cognition, at least to perceptions of improvement (Blumenthal & Gullette, 2002).

In spite of evidence regarding the benefits of physical activity, many older adults remain sedentary. About half of those who start an exercise program stop within 6 months. According to 2000 figures, fewer than a third of people aged 65 to 74 years engaged in 20 minutes of moderate physical activity three or more times a week (Schneider et al., 2004). These figures decrease with age, with only 9% of people over 85 years of age engaging in regular physical activity (Federal Interagency Forum on Aging-related Statistics, 2004). In the United States, less than 6% of older adults meet the national objectives for both physical activity and strength training (Division of Nutrition and Physical Activity, 2004).

Sexuality

Sexuality considerations related to the older population include knowledge, attitudes, values, and behaviors, as well as changes in anatomy and physiology due to the aging process (Johnson, 2004). Research indicates that primary health care providers assume that older clients are asexual and rarely discuss sexual issues with members of the older adult population. Evidence suggests that, despite these perceptions, sexuality continues to be

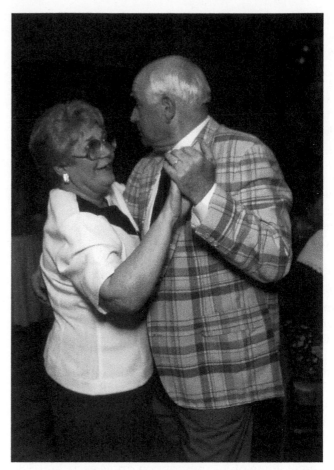

Physical activity is an important element of physical and mental health. (Patrick J. Watson)

an area of importance for many older people. In fact, in the United Kingdom, more than 16,000 people over 50 years of age are seen annually in genitourinary clinics, most of them for sexually transmitted diseases. Similarly, people over 50 years of age constitute 11% of those with AIDS in the UK, most of whom acquired their infection through sexual activity (Gott, Hinchliff, & Galena, 2004).

Older clients may also have concerns regarding sexual dysfunction. Because most older people grew up in an era when sexuality was not a topic for discussion, they may find it difficult to talk about such concerns with health care providers. Many of the medications used to treat chronic diseases common in the elderly cause impotence in men. Similarly, aging may decrease vaginal secretions, making intercourse painful for older women. Both older men and women may experience diminished sexual interest, which may interfere with marital intimacy.

Medication Use

Medication use and misuse are significant factors in the health of the older adult population. Medication use is increasing among the elderly. For example, according to the Federal Interagency Forum on Aging-related

Statistics (2004), older persons in the United States filled an average of 18 prescriptions per year in 1992; by 2000 this figure had increased to 30 prescriptions per person per year. Approximately 94% of women over 65 years of age take at least one prescription medication, 57% take five or more, and 12% take ten or more medications. Among older men, 91% take at least one medication, 44% take five or more, and 12% take ten or more prescription drugs (Logue, 2002). Approximately 40% of all U.S. prescriptions are written for people over 65 years of age (Edlund, 2004). On average, older persons take three times as many prescription medications as younger ones, and the incidence of drug reactions and interactions is two to three times higher than in younger people (Yoon & Horne, 2001).

In addition to taking multiple prescription medications, older adults may also use a variety of over-the-counter (OTC) medications and herbal therapies, compounding the potential for drug interactions and adverse reactions. An estimated 90% of older adults use OTC medications in addition to prescription drugs (Edlund, 2004). In one study, nearly 36% of rural elderly women used some type of self-directed complementary therapy, primarily herbal preparations used for health promotion purposes (Shreffler-Grant, Weinert, Nichols, & Ide, 2005). In another study, 43% of older women used herbal preparations, for an average of 2.5 preparations used per woman. In addition, the women in the study used an average of 3.2 prescription drugs each, and 3.8 nonprescription medications (Yoon & Horne, 2001). A subsequent study by the same authors found that the herbal products most often used were ginger, garlic, glucosamine, ginkgo, and aloe, and that older women frequently used complementary therapies in conjunction with prescription medications (Yoon & Horne, 2004). It is estimated that as many as 3 million U.S. elders may be at risk for herb/vitamin/prescription drug interactions (Edlund, 2004).

In addition to the combination of multiple drugs, OTC medications, and herbal remedies, medication use in the elderly is complicated by the effects of aging. As age increases, lipid compartments increase from 14% of body weight to 30%, which has implications for drug absorption and metabolism (Williams, 2005). These changes in drug metabolism increase the risk of adverse reactions as drug excretion slows and the potential for overdose increases (Caterino, Emond, & Camargo, 2004).

Older clients may also have difficulty taking medications as recommended. An estimated 50% of the elderly have difficulty adhering to medication regimens. Medication misuse and nonadherence have been linked to more than 11% of hospital admissions and 10.5% of emergency department visits by older clients. Overall nonadherence has been found to range from 14% to 77% among older populations, depending on the method used to measure nonadherence. Using electronic monitors, one study found that 43% of clients underdosed,

overdosed, or missed a dose for more than 20% of their medications (Schlenk, Dunbar-Jacob, & Engberg, 2004).

Factors that contribute to medication nonadherence include drug regimen characteristics, health beliefs, side effects, extent of social support, depression, and cognitive function (Schlenk et al., 2004). Drug regimens may be complicated or burdensome in terms of the number of medications, the number and timing of doses, and the number of providers prescribing different medications. In one study, for example, 54% of older clients had more than one prescribing physician, and 36% used more than one pharmacy (Safran et al., 2005). Health beliefs regarding personal self-efficacy or medication efficacy may also affect adherence, as does the occurrence of annoying side effects. In fact, in one study, 57% of older people discontinued prescription medications on their own initiative, 92% of those in response to side effects (Schlenk et al., 2004).

The availability of social support has also been linked to medication adherence. For example, adherence has been found to increase in the presence of assistance with ADLs and to decrease for persons living alone. Depression is also a contributing factor. In one study, depressed clients were nonadherent with medications on 55% of days, whereas nondepressed clients were only nonadherent 31% of days (Schlenk et al., 2004). Cognitive functional ability also affects medication adherence in terms of forgetting to take medications or inability to understand the regimen in terms of dose, timing, route of administration, and other instructions.

Cost of medications is another significant factor in nonadherence. Average annual drug costs per Medicare enrollee in 2000 were $1,340. In a 2003 study conducted by the Kaiser Family Foundation, average annual drug costs per Medicare enrollee had increased to $2,322, and 40% of enrollees had annual drug costs over $2,000 (Brinckerhoff & Coleman, 2005). In another 2003 study, 27% of all seniors studied lacked prescription drug coverage under their health insurance. This figure increased to a third of poor and near-poor elderly. Approximately 26% of participants reported forgoing at least one prescription in the previous year due to cost, and another 12% reported cutting back on basic needs to be able to afford medications. One third of participants reported $100 or more out-of-pocket expenses for medications each month (Safran et al., 2005), and 95% of the U.S. population over 65 years of age had out-of-pocket expenses (Federal Interagency Forum on Aging-related Statistics, 2004). In 2002, out-of-pocket drug costs for older Americans amounted to $87 billion, and this figure was expected to rise to $120 billion by 2005 (Brinckerhoff & Coleman, 2005). Cost may also figure into fears of running out of medications and spacing doses at wider intervals than ordered to conserve medication (Alemagno, Niles, & Treiber, 2004).

During the late 1990s, spending on prescription drugs increased 15% per year for several years. From

1997 to 2001, Medicare expenditures for drugs increased 71.6% more than inflation rates, and this was prior to the advent of Medicare prescription drug coverage. These increasing costs have been the result of a 10% increase in the number of elderly using prescriptions, a 24% increase in the number of prescriptions per person, and a 26% increase in the actual cost of prescription drugs. Using cardiovascular drugs as an example, there has been a 55% increase in spending despite increased use of generic drugs to fill many prescriptions. Similarly, total spending for hormones and psychotherapeutic agents doubled, and spending for analgesics increased by 125%. This latter increase was primarily due to increased use of cyclooxygenase and decreased use of NSAIDS due to safety concerns (Moeller, Miller, & Banthin, 2004).

Inappropriate medication use among the elderly is compounded for cultural minority groups. Cultural factors such as language difficulties, values, and economic status may interfere with medication adherence, as does cultural stereotyping by providers. One study identified four factors influencing medication compliance in ethnic minority groups: difficulty with English, cultural barriers in the health system, lack of health insurance, and failure to consult providers regarding medication discontinuation or use of ancillary therapies (Zhan & Chen, 2004). Inappropriate medication use among older clients, including members of ethnic minority groups, may also be related to deteriorating vision and inability to read prescription labels. The focused assessment provided below can guide evaluation of medication use in elderly clients.

Health System Considerations

The demand for health care services increases sevenfold after 70 years of age compared to that among people under age 60. Most of this increase is due to greater use of expensive technology, but a significant portion of the increase is due to the multiple chronic illnesses experienced by older adults. For these reasons early diagnosis and effective treatment of chronic illness can help to decrease the societal burden of care for the elderly.

The concept of aging in place was conceived as a way of improving the quality of life for older adults and of decreasing the cost burden of their care by maintaining older individuals in their homes whenever possible and providing care in the least expensive setting. Two perspectives are taken on aging in place. In the first, aging in place is conceived as case management to permit provision of care at a consistent level (e.g., with the older adult continuing to reside in their own home). The second perspective views aging in place as provision of a full continuum of services, delivery methods, and policy directions in a system that helps older people successfully navigate various levels of care as they are needed (Bertsch & Taylor-Moore, 2005). Unfortunately, however, a number of health system factors impede effective aging in place. Three of those factors will be addressed here: access to care, prescription drug coverage, and interactions with health care providers.

Health Care Access

Access to health care services for older Americans has improved significantly since the advent of Medicare in the 1960s. In 2003, Medicare provided health insurance coverage for 13.7% of the total U.S. population. Forty-one million Medicare recipients were 65 years of age or over, and another 35 million were disabled. Although only 0.8% of the elderly did not receive Medicare, this still amounted to 286,000 older adults without health insurance coverage (U.S. Census Bureau, 2004a, 2005).

The costs of health care to those without insurance can be prohibitive. For example, hospitalization rates among the elderly in the United States increased by 23% from 1970 to 2000, and the average length of stay in the hospital for people over 65 years of age was 6 days in 2000. Hospitalization costs in 1999 averaged $2,546 for all Medicare beneficiaries, but rose to an average of $7,222 per person for those with Alzheimer's disease (Rosenfeld & Harrington, 2003). Older persons without health insurance cannot afford care at these rates. In some locales, primary health care services may be available from free clinics. Unfortunately, free clinics do not exist in many areas, and, even where they occur, they may not be able to meet the care needs of the uninsured. Similarly, "charity care" or uncompensated care provided by some hospitals may not meet the local needs for care among the elderly. In addition, uncompensated care may threaten the fiscal viability of health care organizations and force their closure, further diminishing access to care for older clients (Pricewaterhousecooper Health Research Institute, 2005).

FOCUSED ASSESSMENT

Assessing Medication Use in Older Clients

- Is the client taking prescribed medications?
- Is the client taking over-the-counter (OTC) medications?
- Are any of the client's medications contraindicated by existing health conditions?
- Do OTC medications potentiate or counteract prescription medications?
- Do prescription medications potentiate or counteract each other?
- Does the client take prescription and OTC medications as directed (e.g., correct dose, route, time)?
- Does the client comply with other directions regarding medications (e.g., not taking with dairy products)?
- Is the client aware of potential food–drug interactions or drug–drug interactions?
- Are medications achieving the desired effects?
- Is the client experiencing any medication side effects?
- What is the client doing about medication side effects, if any?
- Is the client exhibiting symptoms of any adverse medication effects?

Advocacy in Action

Getting into the System

Students working in a student-faculty "miniclinic" held weekly in a local church identified an elderly woman with a blood pressure of 212/184. The woman was uninsured and did not have a regular health care provider. She refused to go to the emergency room even though the students and their instructor strongly urged her to do so. Failing that, the students and faculty member tried to get her an appointment with a physician. Without insurance, however, no one would see her.

The client was eligible for Medicaid. At first she assured the students that she would go to the Medicaid office to apply, but when she was seen week after week with the same high blood pressure and no progress on her Medicaid application, the problem of transportation surfaced. She had no means of transportation herself, and her son, a construction worker, could not—or would not—take time from work to help his mother apply. After many phone calls, the students were able to arrange for an intake worker to come to the woman's home and complete the Medicaid application. The application was approved, and the students found a physician who would care for the woman. She was started on antihypertensive medications and her blood pressure returned to normal.

Even for those with Medicare, access to care may be limited. Medicare pays only 54% of the health care costs for the elderly in the United States. Medicaid pays another 10%, and 15% of costs are covered by private insurance. The remaining 21% of costs are paid for out-of-pocket by the elderly themselves, and the percentage of people with out-of-pocket costs has increased from 83% in 1977 to 95% in 2000 (Federal Interagency Forum on Aging-related Statistics, 2004). Approximately half of the out-of-pocket expenses incurred by Medicare recipients are for Part B premiums. By 2050, Medicare beneficiaries can be expected to spend 30% of their income on health care (AARP, 2002).

In 2002, 40.1 million Americans had Medicare Part A coverage for hospitalization, but only 38 million had Part B coverage for provider fees, outpatient costs, and other costs. Sixty percent of the population also had supplemental insurance through private insurance providers (CDC, 2004a). Many older clients cannot afford either Part B coverage under Medicare or private supplemental insurance due to the cost of premiums. For 6 million of the poorest elderly, Medicaid covers the cost of Medicare Part B premiums as well as prescription drugs and some other expenses not covered under Medicare (Klein, Stoll, & Bruce, 2004), but for others the cost of premiums is prohibitive. Similarly, many older clients cannot afford private supplemental insurance for expenditures not covered under Medicare. Private health insurance coverage may be as much as two to four times more expensive for people aged 50 to 60 years than for the typical 25-year-old, and the extent of supplemental coverage has actually declined from 90% in 1998 to 60% in 2002 (American Association of Retired Persons, 2002; CDC, 2004a). Ethnic minority groups may have particular difficulty obtaining supplemental insurance due to small fixed incomes (Angel, Angel, & Markides, 2002). Lack of supplemental insurance coverage may also affect receipt of health promotion and illness prevention services. For example, in 2003, only 58% of older persons with Medicare coverage alone received influenza immunizations, compared to 71% of those with supplemental insurance coverage (Immunization Services Division, 2005).

In 2000, 5% of Americans over 65 years of age reported delaying needed care because of costs. Although this figure is down from 10% in 1992, it still represents a large segment of the older population who are not receiving appropriate care (Federal Interagency Forum on Aging-related Statistics, 2004).

Cost is not the only factor that may impede access to health care services for older clients. In one study, for example, 12% of older clients reported at least one of several barriers to obtaining care. The most commonly reported barrier was lack of responsiveness on the part of physicians, followed by medical bills, lack of transportation, unsafe streets and neighborhoods, and fear of serious diagnoses or unwanted tests. Some respondents also cited lack of a regular provider as a barrier to care, although 93% of the sample reported seeing the same provider on each visit. Finally, older clients also cited responsibilities for the care of others and work responsibilities as barriers to care (Fitzpatrick, Powe, Cooper, Ives, & Robbins, 2004). Other authors have noted that the health care system is often unresponsive to the needs of older clients as a result of inconvenient office locations, lack of parking, and short encounters that do not allow clients time to voice their concerns (Williams, 2005).

Older clients may also lack access to specific kinds of services. For example, most older clients do not have long-term-care insurance. Currently, Medicaid pays for 46% of nursing home costs in the United States, but many older clients are not eligible for Medicaid (Federal Interagency Forum on Aging-related Statistics, 2004). Medicare pays for short stays in long-term-care facilities, but 25% of nursing home and home health care costs are paid out-of-pocket. Public financing of long-term care is expected to increase 20% to 21% in the United States and the United Kingdom between 2000 and 2020. In the interim, however, many older people are not able to access needed long-term-care services. Due to their emphasis on care of the elderly, Japan's public contribution to long-term care is expected to increase by 102% in the same time period (Division of Adult and Community Health, 2003c).

Older clients may also lack access to care for problems related to substance abuse. In one study, 37% of physicians reported that they do not have time to discuss substance abuse with older clients. Similarly, 20% reported that managed care plans do not cover treatment for alcohol abuse. Medicare coverage for substance abuse treatment is limited to hospital detoxification and 50% of the costs of outpatient care. In addition, providers often lack the knowledge to intervene effectively or are uncomfortable discussing substance abuse with older clients. Finally, few treatment programs are designed to meet the needs of older adults. The author concluded that only 1% of older women in need of treatment for alcohol abuse actually receive the needed services (Finfgeld-Connett, 2004).

Prescription Drugs

Two elements of the health care system related to prescription drugs affect the health of older populations. The first is prescription of inappropriate drugs, and the second is the cost of medications.

In approximately 13% of emergency visits from 1992 to 2000, older clients were given inappropriate medications. This amounted to more than 16 million inappropriate prescriptions provided in emergency departments alone. Six drugs were found to account for 70% of the inappropriate prescriptions: promethazine, meperidine, propoxyphene, hydroxyzine, diphenhydramine, and diazepam. Study findings indicated that as the number of drugs prescribed increased, the number of inappropriate drugs also increased. Many inappropriate drugs are also prescribed in primary care settings

when providers do not attend to the altered risk-benefit ratio for many drugs when taken by the elderly. Certain drugs should not be prescribed for older clients, and others should not be given in specific doses, for extended periods of time, or in the presence of specific comorbid conditions (Caterino et al., 2004). Table 3◆ provides information on selected drugs that are not appropriate for administration to older clients.

As we noted earlier, the cost of prescription drugs is one of the impediments to medication compliance among the elderly. Overall spending on drugs in the United States increased by more than 15% in 2002. A third of this increase was attributed to increased prices of medications rather than increased numbers of prescriptions. Over a 3-year period, the prices of the 30 name-brand drugs most often prescribed for older clients increased 22%, at 4.3 times the rate of inflation from January 2003 to January 2004, and 3.6 times the inflation rate over the previous 3 years (Mahan, 2004).

Prior to initiation of Medicare Part D, an estimated 65 million Americans, including 30% of Medicare beneficiaries, had no insurance coverage for prescription drugs. Some elderly had medication coverage under Medicaid, but this program has increased the amount paid out-of-pocket by recipients. Similarly, employers and private insurance plans that cover prescription drugs have increased copayments or reduced the level of prescription drug benefits. Approximately 28% of Medicare recipients rely on retirement benefits for prescription drug coverage, but many employers have recently eliminated or reduced coverage. For example, in 2003, 57% of firms with retiree coverage increased out-of-pocket costs for recipients, and in 2002, 40% fewer firms offered drug coverage than in 1994 (Mahan, 2004).

Medicare Part D, or the Medicare Prescription Drug, Improvement, and Modernization Act of 1993,

TABLE 3	Hazardous Medications for Elderly Clients	
Drug Classification	**Specific Medications**	**Potential Hazard**
Analgesics	Meperidine, pentazocine, propoxyphene	Confusion, hallucinations
Anticholinergics/antihistamines	Chlorpheniramine, diphenhydramine, hydroxyzine, cyproheptadine, promethazine, tripelennamine, dexchlorpheniramine	Confusion, blurred vision, constipation, dry mouth, lightheadedness, urinary difficulty or incontinence
Antidepressants	Amitriptyline, chlordiazepoxide-amitriptyline, perphenazine-amitriptyline, doxepin	Severe anticholinergic effects, sedation
Barbiturates	All except phenobarbital	Addiction potential
Benzodiazepines, long-acting	Chlordiazepoxide, clindinium-chlordiazepoxide, diazepam, quazepam, halazepam, chlorazepate	Sedation, increased fall risk
GI antispasmodics	Dicyclomine, hyoscyamine, propantheline, belladonna alkaloids	Anticholinergic effects
Muscle relaxants and antispasmodics	Carisoprodol, chlorzoxazone, cyclobenzaprine, metaxalone, methocarbamol, oxybutynin	Anticholinergic effects, sedation, weakness
Nonsteroidal anti-inflammatory drugs (NSAIDS)	Naproxen, oxaprozin, piroxicam	GI bleeding, renal failure, high blood pressure, heart failure

Data from: Wooten, J., & Galavis, J. (2005). Polypharmacy: Keeping the elderly safe. RN, 68(8), 44–50.

was intended to help meet the need for prescription drug coverage for older Americans. When the act is fully implemented in 2006, beneficiaries may choose to enroll in the program with a monthly premium cost of $35. After client payment of an annual deductible of $250 (which will increase to $445 in 2013), Medicare will pay 75% of annual prescription drug costs up to $2,250, with the client responsible for the remaining 25% out-of-pocket or through supplemental insurance. Recipients are responsible for paying 100% of annual drug costs in the "doughnut hole" from $2,250 to $5,100, after which Medicare will pay 95% with a 5% copayment by the recipient (Henley, 2004, Miller, 2004a). Excluding premiums, total out-of-pocket costs for prescription drugs for people with drug use over $5,100 will be $3,600. This figure will rise to $6,400 in 2013 (Henley, 2004). In other nations—the Netherlands, for example—the elderly have extended prescription drug coverage with few copayments (Edwards, 2004). The new law specifically prohibits Medicare from negotiating for blanket drug discounts as other federal health care systems, such as the Veterans Administration, currently do (Mahan, 2004). This means that older clients, as well as the general population, will bear the primary burden for escalating drug costs.

Some local and state jurisdictions have begun contracting with Canadian pharmacies in an effort to control drug costs. For example, a city program in Burlington, Vermont, saved $54,000 in a single year purchasing drugs for employees and retirees from Canada. Similarly, Montgomery, Alabama, saved so much money in purchasing Canadian drugs that they waived copayments for covered citizens. Drug import programs tend to focus on medications used for chronic conditions so prevalent among the elderly. Unfortunately, many of these programs have been threatened with sanctions for violating the Federal Food and Drug Act. Some question has been raised regarding the safety of drugs imported internationally, but many of these drugs are manufactured in the United States and then sold overseas. They can often be resold at lower costs than in the United States because of government regulation of drug prices (Wiebe, 2004).

Client–Provider Interactions

The third major health system consideration that affects the health of older populations is the quality of interactions with health care providers. These interactions are shaped by knowledge and attitudes on the part of providers as well as clients. As reflected in the discussion of inappropriate prescriptions given to older adults, some providers do not have the knowledge or expertise to provide effective care to this population. In one study, for example, nurses had less accurate knowledge of aging and its effects than members of other professions and more anxiety about working with aging clients, and they voiced perceptions that care of the elderly has lower prestige value than work with other populations. The

authors also found that nurses have more positive attitudes toward working with older populations when they work directly for a specific service provider rather than through a "temp" agency, when they had specific geriatric content in their educational programs, and when they worked outside of geriatric residential settings (Wells, Foreman, Gething, & Petralia, 2004).

Difficulties in provider–client interactions may also arise from communication barriers and lack of empowerment of older persons. Guinn (2004) identified three requisites for empowering older clients in health interactions. First, older clients must actively participate in the encounter and in the identification of problems to be addressed. Second, they must contribute to identification of health care goals. A third strategy for empowerment is rehearsal, in which older clients rehearse questions and other forms of input prior to interactions with health care professionals.

Barriers to effective communication between older clients and health care providers may stem from client attitudes and abilities or from provider characteristics. Client attributes that may impede communication include diminished communication abilities due to declining hearing, vision, or cognitive ability; diminished self-worth; and lack of knowledge about health-related issues. Provider-related barriers may include ageist attitudes and discrimination, as well as lack of knowledge and expertise regarding the needs of and interventions appropriate to older clients (Guinn, 2004).

Differences may also arise from the primary foci of providers and clients. According to the National Institute on Aging (2004), providers, especially physicians, focus on disease and its treatment, whereas the primary focus of many older clients is on quality of life. The Institute highlights the need for effective communication to achieve four specific outcomes: preventing errors, strengthening the provider–client relationship and promoting compliance, making efficient use of the time of both, and achieving better client outcomes.

An additional barrier to communication between health care providers and older clients is a phenomenon called "elder speak." Elder speak is an approach to communication with the elderly that conveys a message of incompetence and control and may take one of two forms: excessively nurturing communication and controlling communication. Elder speak may be characterized by a slow rate of speech, exaggerated intonation, elevated pitch and volume, frequent repetition, and the use of simple vocabulary and grammar. Other characteristics may include use of inappropriate terms of endearment (e.g., "honey" or "sweetie"), use of the plural pronoun "we," and use of questions that prompt a specific answer (e.g., "you want to wear this pretty blue sweater, don't you?") such as one might use with a child. An estimated 20% of communication occurring in nursing home settings involves elder speak, and as many as 40% of older clients in both institutional and home settings report caregivers who use speech that they perceive as demeaning, patronizing, or implying their own incompetence (Williams, Kemper, & Hummert, 2004).

Even when providers think they may be communicating effectively, this may not be the case. For example, in one study of primary care physicians caring for clients with Alzheimer's disease and their families, physicians reported providing a variety of information and support that family members reported not receiving. For instance, 80% of the providers believed that Alzheimer's disease can be stabilized, at least temporarily, but only 32% of the caregivers reported having been given this information. Similarly, 74% of the physicians reported that they always provided referrals to community support groups for caregivers, yet only 24% of caregivers said that the providers actually did so (Alzheimer's Association, 2001).

Providers have also been found to neglect to address health promotion activities with older client populations. For example, according to the National Center for Chronic Disease Prevention and Health Promotion (2002b), only 52% of health care providers ask older clients about their activity levels. In the same vein, as we saw earlier, few providers are willing to address issues of substance abuse or sexuality with their older clients.

ASSESSING THE HEALTH OF THE OLDER POPULATION

In the preceding discussion, we have identified a number of factors that influence the health of elderly populations. The task of a given community health nurse working with a given population of elderly individuals is to assess the extent to which these factors are influencing the health of the specific population and the effects of these factors. Here we will focus on assessing the health of older clients as a population group. A tool that can be adapted for use in assessing the health of individual older adults is included in Appendix I on the Companion Website. The *Community Assessment Reference Guide* deigned to accompany this text contains an assessment tool specific to the health status and needs of older clients.

Basic information about the relative proportion of older individuals in the population can be obtained from census figures or other local population figures. Similarly, information on communicable diseases among the elderly will be available from local health department statistics. Health department statistics will also provide information on mortality due to both acute and chronic health conditions. Morbidity data, on the other hand, may be more difficult to obtain. Local acute-care institutions may have data on the number of older persons admitted for specific conditions, or registries may exist for certain selected illnesses (e.g., some forms of cancer). A local Office of Aging and Independence Services may also have figures related to the incidence and prevalence of specific conditions or disabilities.

Such information may also be derived indirectly from the number and type of requests for home care assistance, although these figures are likely to underestimate the true need, since many elders may not request assistance even when it is needed. The focused assessment on page 520 provides guidance for assessing the extent of functional limitations and disabilities in the elderly population. The data included in the assessment will be collected primarily through community surveys.

Churches and other religious groups may also be able to provide some sense of the extent of disability within the congregation or the number of requests for assistance by older members. Community surveys of the older population may also provide information on the extent of acute and chronic illness as well as disability, immunization status, use of health care services, and so on. The effectiveness of pain control or the prevalence of incontinence are other factors that are best assessed in community surveys, as are data on stress, coping, depression, and other psychological factors. Questions for assessing biophysical factors affecting the health of the older population are included on page 520. Some data on rates of treatment for psychiatric disorders may be available from local primary care providers and specific psychiatric services. Emergency department statistics may also provide insights into the kind and frequency of health problems experienced by older adults in the population. Additional areas for consideration in the psychological dimension are reflected in the focused assessment questions provided on the next page.

Much of the information related to physical environmental factors affecting health will be obtained by direct observation and through community surveys. Considerations related to physical environmental influences on the health of older clients are included in the focused assessment questions provided later in this section. Information on many sociocultural factors may also be derived from community surveys, but local social service agencies may also have information related to income levels among the elderly, formal social support available in the community, and so on. Figures related to income, poverty, educational levels, and so on are also available from census data. Information regarding the participation of older clients in the workforce may be available from local employers as well as from census data. Aggregate data regarding family roles and responsibilities among the older population are best derived from community surveys, but local social service agencies may have some data on these factors within segments of the population. Information on elder abuse and violence will most likely be available from local police departments and protective service agencies, although local emergency departments can provide data on the frequency with which older clients are seen for injuries resulting from violence. The focused assessment questions included later in this section can guide community health nurses' exploration of sociocultural factors influencing the health of the older population.

FOCUSED ASSESSMENT

Assessing Disability in the Elderly Population

Basic Activities of Daily Living

What proportion of the population over 65 years of age has difficulty with

- Feeding (feeding self, chewing, or swallowing)?
- Bathing (getting into or out of a bathtub or shower, manipulating soap or washcloth, washing hair, effectively drying all body parts)?
- Dressing (remembering the order in which clothes are put on, dressing self, bending to put on shoes and socks, manipulating fasteners, putting on and removing sleeves, combing hair, applying makeup)?
- Toileting (ambulating to the bathroom, urinary urgency, removing clothing, positioning self on toilet, lifting from a sitting position on toilet, cleaning self after urination or defecation, replacing clothing)?
- Transfer (getting from lying to sitting position, standing from a sitting position, lying or sitting down)?

Instrumental Activities of Daily Living

What proportion of the population over 65 years of age has difficulty with

- Shopping (transporting self to shopping facilities, navigating within shopping facilities, lifting products from shelves, handling money, carrying purchases to and from car, storing purchases)?
- Laundry (collecting dirty clothing, sorting clothes to be washed or dry-cleaned, accessing laundry facilities, manipulating containers of soap, etc., lifting wet clothing into dryer, hanging or folding clean clothes, putting clean clothing away)?
- Cooking (planning well-balanced meals, safely operating kitchen appliances and utensils, reaching dishes and pots and pans, cleaning and chopping foods, carrying food to the table)?
- Housekeeping (identifying the need for housecleaning, light housekeeping, doing heavy chores, doing yard maintenance)?
- Taking medication (remembering medications, opening medication bottles, swallowing medications, giving injections, etc.)?
- Managing money (budgeting effectively, writing checks, balancing checking account, remembering to pay, and recording payment of bills)?

Advanced Activities of Daily Living

What proportion of the population over 65 years of age has difficulty with

- Social activity (maintaining a group of people with whom to socialize, transporting self to social events, seeing and hearing well enough to interact with others, tiring easily, being fearful of incontinence or embarrassed over financial difficulties)?
- Occupation (carrying out occupational responsibilities, if any)?
- Recreation (having the physical strength and mobility to engage in desired recreational activities, maintaining a group of people with whom to pursue recreation, transporting self to recreational activities)?

Most information on behavioral considerations affecting the health status of the older population will be derived from community surveys. Some data may also be available from local police records of arrests for substance abuse–related crimes by older individuals or from local mental health facilities regarding the frequency of hospitalizations for substance abuse among the elderly. Again, however, these data are likely to reflect only the "tip of the iceberg" since many substance abusers in all age groups do not seek treatment. Emergency department data on older clients seen for malnutrition, dehydration, and substance abuse–related health problems may also help to clarify the extent of behavioral factors affecting the older population. Issues related to sexuality, on the other hand, are best addressed with community surveys. Some data related to physical activity by older clients may be derived from observations of physical activity in and around the community, but community surveys may also serve to elicit these data.

Information on medication use among older clients in the community can be derived in a variety of ways. Health care providers may have a sense of the extent of medication noncompliance within this population in their practices. Similarly, pharmacies may provide anecdotal evidence of prescription refills that do not jibe with the dose and frequency of medication prescribed. Some agencies may also use electronic monitors or other devices to monitor medication compliance in individual clients, and some agencies may aggregate

FOCUSED ASSESSMENT

Assessing Biophysical Factors Influencing Older Clients' Health

- What is the age composition of the elderly population?
- What are the primary causes of death in the elderly population?
- What is the incidence and prevalence of acute and chronic disease in the elderly population?
- What is the extent of disability in the elderly population? What types of disability are prevalent?
- What is the immune status of the elderly population? What proportion of the elderly population has received pneumonia vaccine? What proportion has received recent influenza and tetanus immunizations? What is the extent of immunity to other diseases in the elderly population (e.g., pertussis, diphtheria)?

FOCUSED ASSESSMENT

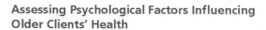

Assessing Psychological Factors Influencing Older Clients' Health

- What sources of stress is the elderly population exposed to? What is the extent of coping abilities in the elderly population?
- What is the prevalence of cognitive impairment in the elderly population? What levels of cognitive impairment are represented in the population (e.g., mild confusion, vegetative states)?
- What is the extent of mental illness in the elderly population? What mental illnesses are prevalent in the population? What are the rates of suicide and attempted suicide in the elderly population?

FOCUSED ASSESSMENT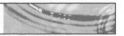

Assessing Physical Environmental Factors Influencing Older Clients' Health

- How adequate is housing available to the elderly population? What is the extent of home ownership in this population? What safety hazards are presented by housing for the elderly? Are rentals and taxes within the budgetary limitations of most of the elderly population?
- Does the physical environment of the community promote or impede physical activity in the elderly population?
- What health effects does environmental pollution have for the elderly population?

this data at the population level. Considerations in assessing behavioral factors influencing the health of the elderly population are reflected in the focused assessment provided at right.

Information on access to health care as well as use of health care services can be obtained from local providers as well as community surveys of the elderly population. The local Social Security and Medicaid offices should have data on the number of older persons enrolled in these

FOCUSED ASSESSMENT

Assessing Sociocultural Factors Influencing Older Clients' Health

- What are societal attitudes toward the elderly? To what extent does the society provide support services for its older members?
- What is the ethnic composition of the elderly population? What languages are spoken among the elderly population? How does culture influence the health of the elderly population?
- What religious affiliations are represented among the elderly population? What health and social services are provided to the elderly population by religious organizations in the community?
- What is the level of economic support available to the elderly population? What is the income distribution within the elderly population? What are the typical sources of income for members of the elderly population? What is the proportion of elderly living in poverty or near poverty?
- What is the typical education level in the elderly population? How does education level influence health?
- What proportion of the elderly population is working? What are the occupations typical of elderly members of the population?
- What retirement planning and assistance are available to older members of the population?
- What proportion of the older population is engaged in caretaking for other family members? What is the effect of caretaking on their health?
- What transportation resources are available to the elderly population? Are they accessible to older clients with mobility limitations? Are they affordable?
- What shopping facilities and other services are available to older members of the population? Are they accessible and affordable?
- What is the extent of social isolation in the elderly population? What resources are available in the community to limit social isolation?

FOCUSED ASSESSMENT

Assessing Behavioral Factors Influencing Older Clients' Health

- What are the typical dietary patterns among the elderly in the population? What is the extent of obesity in the elderly population? What nutritional deficits are prevalent in the elderly population?
- What is the extent of smoking, alcohol, and drug use in the elderly population? What are the treatment rates for alcohol and drug abuse?
- To what extent do members of the elderly population engage in health-related behaviors such as testicular self-examination, mammography, and so on?
- To what extent do members of the elderly population employ safety precautions such as seat belt use?
- What proportion of the elderly population drives? What is the incidence of motor vehicle accidents among this population?
- What prescription and over-the-counter medications are typically taken by elderly clients? What is the incidence of adverse events due to inappropriate medication use in the population?

programs in the local population as well as data on expenditures and types of services for which reimbursement is provided. Finally, community surveys and health institutions can provide information on the extent or lack of health care insurance in the older population. The quality of interactions between providers and older clients, however, is likely to be available only through community surveys or small-scale qualitative studies involving participant observation. Focused assessment questions related to the health system dimension are provided below.

DIAGNOSTIC REASONING AND CARE OF OLDER POPULATIONS

Once the community health nurse has determined the extent to which factors in each of the dimensions of health are affecting the health of the older population and determined what those effects are, he or she would

FOCUSED ASSESSMENT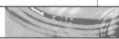

Assessing Health System Factors Influencing Older Clients' Health

- What proportion of the elderly population has a regular source of health care?
- What is the level of insurance coverage among the elderly population (e.g., Medicare A and B, supplementary insurance)?
- To what extent are medication needs covered by insurance plans among the elderly population?
- What preventive and restorative health care services are available to members of the elderly population? To what extent are these services used by the population? How adequate are these services in meeting the needs of the elderly population?
- To what extent are palliative services, end-of-life care, and hospice services available and accessible to the elderly population?

derive community nursing diagnoses related to the population's health status. These diagnoses would reflect the problems identified in the elderly population as well as the availability of resources within the community to address these problems.

Nursing diagnoses may be either positive or negative. An example of a positive diagnosis might be "continued maintenance of older clients in their own homes due to the availability and accessibility of assistance with ADLs." Positive diagnoses usually indicate that no further nursing intervention is needed, but that the health status of the population in this area should continue to be monitored. A negative diagnosis might be "lack of assistance with ADLs for older persons with functional disabilities." In this instance, the diagnosis would indicate the need for intervention by nurses and others in the community to resolve the identified problem.

PLANNING HEALTH CARE FOR OLDER POPULATIONS

Planning to meet the health care needs of older clients may take place at the primary, secondary, and tertiary levels of prevention. Major emphases in planning health care for older clients should be on successful aging and promotion of self-care. As noted earlier, aging can result in loss of functional abilities, stamina, and so on, but these losses can be balanced to achieve successful aging. Health care for older clients should be based on the standards for gerontological nursing practice developed by the American Nurses Association (2001). These standards are included in the Special Considerations Box below.

Primary Prevention

Primary prevention among the elderly is imperative for several reasons. First, they are the fastest-growing segment of the population. In addition, they exhibit the

highest prevalence of chronic illness, and finally, they use the majority of health care services (Wang, 2001). Increasing longevity necessitates a primary prevention focus on health promotion and illness prevention. As noted by members of a global summit on aging, "Because we will be in real trouble if these extra years are not accompanied by more vigor and less disability, we need health policies that support the social, economic, and environmental conditions that promote active aging and give everyone—young and old—access to the best medical and nonmedical resources" (Telling, as quoted in Plese, 2005b, p. 5). The need for prevention among the older population was highlighted in the following comment from the same international forum:

> The short-term thinking about prevention is the most costly policy mistake being made . . . Frailty must be addressed before it happens. Technology is only part of the solution. The solution for polio was not better iron lungs. The solution for healthy aging is not better long-term care institutions; it is prevention, better care early in the disease process, and investment in innovation. (Telling, as quoted in Plese, 2005b, p. 19)

Community health nurses may need to actively advocate for the availability of preventive services to older clients. They may also need to advocate among the elderly population for use of these services.

The Centers for Disease Control and Prevention has identified five roles for which it should be responsible in promoting the health of the older population. These roles are also the responsibility of other jurisdictions (e.g., state and local government), but at a more circumscribed level. These roles and responsibilities are as follows:

- Provide high-quality information and resources to health care providers and members of the general public regarding health promotion activities
- Support prevention activities by local providers and organizations
- Integrate public health prevention expertise with networks of services for the older population
- Identify and implement effective prevention efforts
- Monitor changes in the health status of the older adult population (Division of Adult and Community Health, 2003c)

Primary prevention of disability in the older population requires interruption of the three pathways to disability discussed earlier in this chapter: prevention or delay of fragility; prevention, recognition, and treatment of conditions that contribute to disability; and alteration of the environment to promote independence and prevent disability even in the face of diminished health (Albert et al., 2002). Unfortunately, health promotion and illness prevention are often neglected in the elderly population. For example, Medicare's emphasis on health promotion and illness prevention is piecemeal at best, and Medicare funding only covers a portion of the clinical preventive

---

services recommended for older adults. The Partnership for Prevention (2003) suggested two possible avenues for increasing the focus on promotion and prevention for Medicare beneficiaries. The first is an incremental approach that involves adding coverage for specific services or groups of services. The second approach is to provide a comprehensive examination at age 65 (or when people become eligible for Medicare benefits) that would address existing conditions and provide basic health promotion and illness prevention services and education. This second approach would not, however, address the needs of this population for continuing health promotion and illness prevention services such as annual influenza immunization or continued monitoring of diet, exercise, and other health promotion activities.

Both health promotion and illness prevention in the care of older populations may involve an emphasis on self-care. Leenerts and associates (2002) identified five dimensions of self-care for health promotion in the elderly. The first dimension incorporates the internal and external environment in which self-care occurs. The internal environment includes factors internal to the client him- or herself, such as motivation, self-concept, physical health status, and emotional health. The external environment encompasses the physical, social, and cultural contexts in which self-care takes place. Community health nurses may need to advocate for changes in the external environment that support self-care by older clients. For example, a community health nurse might assist a community to develop a program of assistance with shopping and heavy household chores, allowing frail older clients to remain in their own homes. The second dimension is self-care ability, which involves both knowledge of needed self-care and the physical ability to carry it out. The third dimension, education, provides the link between self-care ability and self-care activity, the fourth dimension of self-care in health promotion. Community health nurses may be particularly helpful in providing older clients with the knowledge required for effective self-care. Self-care activity includes the client's repertoire of activities needed for self-care. The fifth and final dimension is the outcome of self-care, hopefully improved health status.

Health promotion and illness prevention often depend on changes in health-related behaviors. Although we often think about behavioral change as occurring at the individual client level, behavior-related interventions should actually occur at three levels: individual, community, and national (Cutler, 2004). Community health nurses can be particularly active in promoting activity at each of these levels. At the individual level, community health nurses can educate clients to take steps to modify factors that place them at risk for disease and injury. At the community level, initiatives can be undertaken to change environmental factors that influence health-related behaviors. These initiatives may include public policy interventions such as designing communities to promote safe opportunities for exercise by all age groups, but particularly for the elderly. At the national level, comprehensive campaigns can be undertaken to address widespread behavior change among either clients (e.g., the recent campaign on weight control and physical activity) or health care providers (e.g., the development of national guidelines for preventive activities). In the next few sections, we will examine some of the major considerations in primary prevention among older adults.

Nutrition

Adequate nutrition is important for the older population to maintain health, prevent disease, and prevent further effects of existing chronic conditions. Adequate nutrition for health promotion frequently entails a reduction in caloric intake. For example, caloric needs decrease roughly 7% for each decade after 30 years of age for men and 10% for women. Specific caloric needs vary from person to person: older persons engaged in physical activity and resistance training do not experience such a marked reduction in caloric needs (Tabloski, 2006).

Despite reduced caloric needs, older adults continue to require a balance of all other nutrients. Nutritional deficits are most frequently noted for calcium; iron; vitamins A, D, and C; the B vitamins riboflavin and thiamine; and dietary fiber. Care should be taken, however, in the use of fat-soluble vitamins A, D, E, and K, which are stored in the body more readily than water-soluble vitamins and may lead to vitamin toxicity in the older population due to diminished metabolism (Tabloski, 2006). Community health nurses can promote the health of older clients by educating this population regarding their nutritional requirements.

Other, more general interventions may also be needed to improve older clients' nutritional status by eliminating impediments to good nutrition. For example, social isolation may need to be addressed because people tend to eat better in company with others. Older clients can be referred to senior nutrition centers, or family members can be encouraged to drop by at mealtimes to eat with older clients who live alone. Interventions may also be required to deal with nausea, poorly fitting dentures, or other factors that may impede good nutrition. Community health nurses may also need to be active in the development and implementation of programs to meet the nutritional needs of the older population where these services do not already exist, or in increasing access to existing services for underserved segments of the population.

Safety

Safety is an area of significant concern in the care of the older population. Injuries are the eighth leading cause of death in people over 65 years of age in the United States (Division of Unintentional Injury Prevention, 2003), and the fifth leading cause in countries such as Finland (Kannus, Parkkari, Niemi, & Palvanen, 2005) and China

(You et al., 2004). The majority of these deaths are related to falls resulting in hip fractures. An estimated 16% of White U.S. women will experience a hip fracture sometime in their lives. Seventeen percent of these women will die within one year, and half will never regain their independence. Hip fracture incidence has actually been found to be increasing with recent birth cohorts (Samelson, Zhang, Kiel, Hannan, & Felson, 2002). Risk factors for falls in the elderly include arthritis, problems with gait or balance, poor muscle strength, and vision problems. The risk of falls also increases with the number of medications taken. On average, 3,000 falls among the elderly each year in the United States require hospitalization for traumatic brain injury, with an annual cost of $50 million (Division of Surveillance and Informatics, 2003). Cognitive ability also affects falls and fracture mortality (Williams & Jester, 2005). In fact, therapeutic interventions in dementia may actually increase the potential for falls. For example, hypnotics used for agitation may increase gait disturbances or drowsiness, leading to falls and other accidental injuries (Hurley et al., 2004).

Exercise by older adults can reduce the risk of falling by as much as 15% (Division of Unintentional Injury Prevention, 2003). In one study, for example, biweekly exercise sessions in community settings combined with at-home exercise significantly improved balance and mobility in elderly clients (Robitaille et al., 2005). Interventions may also be aimed at reducing environmental risks for falls and effective medication management. Individualized risk assessments have been shown to increase self-efficacy related to falls, environmental safety, and knowledge of medication safety (Huang & Acton, 2004).

Another area of concern is that of driving by older clients with sensory impairments or diminished reaction times. From 1990 to 1997, the number of motor vehicle deaths among older clients increased 14%, and nonfatal motor vehicle injuries increased by 19% (National Center for Injury Prevention and Control, 2005b). Drivers over 65 years of age have threefold higher crash rates per mile driven than any other group except teenagers. Because they drive fewer miles, however, motor vehicle accident rates per number of drivers are comparable. Men over 65 years of age drive an average of 10,000 miles per year (a 74% increase in the last 30 years), and women average 5,000 miles per year (a 31% increase). Most older drivers decide for themselves when it is appropriate to stop driving, although women are 78% more likely to stop than men. Each year more than 600,000 older drivers decide to stop driving, and this decision is often associated with depression and social isolation. Based on longevity projections, older men can anticipate 7 years of needing other sources of transportation and women 10 years (Foley, Heimovitz, Guralnik, & Brock, 2002). Unfortunately, transportation services for the elderly are often lacking, leaving older populations with decreased mobility and diminished opportunities for social interaction.

Motor vehicles are also problematic when older people are pedestrians. In many areas, the bulk of pedestrian fatalities occur among elderly individuals. In areas where there are large numbers of elderly, nurses can campaign for traffic signals at heavily used crossings, strict enforcement of speed limits, and public awareness of the presence of older adults.

Community health nurses can initiate and participate in education campaigns related to safety issues for the older population. In addition, they can support initiatives that promote safe environments for the elderly. Finally, they may need to engage in activity to promote access to public transportation to meet the needs of the elderly, particularly those with disabilities that may limit their ability to use existing public transportation systems.

Home and neighborhood safety and prevention of elder abuse are two other safety concerns with older populations. Community health nurses can be active in promoting police activity to make neighborhoods safe for older clients to move about in them. They may also be involved in the development of neighborhood watch programs and in programs to alert public safety officials that older clients are residing in particular places. This is particularly important for older disabled individuals in the community. For example, nurses can participate in the development of programs to identify homes with older residents so fire and police personnel can meet their special needs in the event of an emergency.

The last area of concern in promoting the safety of older clients is preventing abuse and neglect. Elder abuse and neglect frequently occur when those caring for elderly clients are unable to cope with the resulting stress. Providing support for these caretakers, teaching positive coping skills, and providing periodic respite care may help to prevent abuse. Assisting older clients to maintain their independence may also help prevent the development of a potentially abusive situation.

Immunization

The Advisory Committee on Immunization Practices (ACIP) (2004) recommends tetanus and diphtheria immunization every 10 years, annual influenza immunization, and one dose of pneumococcal vaccine for all older adults in the United States. Additional recommendations for older adults at particular risk of disease include three doses of hepatitis A, two doses of hepatitis B, and two doses of varicella vaccine for susceptible persons of all ages. In addition, adults with medical or exposure indications should receive meningococcal vaccine. It is estimated that for every million persons who receive influenza vaccine, 900 deaths and 1,300 hospitalizations are prevented (Centers for Medicare and Medicaid Services [CMS], 2004). Similar, but less pronounced, effects are noted for other immunizations.

Unfortunately, immunization is an often neglected intervention among older clients. For example, only 40% of people over 65 years of age have had a tetanus booster in the last 10 years (Matthews et al., 2004). Similarly, as of 2003, only 55% of this population had received pneumococcal vaccine (Centers for Disease Control and Prevention, 2003). During the 2004–2005 influenza season, only 63% of people over age 65 received influenza vaccine (Division of Adult and Community Health, 2005). Immunization levels are often lower in certain subsegments of the elderly population. For example, in 2003, only 54% of older people with incomes below poverty level received influenza immunizations, compared to 58% of the total Medicare population and 71% of those with both Medicare coverage and supplemental health insurance (Immunization Services Division, 2005). The three reasons most often given for not receiving influenza immunizations, which also have relevance for failure to receive other recommended immunizations, are lack of knowledge of the need for immunization, concerns regarding potential side effects, and lack of vaccine availability (CMS, 2004).

Community health nurses can be active in providing immunization services for older adults as well as in educating the older population regarding the need for immunizations. Nurses may also be involved in the design of programs and services to meet the immunization needs of the older population, making sure that all segments of the population have access to services. In 2003, ACIP recommended that nurses and pharmacists be allowed to provide influenza and pneumonia immunizations under standing orders without a physician's signature. CMS also published rules removing the requirement for a physician's signature for immunizations as part of the Conditions of Participation for hospitals, nursing homes, and home health agencies receiving Medicare and Medicaid funding (Centers for Disease Control and Prevention, 2003).

Rest and Exercise

Many people believe that the need for exercise decreases with age; however, older people need exercise as much as their younger counterparts. Thirty minutes of aerobic exercise 5 days a week is recommended for older adults (Resnick, 2005). Exercise sessions should also include 10 to 15 minutes of warm-up exercises and a 10- to 15-minute cool-down period (Resnick, 2004). The American College of Sports Medicine also recommends strength training at least twice a week as part of a comprehensive physical activity program. Strength training has been associated with improved health and fitness, increased muscle strength and endurance, increased bone density, improved insulin sensitivity and glucose metabolism, decreased fall risk, and continued independent living (Division of Nutrition and Physical Activity, 2004). Unfortunately, members of the older adult population often fail to engage in recommended physical activity. Barriers to physical activity among the elderly include lack of time, pain, boredom, fatigue, unsafe environments, fear of injury, lack of awareness of the need to exercise, environments not conducive to physical activity, and failure to set reasonable exercise goals (Resnick, 2005). Community health nurses can help design and provide physical activity programs for older adults that address these barriers. As we saw earlier, community-based exercise programs can have positive effects on physical activity among older clients. Similarly, a cognitive behavioral intervention designed to promote exercise in this age group was found to result in moderately increased overall exercise behavior in experimental subjects as compared to a control group (Schneider et al., 2004).

The quality of rest is another consideration in caring for the older adult population. Many older adults experience insomnia that may be due to underlying disease states, medications, or use of alcohol, tobacco, or caffeine. Interventions that may assist clients with insomnia include treating underlying diseases, keeping a sleep log to determine possible triggers to wakefulness, adjusting medication regimens as needed, and promoting good sleep hygiene. The last can be accomplished by promoting exercise (particularly outdoor activity); increasing exposure to light; avoiding alcohol, tobacco, and caffeine after midafternoon; napping for 30 minutes or less, if at all, during the day; and not working or reading in bed. Other possible interventions include developing a relaxing bedtime routine, promoting pain control, and keeping the environment bright during the day and dark at night (Williams, 2004). Community health nurses can educate clients with sleep problems regarding these strategies. They may also refer them for medical care of underlying diseases or for changes in medications that may be contributing to wakefulness.

Smoking Cessation

Smoking cessation is another primary prevention activity that may be beneficial for the older population in preventing smoking-attributable health problems. As we saw earlier, it is never too late to stop smoking. In addition to the obvious cardiovascular and respiratory effects, not smoking has been associated with decreased risk for colorectal cancer (Kather, 2005). A five As model has been developed to assist with smoking cessation in older adults. Elements of this model are:

- **A**sking about smoking behaviors
- **A**dvising clients regarding the need to stop smoking
- **A**ssessing clients' willingness to stop smoking
- **A**ssisting them with smoking cessation strategies or referral to smoking cessation programs
- **A**rranging for follow-up to support smoking cessation and monitor its effectiveness (Andrews et al., 2004)

Community health nurses can refer older clients who smoke to smoking cessation programs. They can also campaign for access to such programs and coverage of smoking cessation under health insurance plans.

Maintaining Independence

Because of physical and economic limitations, it is sometimes difficult for older persons to maintain their independence. Decreased income and physical inability to care for themselves sometimes force older clients to give up their own residence and live with family members. Whatever the living arrangements of the older client, community health nurses should assist them to maintain the highest degree of independence possible. Some older clients may be able to continue to live alone if referred to supportive services such as homemaker aides, transportation services, and Meals-on-Wheels. When older persons are living with family members, the nurse can encourage family members to foster independence in the client. This may mean encouraging families to assign specific roles within the household to the older family member. Community health nurses can also be actively involved in designing and implementing programs intended to assist older clients to age in place.

Life Resolution

Creating meaning for one's life is one of the developmental tasks to be accomplished by older adults. This entails developing a personal set of goals and the ability to view one's life as having been productive. Reminiscence is one way of accomplishing life resolution and achieving positive feelings about one's own life. The community health nurse must recognize and foster older clients' need to reminisce and should encourage family members to do so as well. This is sometimes difficult given the nurse's busy schedule and the number of clients who need to be seen; however, nurses should be able to find some time during interactions with older clients to listen to these reminiscences and to help clients reflect on their lives. In spite of cognitive losses, reminiscence or "life review" has also been shown to be effective with some clients with Alzheimer's disease (Haight, 2001). Primary preventive interventions for older adult populations are summarized in Table 4◆.

Secondary Prevention

As with other population groups, secondary prevention with older adults focuses on screening and treatment of disease. Because of the prevalence of chronic illness, self-management of disease is another important area of emphasis in secondary prevention.

Screening

Screening for older clients is another aspect of care that is often neglected. Many people believe that it is not necessary to engage in early detection of disease because the benefits of treatment are minimal among the elderly.

TABLE 4	Primary Prevention Strategies for Older Adult Populations
Area of Concern	**Primary Prevention Strategies**
Diet and nutrition	Educate public regarding nutritional needs of older adults.
	Assure access to nutritional foods.
	Eliminate social and environmental barriers to good nutrition.
Safety	Educate public regarding safety issues for older adults.
	Promote exercise to strengthen muscles, bones, and joints.
	Eliminate environmental safety hazards.
	Educate older drivers regarding the hazards of driving.
	Promote alternative forms of transportation for older adults.
	Initiate or promote programs to alert fire and police personnel to older clients in specific residences.
	Promote family coping abilities and relieve stress to prevent abuse of older persons.
Immunization	Educate older populations regarding the need for immunizations.
	Provide immunization services and assure their accessibility to all segments of the older population.
	Develop immunization programs in places where older clients are frequently found.
Rest and exercise	Educate the older population on the need for exercise.
	Participate in the development of physical activity programs that address the most common barriers to exercise among older clients.
	Develop programs to deal with insomnia in the elderly.
Smoking cessation	Assist in the development of programs to assist older clients with smoking cessation.
	Educate the older population on the need for and benefits of smoking cessation.
Maintaining independence	Participate in the development of services that allow clients to live independently as long as possible.
	Promote environments that support independent living by the older population.
Life resolution	Encourage reminiscence. {(TR 13 0)}

A number of disease conditions can still be effectively treated in the older population, however, if found early enough. For example, older adults are perceived to have a poor prognosis for colorectal cancer, yet surgery is quite effective following early detection of disease. An estimated third of deaths due to colorectal cancer could be prevented with screening in persons over the age of 50 (Kather, 2005). Unfortunately, in 2001, 69% of people in this age group had not had a test for fecal occult blood in the previous 2 years (CDC, 2004b), and only 34% of adults over age 50 have ever had a sigmoidoscopy (Matthews et al., 2004). Similarly, risk reduction for breast cancer fatality is greatest among women over 50 years of age, and early detection can reduce mortality by 25% to 30% (CDC, 2004b), yet from 2000 to 2002, 16% of women between 65 and 74 years of age and 23% of those 75 years of age and older had not had a mammogram in the previous 2 years (Division of Cancer Prevention and Control, 2005).

A number of routine screening procedures are recommended for the older adult population. These procedures are summarized in Table 5◆. As noted in the table,

general recommendations are to discontinue annual Papanicolaou smears at age 65 or 70 years. Some authors, however, note a need to continue this screening test in older women who are sexually active due to the potential for human papilloma virus (HPV) infection (Neher, 2004). As noted above, many of the recommended screening practices are not provided to older clients.

Community health nurses can educate older clients regarding the need for routine screening and refer them for screening services. Clients with particular risk factors or symptoms of possible disease should also be referred for screening and diagnostic services as appropriate. For example, a community health nurse might refer an older immigrant woman with a persistent productive cough for tuberculosis screening or refer a client with an elevated blood pressure for possible diagnosis and treatment of hypertension. Community health nurses may also need to advocate for access to screening services for older clients. For example, a nurse might advocate expanding breast cancer education and screening programs to target older women.

TABLE 5	Routine Screening Recommendations for Older Adult Populations
Type of Screening	**Recommendation**
Abdominal aortic aneurysm	**U.S. Preventive Services Task Force:** One-time screening in male smokers aged 65 to 75 years; recommend against routine screening in older women
Colorectal cancer	**U.S. Preventive Services Task Force:** All adults over age 50 (fecal occult blood and/or sigmoidoscopy); no evidence of effectiveness of screening colonoscopy
Depression	**U.S. Preventive Services Task Force:** Older adults in practice settings where follow-up is available
Elder abuse	**U.S. Preventive Services Task Force:** Insufficient evidence for effectiveness of routine screening
Hearing impairment	**U.S. Preventive Services Task Force:** All older adults
Hypertension	**U.S. Preventive Services Task Force:** All older adults
Lipid disorders (total cholesterol and HDL-C)	**U.S. Preventive Services Task Force:** All adults over age 45 (total cholesterol and HDL-C)
Mammogram	**U.S. Preventive Services Task Force:** Women over age 40 (with or without clinical breast examination)
Osteoporosis	**U.S. Preventive Services Task Force:** All adults over age 65 (over age 60 for those with risk factors) **Scientific Advisory Council of the Osteoporosis Society of Canada:** All women over age 65
Papanicolaou smear	**American Cancer Society:** Not recommended for women over age 70 with three consecutive normal smears **American College of Obstetricians and Gynecologists:** An individual decision between provider and client **Canadian Task Force on Preventive Health Care:** Not recommended for women over age 70 with four consecutive normal smears **U.S. Preventive Services Task Force:** Not recommended for women over age 65 with previous normal smears
HIV infection	All men at risk of infection
Obesity	All adult men
Syphilis	All men at risk
Tobacco use	All adult men

Data from: Curran, D. R. (2004). Should we discontinue Pap smear screening in women aged > 65 years? Journal of Family Practice, 53, 308–309; Shepherd, A. J. (2004). *An overview of osteoporosis.* Alternative Therapies, 10(2), 26–33; U.S. Preventive Services Task Force. (2005). The guide to clinical preventive services, 2005. *Retrieved August 13, 2005, from http://www.ahrq.gov/clinic/pocketguide.htm; U.S. Preventive Services Task Force. (2005). Screening for abdominal aortic aneurysm. Retrieved August 13, 2005, from http://www.ahrq.gov/clinic/uspsaneu.htm*

Disease Self-management

Effective chronic disease control requires a combination of supportive care, self-management, maintenance of function, and prevention of further disability. Over time, chronic illness requires an increasing burden of self-management. The ability to cope with the demands of self-management are complicated by three features of chronic illness: interference with functional abilities, limited effectiveness of treatment modalities, and disruption of one's daily routine. As noted by one author, life is often "consumed with the demands imposed by the coping strategies expected" in dealing with chronic illness (Tanner, 2004, p. 313). One's ability to cope with chronic illness is based on perceptions of four factors: the severity of the condition, one's personal responsibility for dealing with it, the controllability of its effects, and the changeability of the situation.

Tanner (2004) described three requisites for self-management of chronic disease. The first requisite is the presence of physical, environmental, mental, and socioeconomic factors that promote effective disease management. For example, one must have the cognitive ability, economic resources, and knowledge of and access to a variety of community services needed to manage the chronic condition. Depression is an emotional factor that may preclude an environment conducive to self-management of disease.

The second requisite for effective self-management of disease is the knowledge and skills required to discontinue unhealthy behaviors, learn and execute replacement behaviors, and learn and execute related behaviors. The final, and perhaps most critical, requisite is the desire to cope with one's illness and take action.

Self-management of chronic disease involves a number of activities, including symptom response and monitoring, compliance with complicated medical and lifestyle regimens, and developing the skills needed for self-management. Steps that can promote self-management of disease among older clients mirror the nursing process and include establishing treatment goals, identifying alternative methods to achieve these goals, planning short-term interventions to achieve goals, implementing the plan, and evaluating and revising the plan (Tanner, 2004).

Managing medications is an important element of self-management of chronic illness. Community health nurses may assist with this task by encouraging providers to simplify medication regimens as much as possible for older adults. Targeted interventions that assist older adults with medication compliance may also be helpful. Technological interventions such as prompting devices, electronic dispensers, monitoring devices, and data management systems may be effective for clients who can afford them, but research is needed to test their effectiveness in practice (Logue, 2002). In one study, electronic monitors increased medication compliance among older women from various ethnic backgrounds.

Other research has indicated that expanded instructions in simple language also improves adherence (Robbins, Rausch, Garcia, & Prestwood, 2004). Results of another study indicated that the MD.2® automated medication dispensing system resulted in decreased time spent in nursing visits on medication review as well as fewer missed doses, lower hospitalization rates and fewer emergency department visits, and a decrease in the overall number of prescription medicines required (possibly due to better compliance and, therefore, increased effectiveness) (Buckwalter, Wakefield, Hanna, & Lehmann, 2004). Unfortunately, many elderly clients cannot afford these technological advances. Other, less expensive, strategies include pill organizers (Alemagno et al., 2004; Miller, 2004b) and telephone reminders (Buckwalter et al., 2004), and community health nurses can advocate the use of such strategies with low-income clients. Some automated reminder or dispensing systems are available via the Internet (http://www.epill.com, http://www. ontimrx.com, http://www.medpromot. com) (Miller, 2004b).

With increasing drug advertising, clients may request specific drugs, and community health nurses need to be knowledgeable in answering clients' questions about drugs for their conditions. Community health nurses can also refer clients to Web sites that provide comparisons of the effectiveness of specific medications. Effectiveness comparisons for multiple categories of drugs are available from the Drug Effectiveness Review Project (2005) or from AARP (2005) (http://www.ohsu.edu/drugeffectiveness/reports/final. cfm, http://www.aarp.org/health/comparedrugs).

Clients may also have questions about Medicare part D prescription drug coverage benefits, and community health nurses can either educate clients themselves

EVIDENCE-BASED PRACTICE

Logue (2002) described a variety of technology-based devices that may help improve medication compliance among older clients. She also noted a lack of evidence on the effectiveness of such devices for promoting compliance and suggested a number of self-medication outcomes that could be used in such research. These included (a) objective symptom measurement and physical examination (e.g., blood pressure monitoring), (b) direct indicators (e.g., blood glucose levels, or blood serum levels of medications), (c) indirect indicators (e.g., pill counts, prescription refills, pill diaries), subjective report of clients and families, and the frequency of visits to primary care providers and emergency departments.

Examine the health care literature. To what extent have these outcome measures been used to evaluate the effectiveness of technology-based interventions in promoting medication compliance among the elderly? What conclusion can be drawn from these studies? What other factors related to their effectiveness in the general population have not been addressed (e.g., the cost of technology for some segments of the population)? How might research be designed to address these additional factors?

or refer them to other sources of information. Community health nurses may also need to advocate for effective drug coverage for older clients and assist them to select prescription drug plans that best meet their personal needs. For example, during the transition to Medicare part D, many community health nurses found themselves battling drug plans to assure that clients' needs for medications were met. This was particularly true for clients with dual eligibility for Medicare and Medicaid who were used to having prescription drugs covered by Medicaid at low copayment rates. Following initiation of Medicare part D, some clients found that higher copayments were required or that some previously covered drugs were not covered under specific plans. Community health nurses worked with the Social Security Administration, local offices of Aging and Independent Services, prescription drug plans, and local pharmacies to assure continued medication access for these clients. At the aggregate level, community health nurses also need to advocate coverage of a set of drugs most commonly used by older clients under all Medicare-approved prescription drug plans.

The effectiveness of self-management of chronic illness may be evaluated based on symptom assessment and physical examination, direct indicators of disease processes (e.g., blood glucose levels), or indirect indicators of medication compliance (e.g., pill counts, prescription refills). Additional measures of effectiveness include subjective reports of clients or family members or the frequency of visits to primary health care providers or emergency departments (Logue, 2002).

Dealing with Common Health Problems

As noted earlier, older clients experience a variety of health problems related to the effects of aging. They are also subject to problems stemming from chronic and communicable diseases. Here we will address interventions for some of the health problems commonly found in older populations. Community health nurses can assist individual clients in dealing with these problems or educate the older population in general. Some of the common problems encountered in caring for older clients include skin breakdown, constipation, urinary and fecal incontinence, sensory loss, mobility limitations, pain, and cognitive impairment. Additional problems that may be encountered by community health nurses working with this population include depression, social isolation, abuse and neglect, and substance abuse. Inadequate financial resources and the need for advocacy at individual and population levels are also areas that may be addressed by means of community health nursing interventions.

Some problems, like fecal and urinary incontinence, chronic pain, and cognitive impairment, are particularly

distressing to clients and their caregivers and warrant specific consideration here. Urinary incontinence occurs in approximately 15% of older men and 30% of older women (National Institute on Aging, 2004). Generally speaking, behavioral approaches have proven more effective than medication in reducing urinary incontinence (Teunissen et al., 2004). Recommended interventions include decreasing fluid intake after the evening meal, urinating every 2 to 3 hours during the day, Kegel exercises, and eliminating constipation. Additional approaches may include treatment of underlying physical causes, use of prescription drugs, or modification of existing drug regimens (Dash et al., 2004).

Treatment of fecal incontinence may also employ a variety of strategies depending on its cause and severity. Community health nurses should encourage clients with incontinence to be examined by their primary care provider to identify any underlying medical conditions. In addition, community health nurses can suggest several dietary changes that may improve continence. For example, if incontinence is due to watery stools or to constipation, increasing bulk in the diet may contribute to stools that are more formed and easier to control. Conversely, for some people, high-fiber diets may have a laxative effect, increasing the problem of incontinence. Specific foods that relax the internal anal sphincter (e.g., caffeine-containing beverages and foods such as coffee, tea, and chocolate) may need to be avoided. Other foods that may contribute to fecal incontinence include cured meats, spicy foods, alcohol, dairy products, fruits (e.g., peaches and pears), fatty foods, and artificial sweeteners (National Digestive Diseases Information Clearinghouse, 2004).

Keeping a food diary may allow the client to identify other foods that cause problems. Community health nurses can educate clients about other dietary strategies that may help, including:

- Eating smaller, more frequent meals
- Eating food and drinking liquids at different times
- Eating an appropriate amount of fiber and focusing on foods with soluble fiber (e.g., bananas, rice, bread, potatoes, applesauce, cheese, smooth peanut butter, yogurt, pasta, oatmeal)
- Drinking sufficient fluids (64 ounces per day unless fluids are otherwise contraindicated) (National Digestive Diseases Information Clearinghouse, 2004)

Medications may also be used in the control of fecal incontinence, but clients should be encouraged to consult their primary care providers rather than use over-the-counter remedies. Bowel training using Kegel exercises or developing regular bowel patterns has also been found to be helpful in dealing with fecal incontinence (International Foundation for Functional Gastrointestinal Disorders, 2006b).

Community health nurses can also assist older clients with fecal or urinary incontinence to address the psychological effects of these problems. Some easy suggestions are to carry a backpack with cleanup supplies and a change of clothing whenever one leaves the house, locate restrooms before they are needed, use the toilet before leaving home, wear disposable undergarments or sanitary pads if needed, or use oral fecal deodorants for frequent episodes of incontinence.

Chronic pain in the elderly is often overlooked or undertreated. As we saw earlier, a significant proportion of older clients experience ongoing pain that is perceived by them and by their providers and caretakers to be a normal part of aging. Others experience pain as a result of a variety of chronic illnesses. A number of barriers exist to effective pain control in the older population. These barriers may relate to providers, to clients and/or their families, or to the health system in general (Hanks-Bell et al., 2004). Provider-related barriers include lack of expertise in pain assessment and management with older clients, concerns related to regulatory scrutiny in the prescription of pain medication, fear of opioid side effects, inability to assess pain in clients with cognitive impairment, and the previously mentioned perception that pain is normal in the aged. Client/family barriers include fear of medication side effects and addiction, reluctance to be considered a "bad patient," and, again, the fatalism exemplified in the belief that pain is part of aging, to be accepted. Health system barriers include the cost of pain medication, insufficient time to adequately assess pain and its management during client encounters, and cultural biases in the health professions against opioid use. Community health nurses can help educate the general public, as well as health care providers, regarding the need for appropriate pain control in the elderly. In addition, they can assist in the development of alternative options for pain control (e.g., development of and insurance coverage for acupuncture, guided imagery, and other pain relief services). Community health nursing advocacy may be required with health care providers, with family members, or within the health system to develop attitudes and services that support effective pain control for older clients. For example, the community health nurse might educate family members, or even clients themselves, regarding the improbability of addiction. Or, the nurse may need to advocate for access to pain-control services for low-income elderly clients.

The shortness of breath characteristic of advanced COPD can also be very disabling for older clients. In addition to referring clients for medical evaluation and possible therapy with bronchodilators, steroids, and oxygen, community health nurses can assist clients with COPD in implementing a variety of strategies that may improve lung function and limit disability. The primary intervention among smokers is, of course, smoking cessation. Clients with COPD who stop smoking have slower progression of disease than those who do not (Rennard, 2005). Community health nurses can refer clients who smoke to smoking cessation programs. They

may need to advocate with insurance plans for coverage of such services as necessary therapy for COPD.

Community health nurses can also suggest that clients refrain from excessive use of cough medicines to control the chronic cough characteristic of COPD because they decrease clearance of secretions, making clients more susceptible to respiratory infection. The nurse can also refer clients for pneumonia vaccine as well as annual influenza immunization to prevent infection. Nutrition is another important aspect of COPD control; more than 30% of patients with severe COPD exhibit malnutrition (Rennard, 2005). Suggestions for improving the nutritional status of clients with COPD include the following:

- Clearing airways and resting before eating
- Eating slowly and taking small bites that are chewed thoroughly
- Choosing foods that are easy to prepare and to chew
- Asking family members to help with meal preparation
- Eating smaller, more frequent meals
- Drinking fluids at the end of the meal instead of before or with food
- Sitting up straight while eating and using pursed-lip breathing during the meal
- Obtaining meals from a local Meals-on-Wheels program
- Eating the main meal early in the day to provide energy for the rest of the day (Cleveland Clinic, 2005c)

Pulmonary rehabilitation is another approach to controlling the debilitating effects of COPD. Comprehensive pulmonary rehabilitation may include education, exercise, psychosocial support, and the use of specific breathing techniques such as pursed-lip breathing, diaphragmatic breathing, and controlled coughing (Cleveland Clinic, 2005a, 2005b, 2005d). Easy-to-follow client instructions for these breathing techniques are available at the Web site of the Cleveland Clinic at http://www.clevelandclinic.org/health. Community health nurses can teach these strategies to clients with COPD as well as advocate for access to necessary diagnostic and treatment services.

As we saw earlier, the number of older adults with cognitive impairment is expected to increase significantly in the next few decades. In older clients, it is particularly important to distinguish among depression, dementia, and delirium, as each of these conditions may produce similar effects. Depression can be effectively treated in most older clients. Treatment goals for depression in the elderly include reduction of suicide risk, improved level of function, and improved quality of life. Older antidepressant medications (e.g., tricyclic antidepressants, or TCAs) are cardiotoxic and may be less well tolerated in the elderly than newer drugs, leading to increased risk of overdose and mortality. For this reason, these drugs should not be routinely used to treat depression in older clients. Instead, "novel antidepressants" (e.g., selective serotonin reuptake inhibitors,

SSRIs) are recommended with close monitoring of treatment and adverse effects. Older clients are also more likely than younger ones to experience "discontinuation syndrome," a temporary condition that may include severe cognitive impairment, so they should be cautioned against abruptly stopping their medications (Antai-Otong, 2004). Community health nurses may advocate with health care providers for recognition and treatment of depression in elderly clients. They may also engage in political advocacy to assure access to treatment services for the older population.

Delirium is usually characterized by a sudden onset and is generally reversible if the underlying cause is identified and treated. Some possible causes of delirium in the elderly include drug toxicity, infectious diseases, problems with elimination, exacerbation of chronic illness, or development of new disease processes. Other potential causes of delirium include changes in the psychosocial context such as a recent loss, a move to a new residence, or hospitalization. Dementia, on the other hand, is characterized by a gradual onset, progressive decline, and irreversibility (Henry, 2002; Naylor, 2003).

Recently, there has been progress in the development of drug therapies to retard the progression of Alzheimer's disease. Until a truly effective treatment is found, however, early detection and advance planning for progressive decline are the best modes of control for this condition (National Institute on Aging, 2002). The most effective approaches to care of individual clients with Alzheimer's disease combine medication, lifestyle changes, and supportive services for both clients and their families (Alzheimer's Association, 2001).

The goal of treatment in the face of cognitive impairment is to maintain the client's quality of life as much as possible. Specific medications such as donepezil, galantamine, and rivastigmine may be helpful in slowing cognitive decline in clients with Alzheimer's disease, particularly when initiated early in the disease process. Antidepressants, mood stabilizers, and antipsychotics may also be warranted for some clients (Vogel, 2003), although, as we saw earlier, use of these medications may lead to accidental injury in some clients. Activities that enhance memory capabilities may also be of some help. Similarly, exercise, hand massage, and therapeutic touch have been shown to be of some benefit (Bates, Boote, & Beverly, 2004; Vogel, 2003). Consistent routines, reduction of environmental stimulation and triggers for agitated or aggressive behavior, and adequate rest are other interventions that may assist the cognitively impaired client (Vogel, 2003).

In the past, reality orientation was recommended as a strategy for dealing with confusion in older people, particularly those with dementia. Reality orientation was a practice of reminding the client of "reality" when they strayed too far from it. For example, the nurse might persistently inform a client with dementia that

her husband would not be coming to visit her because he died 3 years ago or that she cannot find the closet because she is no longer living in her old home. Research has indicated, however, that the effect of reality orientation was not to reorient the client to the present but to create anxiety and distress (Allen, 2000).

A more recent approach is termed **validation therapy**, a therapeutic approach to dealing with dementia by *validating* and accepting what the client perceives as reality. Validation therapy is based on the theory that people attempt to resolve unfinished life issues and that retreat into a specific *unreality* is an attempt to do that. It also presupposes that there is a reason for the behavior exhibited. Validation classifies dementia behaviors into four progressive stages: malorientation, time confusion, repetitive motion, and vegetation (Validation Training Institute, 2003). In the malorientation stage, the client expresses past conflicts in "disguised forms." For example, a client may believe that her daughter is her mother and reenact conflicts from the past. In the time confusion stage, the client retreats inward and may not be in touch with reality, but still attempts to resolve old life issues. In the repetitive motion stage, movements replace words in the attempt to resolve past conflicts, and finally, in the vegetation stage, the client gives up trying to resolve life issues and retreats from the world. In the validation approach, the caregiver (nurse or family member) accepts what the client perceives as reality and tries to redirect them without engaging in confrontations aimed at orienting them to reality. For example, a confused client may be asking when her dead husband will arrive. Rather than reminding her that he will never arrive because he is dead, the caretaker might just say, "Oh, not for a while yet, let's have lunch while we wait," redirecting the client's attention to a positive activity without causing distress.

Although validation therapy was developed between 1963 and 1980, there is limited research examining its effectiveness in addressing the problems of dementia. A recent meta analysis of research in this area found only three studies that met inclusion criteria. Based on the results of the analysis, the author concluded that there was "insufficient evidence from randomized trials to allow any conclusion about the efficacy of validation therapy for people with dementia or cognitive impairment" (Briggs, 2006, p. 3).

Advocacy may be required to be sure that treatment and supportive services are available in the community for older clients with impaired cognitive function and their families. Advocacy for respite care for caregivers is particularly important, and community health nurses may even advocate with caregivers themselves to take advantage of such services. Finally, advocacy is needed to support continuing research on the effectiveness of therapeutic approaches in dealing with the issues of dementia and cognitive impairment in the elderly. Secondary prevention interventions for these and other problems common among older clients are presented in Table 6◆.

TABLE 6	Secondary Prevention Strategies for Common Problems in the Older Population
Client Problem	**Secondary Prevention Strategies**
Skin breakdown	Inspect extremities regularly for lesions.
	Keep lesions clean and dry.
	Eliminate pressure by frequent changes of position.
	Refer for treatment as needed.
Constipation	Encourage fluid and fiber intake.
	Discourage ignoring urge to defecate.
	Encourage regular exercise.
	Encourage regular bowel habits.
	Use mild laxatives as needed, but discourage overuse.
	Administer enemas as needed; discourage overuse.
	Administer bulk products or stool softeners as indicated.
Urinary incontinence	Refer for urological consult or treatment of underlying physical causes.
	Refer for modification of medication regimen as needed.
	Encourage frequent voiding.
	Teach Kegel exercises.
	Decrease fluids after the evening meal.
	Assist with bladder training.
	Encourage use of sanitary pads, panty liners, etc., with frequent changes of such aids.
	Keep skin clean and dry; change clothing and bed linen as needed.
	Offer bedpan or urinal frequently or assist to bedside commode at frequent intervals.
Fecal incontinence	Refer for medical treatment of underlying causes as needed.
	Educate for dietary changes to address contributing factors.
	Encourage avoidance of caffeinated beverages and chocolate.
	Suggest smaller, more frequent meals.
	Suggest eating and drinking at different times.
	Encourage consumption of soluble fiber.
	Encourage sufficient fluid intake.
	Teach Kegel exercises or bowel training.
	Suggest strategies to decrease embarrassment.
Sensory loss	Provide adequate lighting.
	Keep eyeglasses clean and hearing aids functional.
	Eliminate safety hazards.
	Use large-print books or materials.
	Use multisensory approaches to communication and teaching.
	Avoid using colors that make discrimination difficult.
	Speak clearly and slowly, at a lower pitch.
	Eliminate background noise.
	Assist clients to obtain voice enhancers for phone.
	Use additional herbs and spices, but use with discretion.
	Purchase small amounts of perishable foods.
	Check pilot lights on gas appliances frequently.
	Encourage the use of smoke detectors.
Mobility limitation	Provide assistance with ambulation, transfer, etc.
	Assist clients to obtain equipment such as walkers and wheelchairs.
	Install ramps, tub rails, etc., as needed.
	Promote access to public facilities for older persons.

Continued on next page

TABLE 6	Secondary Prevention Strategies for Common Problems in the Older Population *(continued)*
	Assist clients to find alternative sources of transportation.
	Make referrals for assistance with personal care or instrumental activities as needed.
Pain	Plan activities for times when pain is controlled.
	Encourage warm soaks.
	Encourage adequate rest and exercise to prevent mobility limitations.
	Encourage effective use of analgesics.
	Refer for assistance with alternative pain control measures.
COPD (shortness of breath)	Refer for medical therapy (e.g., bronchodilators, steroids, oxygen), as needed.
	Educate regarding safety precautions with oxygen therapy.
	Encourage smoking cessation, as needed.
	Advocate for coverage of smoking cessation under health insurance plans.
	Encourage and refer for pneumonia and influenza immunization.
	Promote adequate nutrition.
	Encourage small, easily prepared and eaten meals or ask for assistance in meal preparation from family members.
	Discourage use of cough suppressants.
	Suggest taking fluids at the end of the meal rather than before or with foods.
	Refer to Meals-on-Wheels, if appropriate.
	Suggest sitting upright to eat.
	Educate client for pursed-lip breathing, diaphragmatic breathing, and controlled coughing.
	Promote physical activity as tolerated.
	Advocate for access to necessary diagnostic and treatment services.
Cognitive impairment	Apply principles of validation therapy, if helpful.
	Refer for Alzheimer's drug therapy as indicated.
	Refer for antidepressant, mood-stabilizing, or antipsychotic medications as needed.
	Promote exercise (register wanderers with national registry if appropriate).
	Promote activities to enhance memory (e.g., discussion of current events, games, puzzles, etc.).
	Educate families and caregivers regarding the progression of disease.
	Provide hand massage or therapeutic touch services or teach these interventions to caregivers.
	Establish consistent daily routines.
	Reduce environmental stimulation and triggers for aberrant behavior.
	Provide adequate rest.
Depression	Accept feelings and reflect on their normality; encourage client to ventilate feelings.
	Refer for counseling or medications as needed.
Social isolation	Compensate for sensory loss; enhance communication abilities.
	Improve mobility; provide access to transportation.
	Assist client to obtain adequate financial resources.
	Refer client to new support systems.
	Assist client to deal with grief over loss of loved ones.
Abuse or neglect	Assist caretakers to develop positive coping strategies.
	Assist families to obtain respite care or day care for older members.
	Refer families for counseling as needed.
	Arrange placement in temporary shelter.
	Assist families in making other arrangements for safe care of older clients.
	Advocate for laws and protective services systems that protect older clients from abuse.
Substance abuse	Identify problem drinking by older clients.
	Refer for therapy, Alcoholics Anonymous, or Al-Anon as appropriate.

Continued on next page

TABLE 6	Secondary Prevention Strategies for Common Problems in the Older Population *(continued)*	
	Observe for toxic effects of alcohol ingestion.	
	Maintain hydration and nutrition.	
Inadequate financial resources	Refer for financial assistance.	
	Assist with budgeting and priority allocation.	
	Educate for less expensive means of meeting needs.	
	Function as an advocate as needed.	

Tertiary Prevention

Tertiary preventive activities for older clients focus on preventing complications of existing conditions and preventing their recurrence. Tertiary prevention for the individual client depends on the problems experienced by the client. For example, tertiary prevention for an abused older client may include long-term counseling for family members, whereas prevention related to financial inadequacies may involve assistance with budgeting. Four specific areas of tertiary prevention in the care of older populations will be addressed here. These include monitoring health status, palliative care, end-of-life care, and caring for caregivers.

Monitoring Health Status

As we saw earlier, the majority of older clients will experience one or more chronic health conditions, and the prevalence of these conditions increases with increasing age. Community health nurses can be actively involved in monitoring the continuing health status of individual older clients and in the development and implementation of programs to monitor the effectiveness of provider intervention and self-management. For example, community health nurses may advocate for the initiation of community programs to support the needs of clients with diabetes or pain control for populations with arthritis. Monitoring of hypertension is another important role for community health nurses. In one study, older clients perceived ongoing blood pressure monitoring as reassuring and contributing to effective decisions regarding self-management. Monitoring provided opportunities to educate clients regarding their conditions and treatment regimens, as well as ensuring regular social contact and demonstration of concern (Vivarai-Dresler & Bakker, 2004). Community health nurses should advocate for, and in some cases provide, disease management and monitoring services available to all segments of the older population, particularly low-income older clients.

Palliative Care

Palliative care is another important consideration in tertiary prevention with the older adult population. Because of the incurability of many chronic conditions, the only avenue open for intervention is symptom management. **Palliative care** is care that addresses pain and symptom relief without attempting to cure the underlying disease process. The intent of palliative care is to decrease suffering and improve quality of life for both clients and families (Zerwekh, 2006). Although often viewed in the context of end-of-life care, as indicated in this definition, palliative care is also warranted when symptom control is the primary goal of care. Important features of palliative care include relief of pain and other symptoms, effective communication with health care providers, and achievement of a sense of completion. Goals for palliative care include the following:

- Sustained relationships with client and family
- Continued independence and function as long as desired by the client
- Aggressive symptom relief
- Physical, psychosocial, and spiritual support
- Attention to client needs in the context of the family and community
- Family involvement in care
- Incorporation of cultural and spiritual perspectives in care
- Determination of goals based on client and family values and choices
- Care provided through a multidisciplinary approach
- Acknowledgment and relief of caregiver burden
- Development of support systems in home and community (Zerwekh, 2006)

Palliative care often takes place in hospice settings. Unfortunately, Medicare's requirement for hospice care includes forgoing all further curative measures and a projected life expectancy of less than 6 months, leading to initiation of hospice care too late in the trajectory of disease (Matesa, 2002). Some hospices, particularly those in managed care systems, are now instituting separate palliative services that may be initiated prior to actual hospice care. In 2002, however, only 26% of hospitals provided palliative care programs, primarily due to lack of insurance coverage for such programs (Plese, 2002). Some managed care organizations cover the cost of palliative care, but costs are often borne as out-of-pocket expenses by older clients or their families.

Last Acts (2002), an advocacy group for end-of-life care, identified five principles of palliative care:

- Respect for the goals, likes, and choices of clients
- Attention to the medical, emotional, social, and spiritual needs of clients
- Support for family members

- Promotion of access to necessary health care providers and settings
- Promotion of excellent end-of-life care through support and assistance to caregivers

Community health nurses may be involved in providing palliative care to older clients and others with incurable conditions. Such care presents a number of challenges, including provision of pain relief and holistic care and dealing with symptoms such as fatigue and breathlessness, among others. In one study, community health nurses reported being unprepared to discuss death with clients' families or to deal with other areas of communication. For example, community health nurses experienced difficulty regarding disclosure of the client's condition or prognosis to the client or to family members. Community health nurses also reported being unprepared to deal with the emotional reactions of family members (particularly anger) and with their own personal emotional reactions to caring for these clients (Dunne, Sullivan, & Kernohan, 2005). In addition to providing care to individual clients, community health nurses may be actively involved in developing palliative care services and in advocating coverage of these services under both public and private health insurance programs.

End-of-life Care

Three specific considerations must be addressed in providing effective end-of-life care to older clients. These include formulation of advance directives, personal preparation for death, and actual care of the dying client.

In 1990, the Patient Self-determination Act required hospitals, nursing homes, hospices, managed care organizations, and other agencies receiving Medicare and Medicaid funds to inform clients of their right to refuse treatment and formulate advance care directives (Kleespies, 2004). Advance care planning is defined as "a process of discussion between professionals, families, and patients aimed at quality of care at the end of life" (Laakkonen, Pitkala, Strandberg, Berglind, & Tilvis, 2004, p. 247). Advance care planning may result in specific documents such as living wills or health-related powers of attorney. These documents specify circumstances in which life-sustaining treatment is or is not to be provided and appoint a surrogate to make decisions regarding life-sustaining treatments in the event of the client's incapacitation (Last Acts, 2002). **Life-sustaining treatment** is defined as "any medical intervention that would have little or no effect on the underlying disease, injury, or condition, but is administered to forestall the time of death or to reinstate life when death can be regarded as having occurred" (Kleespies, 2004, p. 57).

Three assumptions form the underlying premise for advance care directives: (a) people complete them, (b) the treatment preferences expressed are accurate and current, and (c) surrogate decision makers are able to interpret advance directives in light of the circumstances of a given situation. Unfortunately, research suggests that none of these assumptions is consistently met (Kleespies, 2004). For example, in one study in Finland, only 12% of the population studied had executed a living will. Among those who had a living will, 46% indicated that they would want to have cardiopulmonary resuscitation performed if needed, in contrast to the declarations in their living will documents (Laakkonen et al., 2004). In another study, subjects perceived both advantages and disadvantages to advance directives. Advantages included protection of personal integrity and support for family decision making; however, participants also saw advance directives as opening the possibility of euthanasia. They also voiced concerns that changes in perspective after executing an advance directive would not be taken into consideration and 57% of them indicated that they might not want to adhere to advance directives during dying (Seymour, Gott, Bellamy, Ahmedzai, & Clark, 2004). Studies of clients with cancer in intensive care units have also indicated that the presence of advance directives did not influence whether or not life-support interventions were initiated (Last Acts, 2002).

To be effective, advance care planning documents must be supported by state policies, usually legislation, that promote their implementation. Last Acts (2002) has identified six criteria for such state-level policies. The first criterion is that policies recommend one advance directive to address foreseeable circumstances. Second, states should avoid mandating a specific format for advance directives. The third criterion is that state policy gives precedence to the designated surrogate decision maker that overrides the written document or to the most recent directive. Fourth, state policies should authorize specific default surrogate decision makers in the event that none have been named. Fifth, close friends, as well as family members, should be recognized as possible surrogates. Finally, states should establish a statewide do-not-resuscitate (DNR) order for emergency medical services in the state. Unfortunately, by 2002, only seven states had laws related to advance directives that addressed all criteria (Last Acts, 2002).

Based on the difficulties noted with formal documents, some authors suggest that, in advance care planning, it "now seems more important to investigate the process of advance care planning in the doctor-patient relationship and to explore the poorly understood values and motives behind the expressed preferences" (Laakkonen et al., 2004, p. 248). The same need for exploration of desires and the values underlying them would seem to exist for families as well, and community health nurses may need to advocate for such discussions. They may also need to advocate compliance with advance directives by family members or health care providers when these directives have been written.

Preparation for death usually also entails a number of practical activities involved in getting one's affairs in order. Older clients may need to make decisions about funeral arrangements or the disposition of their belongings. Both nurses and family members should be encouraged to listen to clients in their reflections on such matters, rather than put them off with assurances that they "won't die for a long time yet." Community health nurses may need to advocate with family members to encourage them to address older clients' concerns about dying. Nurses may also need to refer clients for legal assistance with wills, burial plans, and other financial arrangements. Many communities have low-cost legal aid services available to elderly clients. Community health nurses should keep in mind, however, the cultural differences in preparation for death that clients may exhibit (Mitty, 2001). For example, in many cultures, such decisions are believed to be the responsibility of children, and the dying client should not be bothered. In others, discussion of death is believed to hasten its occurrence, so clients are not willing to explore plans related to their deaths.

"End-of-life care begins the moment there is a shift from trying to challenge the illness to trying to challenge the suffering of the human who is experiencing serious life-threatening illness" (Plese, 2002, p. 7). End-of-life care includes five essential services: assessment of the living situation, management of symptoms and promotion of quality of life, promotion of advance care planning, counseling for client and family, and provision of continuity, communication, and coordination of care. The Palliative Care Task Force (Henderson, 2004) has identified five principles of end-of-life care. These principles are as follows:

- Respect for client and family goals, preferences, and choices
- Provision of comprehensive care
- Use of interdisciplinary expertise
- Attention to caregiver concerns
- Use of systems and mechanisms that support dying clients and their families

At present, more than half of older Americans die in hospitals, although 70% express the desire to die at home. Approximately half of dying clients do so in pain, and only 42% of U.S. hospitals have formal pain management programs and 23% provide hospice services. Only seven states have high-quality pain management policies. In addition, no state has more than 1% of primary care providers who are certified in palliative care, and only 15 states have more than 1% of full-time-equivalent registered nurses with certification (Last Acts, 2002). Community health nurses can be active in promoting effective end-of-life policies through legislative advocacy. Locally, they can help to ensure that advance directives will be implemented and support clients and family members in their execution.

End-of-life care also includes care for family members of the dying client. Community health nurses can assist families with both anticipatory grief and grief after the death of a loved one. In addition, they can advocate for effective services that assist with the management of grief. As many as 35% of bereaved family members have been found to meet the criteria for major depression, yet their depression is often unrecognized and few services are available to them. Anticipatory grief is defined as "any grief occurring prior to a loss, as distinguished from the grief that occurs at or after a loss" (Aldrich, as quoted in Lewis & McBride, 2004, p. 45). Anticipatory grief is experienced in response to an impending loss, and may be characterized by withdrawal, detachment, or caring and love. Community health nurses can assist families to share information and feelings and to resolve unfinished business in either practical or relational realms. Community health nurses may also need to help families adjust to changes in roles, particularly in cultural groups in which loss of people in specific designated roles may have a greater impact on the family (Lewis & McBride, 2004).

Caring for Caregivers

The last major consideration in tertiary prevention with the older population is caring for those who provide care to this group. The National Family Caregiver Support Program (NFCSP) has identified five core services needed by caregivers. These include information, referral to needed assistance, counseling, respite, and help with supplies, assistive devices, and so on (Plese, 2005a). Caregivers need information regarding the older client's condition and treatment regimen as well as the availability of services in the local community and how to obtain them. Information may also be needed on managing life changes and on dealing with financial and legal issues, particularly in the face of increasing cognitive impairment in the recipient of care (Alzheimer's Association, 2001). Many caregivers lack information about resources available to them. In some instances, services may be perceived as unable to meet the religious and cultural needs of some segments of the population (Merrell et al., 2005). Caregivers may also benefit from counseling services that help them to cope with the physical and emotional burdens of caregiving. Counseling may prevent caregivers from being "engulfed" by their caregiving role (Brown & Alligood, 2004). **Respite**, the provision of temporary relief from caregiving responsibilities, is often lacking for many caregivers who have 24-hour, 7-day-a-week responsibilities for the care of their aging family members. When available, respite may be provided by informal (other family members and friends) or formal support networks. Finally, caregivers may need help with obtaining needed supplies and assistive devices or in dealing with the financial burden of caregiving.

Both health care systems and caregivers themselves give rise to barriers to caregiver empowerment. Caregiver-related barriers may include an absence of focus on self, reluctance to share caregiving duties with

TABLE 7	Tertiary Prevention Strategies in the Care of Older Populations
Focus	**Tertiary Prevention Strategies**
Monitoring health status	Monitor health status and treatment effects for individual older clients.
	Design and implement programs to monitor health status in older client.
Palliative care	Provide palliative care or refer individual clients for palliative care services.
	Advocate for accessible palliative care services for population groups.
End-of-life care	Assist individual clients and families with advance care planning.
	Advocate for adherence to advance directives within health care systems.
	Advocate for effective state and national policies related to advance directives.
	Provide culturally sensitive and appropriate end-of-life care to individual clients.
	Advocate for access to hospice and other end-of-life services.
	Advocate for changes in reimbursement for end-of-life services.
Caregiver support	Provide support to individual caregivers, including referral to available support services.
	Educate the public and caregivers regarding their own needs.
	Promote caregiver empowerment.
	Advocate for support services for caregivers.
	Advocate for insurance coverage of supportive services needed by caregivers.

others, reluctance to consider or discuss the effects of caregiving on their own health, and lack of awareness of caregiver support services (Plese, 2005a). Caregivers may focus on the needs of the care recipient to the exclusion of their own needs. They may also feel a duty and responsibility for caregiving as part of their relationship with the recipient. In addition, as we saw earlier, many caregivers do not perceive themselves as such and do not realize that they are eligible for whatever supportive services may exist. Barriers related to the health system include a lack of attention to the needs of caregivers and lack of availability of and funding for caregiver support services. Specific services that may be needed to support caregivers include domiciliary assistance with personal care, social work services to maintain clients in home settings without undue burden on caregivers, respite care, support groups, and interactions with multidisciplinary teams that can address the multiple needs of clients and their caregivers (Hoskins et al., 2005). Community health nurses can be actively involved in supporting individual caregivers and referring them for needed assistance, including respite services and counseling. They can also function as advocates to assure that such services are provided and that caregivers in all segments of the population have access to culturally sensitive and appropriate support. Selected strategies for tertiary prevention in the care of older populations are presented in Table 7◆.

IMPLEMENTING CARE FOR OLDER POPULATIONS

Two major considerations in implementing care for older populations are health education directed at this group and political advocacy. Information sources for educating clients and the general public on health issues of concern to older populations are presented on the next page.

Health education initiatives are based on general principles of teaching and learning, but there are also some unique considerations in implementing education programs for the older adult population.

Older adults may exhibit some decline in linguistic skills with age. Auditory communication may be too fast-paced for comprehension or contain too much information to be easily comprehensible (Qualls, Harris, & Rogers, 2002). Sensory losses also need to be considered when teaching the older client population. Strategies to circumvent hearing loss include using a lower-pitched voice; facing the listener while speaking; employing nonverbal teaching techniques; using clear, concise terminology; and having the client use a hearing aid if needed. The effects of hearing loss can also be minimized by limiting background noise, reemphasizing important points, and supplementing verbal with written materials.

The use of glasses, a magnifying glass, and large print may help to minimize visual deficits. Learning can also be enhanced by visual materials using black lettering on white or yellow paper, providing adequate lighting, and eliminating glare in the learning environment.

In implementing health education plans for older adults, the nurse may need to repeat material more frequently. Because of decreases in short-term memory, it may take longer for some older clients to learn new material. Once material is learned, however, older clients retain it as well as younger ones. Multisensorial presentation, multiple repetitions, reinforcement of verbal content with written materials, and use of memory aids (e.g., a calendar for taking medications) may also assist learning in older clients.

Because response times are longer for older people than for their younger counterparts, lessons should proceed at a slower pace, and the nurse should allow more time for responses on the part of the client. Self-paced

CLIENT EDUCATION — Information Resources for Older Clients

Information Category	Agency/Organization	Information Category	Agency/Organization
Abuse	National Center on Elder Abuse	Exercise and nutrition (cont.)	Healthy Aging Campaign
	http://www.elderabusecenter.org		http://www.healthyaging.net
Advanced care directives	Aging with Dignity		National Institute on Aging
	http://www.agingwithdignity.com		http://www.niapublications.org
	Partnership for Caring		http://www.nia.nih.gov/exercisebook
	http://www.partnershipforcaring.org		National Policy and Resource Center on Nutrition and Aging
Alzheimer's disease	Alzheimer's Association		http://www.fiu.edu
	http://www.alz.org		USDA Food and Nutrition Information Center
	Alzheimer's Disease Education and Referral Center (ADEAR)		http://www.nal.usda.gov/fnic
	http://www.alzheimers.org	Financial barriers to care	Medicare Rights Center
Caregiving	American Association of Retired Persons (AARP)		http://www.medicarerights.org
	http://www.aarp.org/life/caregiving		National Council on Aging
	Family Caregiver Alliance		http://www.benefitscheckup.org
	http://www.caregiver.org		Pharmaceutical Research and Manufacturers of America
	National Alliance for Caregiving		http://www.helpingpatients.org
	http://www.caregiving.org	Immunization	National Immunization Program
	National Family Caregivers Association		http://www.cdc.gov/nip/recs/adult-schedule.htm
	http://www.nfcacares.org	Mental health/ substance abuse	American Association for Geriatric Psychiatry
Cultural competence	National Council on Interpreting in Health Care		http://www.aagponline.org
	http://www.ncihc.org/index.htm		National Clearinghouse for Alcohol and Drug Information (NCADI)
	National Institutes of Health (NIH)		http://www.health.org
	http://www.salud.nih.gov		National Institute of Mental Health (NIMH)
	U.S. Office of Minority Health		http://www.nimh.nih.gov
	http://www.omhrc.gov	Sexuality	Sexuality Information and Education Council of the United States
Driving/safety	American Association of Retired Persons (AARP)		http://www.siecus.org/pubs/biblio/bibs0012.html
	http://www.aarp.org/drive	Social services	Eldercare Locator
	Getting Around Safe & Sound and Granddriver		http://www.eldercare.gov
	http://www.aamva.org/drivers/drv_AgingDrivers.asp	Urinary incontinence	American Foundation for Urological Diseases
	http://www.granddriver.info		http://www.afud.org
End-of-life care	National Hospice and Palliative Care Organization		National Institute of Diabetes and Digestive and Kidney Disorders (NIDDK)
	http://www.nhpco.org		http://www.niddk.nih.gov
Exercise and nutrition	Centers for Disease Control and Prevention		The Simon Foundation for Continence
	http://www.cdc.gov/agomg/index.htm		http://www.simonfoundation.org/html
	http://www.cdc.gov/nccdphp/dnpa/index.htm		
	http://www.cdc.gov/nccdphp/dnpa/physical/growing_stronger/growing_stronger.pdf		

instruction is helpful. Motivation to learn can be heightened by increasing client participation in the lesson and by setting easily attainable, progressive goals that enhance success and satisfaction. Irrelevant material can confuse clients and should be eliminated from the presentation.

Endurance may be somewhat limited in older clients, so teaching sessions should be kept short (10 to 15 minutes per session). Lessons should be scheduled at times of the day when learners are rested and comfortable. Health education for older clients should not be time limited, as they may need more or less time to learn specific material. Again, learning should be broken down into small, progressive steps so that periodic success will continue to motivate older learners.

The teaching-learning process should also allow for rest periods as needed.

Political advocacy may be needed to implement primary, secondary, and tertiary prevention strategies with older populations. Political advocacy may require more effort than advocacy for other population groups in countries like the United States that are affected by pervasive ageism. Advocacy efforts may need to start at local levels, with research that documents the cost savings of health promotion strategies and effective end-of life care. For example, it has been demonstrated that every Medicare dollar spent on hospice services actually saves $1.52 in hospitalization costs and that expenditures for hospice clients in the last month of life are two thirds lower than those for clients who do not receive hospice services (Plese, 2002). Similarly, the cost savings associated with family caregiving versus formal care can be used as justification for services to support caregivers.

EVALUATING HEALTH CARE FOR OLDER POPULATIONS

Evaluating the effectiveness of health care for older members of the population can occur at the individual or aggregate level. At the individual level, the community health nurse would assess the client's health status and the effects of primary, secondary, and tertiary interventions in improving health status. On occasion, the effectiveness of care would be measured in terms of a peaceful death and the physical and emotional health of family members and caregivers.

At the aggregate level, evaluation of the effects of care on the health of the elderly can be measured, in part, by the level of accomplishment of relevant national health objectives. The status of selected national objectives for the year 2010 related to the health of older clients is reflected below. As we can see, only one of the objectives for this age group has been met, and four objectives are actually moving away from their targets. These data indicate that more effort is required to promote the health of the older U.S. population.

Because older clients frequently have multiple health problems, many people consider care for older individuals as incongruent with the population-focused health promotion emphasis of community health nursing. Primary, secondary, and tertiary prevention efforts by community health nurses, however, can decrease the burden of illness experienced by older clients themselves as well as by society.

HEALTHY PEOPLE 2010
Goals for Population Health◆

OBJECTIVE	BASELINE	MOST RECENT DATA	TARGET
■ 1-9c. Reduce hospitalization rates for immunization-preventable pneumonia (per 10,000 persons over 65)	10.6	11.2	8#
■ 2-9. Reduce cases of osteoporosis in adults 50 years of age and older	10%	NDA	8%
■ 2-10. Reduce hospitalization for vertebral fractures due to osteoporosis (per 10,000 persons over 65)	17.5	14.1	14.0
■ 3-12. Increase colorectal cancer screening with fecal occult blood in persons 50 years of age and older	35%	33%	50%#
■ 12-6. Reduce hospitalization for heart failure in:			
a. Adults 65 to 74 years of age (per 1,000 people)	13.2	12.3	6.5
b. Adults 75 to 84 years of age (per 1,000 people)	26.7	27.1	13.5#
c. Adults 85 years and older (per 1,000 people)	52.7	50.4	26.5
■ 14-5. Reduce invasive pneumococcal infections (per 100,000 people)	62	51	42
■ 14-29. Increase immunization among those 65 years of age and older for:			
a. Influenza	64%	66%	90%
b. Pneumococcal disease	46%	56%	90%
■ 15-15. Reduce motor vehicle crash deaths (per 100,000 people over 70 years of age)	23.7	23.1	9.2
■ 15-16. Reduce pedestrian deaths (per 100,000 people over 70 years of age)	3.9	2.7	1
■ 15-28. Reduce hip fractures (per 100,000 people over 65 years of age			
a. Females	1,055.8	1029.2	416.0
b. Males	592.7	484.2	474.0
■ 19-1. Increase the proportion of people over 60 years of age at healthy weight	36%	28%	60%#
■ 21-4. Reduce the proportion of older adults who have lost all of their teeth	26%	24%	20%

Continued on next page

■ 22-1. Reduce the proportion of adults with no leisure-time physical activity as follows:			
a. 65 to 74 years of age	51%	47%	20%
b. Over 75 years of age	64%	61%	20%
■ 24-4. Reduce hospitalizations for asthma (per 10,000 people over 65 years of age)	17.7	21.4	11#
■ 24-10. Reduce activity limitation due to COPD in:			
a. Men over 65 years of age	4.4%	4.4%	1.5%
b. Women over 65 years of age	3.3%	3.2%	1.5%
■ 27-1. Reduce tobacco use (older adults)	11%	9%	12%*

NDA—No data available

* Objective has been met

 # Objective moving away from target

Data from: Centers for Disease Control and Prevention. (2005). **Healthy people data.** *Retrieved September 5, 2005, from http://wonder.cdc.gov/data2010*

Case Study

Caring for an Elderly Woman

Henrietta Walker is a 68-year-old African American woman who has been referred for community health nursing services following her discharge from the hospital. She was hospitalized after being found unconscious in her room by her 50-year-old daughter. A diagnosis of diabetes mellitus was made, and Mrs. Walker was placed on 15 units of NPH insulin daily. She and her daughter were instructed on injection technique and a diabetic diet at the hospital.

Mrs. Walker lives with her daughter and son-in-law and their three teenage boys (ages 18, 15, and 13). They live in a lower-class neighborhood, and the son-in-law works at the local textile plant. His income is barely enough for the family to live on. Mrs. Walker does not know how she will pay her hospital bill. She has Medicare, Part A, and a small Social Security income, but she does not have any supplemental health insurance.

Mrs. Walker's vision is failing, probably as a result of undiagnosed diabetes of long standing. She hears well but is 80 pounds overweight, so is unsteady on her feet. The family lives in a second-floor apartment, and there is no handrail on the stairs outside the apartment. Mrs. Walker tries to help out around the house because her daughter works. She says she does not want to be a burden to her daughter and her son-in-law. Mrs. Walker's husband died of a heart attack 8 months ago, and that was when she came to live with her daughter. Mrs. Walker's daughter says that her mother's presence has caused some friction among the boys because the two younger ones now have to share a room.

1. What are the biophysical, psychological, physical environmental, sociocultural, behavioral, and health system factors influencing Mrs. Walker's health?
2. What nursing diagnoses can be derived from the information presented in the case study? Be sure to include the etiology of Mrs. Walker's problems where appropriate.
3. How would you prioritize these diagnoses? Why?
4. How would you go about incorporating client participation in planning interventions for Mrs. Walker's health problems?
5. List at least three client care objectives that you would like to accomplish with Mrs. Walker.
6. Describe some of the primary, secondary, and tertiary prevention strategies that would be appropriate in resolving Mrs. Walker's health problems. Why would they be appropriate?
7. How would you evaluate your nursing intervention? What criteria would you use to evaluate care?

Test Your Understanding

1. What are the three categories of theories of aging? What theories fit within each category?

2. What are some of the biophysical, psychological, physical environmental, sociocultural, behavioral, and health system factors that affect the health of older clients?

3. What are the major emphases in primary prevention in the care of older clients? Give examples of community health nursing interventions related to each.

4. Describe at least one secondary preventive measure in each of four common health problems encountered among older clients.

5. Identify at least one tertiary prevention measure in each of the four emphasis areas discussed in this chapter.

6. What are two major considerations in implementing health-related interventions with older adults? In what ways are these considerations similar to and different from care of other age groups?

EXPLORE MediaLink

http://www.prenhall.com/clark
Resources for this chapter can be found on the Companion Website.

Audio Glossary
Appendix I: Adult Health Assessment and
  Intervention Guide
Exam Review Questions

Case Study: Caring for the Aged
MediaLink Application: Defying
  Ageism (video)
Media Links

Challenge Your Knowledge
Update *Healthy People 2010*
Advocacy Interviews

References

Advisory Committee on Immunization Practices. (2004). Recommended adult immunization schedule—United States, October 2004–September 2005. *Morbidity and Mortality Weekly Report, 53*, Q1–Q4.

Albert, S. M., Im, A., & Raveis, V. H. (2002). Public health and the second 50 years of life. *American Journal of Public Health, 92*, 1214–1216.

Alemagno, S. A., Niles, S. A., & Treiber, E. A. (2004). Using computers to reduce medication misuse of community-based seniors: Results of a pilot intervention program. *Geriatric Nursing, 25*, 281–285.

Allen, J. (2000). *Using validation therapy to manage difficult behaviors.* Retrieved March 16, 2006, from http://www.ec-online.net/ Community/Activists/difficultbehaviors.htm

Alzheimer's Association. (2001). *The Alzheimer's disease study: Communication gaps between primary care physicians and caregivers.* Retrieved December 20, 2001, from http://www.alz.org

American Association of Colleges of Nursing & the John A. Hartford Foundation Institute for Geriatric Nursing. (2000). *Older adults: Recommended baccalaureate competencies and curricular guidelines for geriatric nursing care.* Washington, DC: American Association of Colleges of Nursing.

American Association of Retired Persons. (2002). *Beyond 50.02: A report to the nation on trends in health security.* Washington, DC: Author.

American Association of Retired Persons. (2005). Effective and safe prescription drugs. Retrieved October 18, 2005, from http:// www.aarp.org/health/comparedrugs

American Nurses Association. (2001). *Scope and standards of gerontological nursing practice* (2nd ed.). Washington, DC: American Nurses Publishing.

Andrews, J. O., Heath, J., & Graham-Garcia, J. (2004). Management of tobacco dependence in older adults. *Journal of Gerontological Nursing, 30*(12), 13–24.

Angel, R. J., Angel, J. L., & Markides, K. S. (2002). Stability and change in health insurance among older Mexican Americans: Longitudinal evidence from the Hispanic Established Populations for Epidemiologic Study of the Elderly. *American Journal of Public Health, 92*, 1264–1271.

Antai-Otong, D. (2004). Antidepressants and older adults. *Advance for Nurses, 1*(7), 15–17.

Baine, W. B., Yu, W., & Summe, J. P. (2001). Epidemiologic trends in the hospitalization of elderly Medicare patients for pneumonia, 1991–1998. *American Journal of Public Health, 91*, 1121–1123.

Balfour, J., & Kaplan, G. (2002). Neighborhood environment and loss of physical function in older adults: Evidence from the Alameda County study. *American Journal of Epidemiology, 155*, 507–515.

Bates, J., Boote, J., & Beverly, C. (2004). Psychosocial interventions for people with a milder dementing illness: A systematic review. *Journal of Advanced Nursing, 45*, 644–658.

Beltran-Aguilar, E. D., Barker, L., K., Canto, M. T., Dye, B. A., Gooch, B. F., Griffin, S. O., et al. (2005). Surveillance for dental caries, dental sealants, tooth retention, edentulism, and enamel fluorosis—United States, 1988–1994 and 1999–2002. *Morbidity and Mortality Weekly Report, 53*(SS-3), 1–43.

Benjamins, M. R., & Brown, C. (2004). Religion and preventative health care utilization among the elderly. *Social Science & Medicine, 58*, 109–118.

Bennett, J. A., Thomas, V., & Riegel, B. (2004). Unrecognized chronic dehydration in older adults: Examining prevalence rates and risk factors. *Journal of Gerontological Nursing, 30*(11), 22–28.

Bennett, S. J., Suave, M. J., & Shaw, R. M. (2005). A conceptual model of cognitive deficits in chronic heart failure. *Journal of Nursing Scholarship, 37*, 222–228.

Bertsch, D. K., & Taylor-Moore, P. C. (2005). Elderly want to "age in place." *NurseWeek, 18*(14), 17–18.

Blazer, D. G., Sachs-Ericsson, N., & Hybels, C. F. (2005). Perception of unmet basic needs as a predictor of mortality among community-dwelling older adults. *American Journal of Public Health, 95*, 299–304.

Blumenthal, J. A., & Gullette, E. C. D. (2002). Exercise interventions and aging: Psychological and physical benefits in older adults. In K. W. Schaie, H. Leventhal, & S. L. Willis (Eds.), *Effective health behavior in older adults* (pp. 157–177). New York: Springer.

Briggs, N. M. (2006). *Validation therapy for dementia.* Retrieved March 16, 2006, from http://www.cochrane.org/reviews/en/ ab001394.html

Brinckerhoff, J., & Coleman, E. A. (2005). What you need to know about the Medicare Prescription Drug Act. *Family Practice Management, 12*(3), 49–52.

Brown, J. W., & Alligood, M. R. (2004). Realizing wrongness: Stories of older wife caregivers. *Journal of Applied Gerontology, 23*, 104–119,

Buckwalter, K. C., Wakefield, B. J., Hanna, B., & Lehmann, J. (2004). New technology for medication adherence: Electronically managed medication dispensing system. *Journal of Gerontological Nursing, 30*(7), 5–8.

Burholt, V., & Wenger, G. C. (2005). Migration from South Asia to the United Kingdom and the maintenance of transnational intergenerational relationships. In M. Silverstein & K. W. Schaie (Eds.), *Annual review of gerontology and geriatrics (Vol. 24), Focus on intergenerational relations across time and space* (pp. 153–176). New York: Springer.

Calabrese, D. A. (2004). Prostate cancer in older men. *Urologic Nursing, 24*, 258–269.

Calandra, J. (2003). Mental health & older adults: Mental illness in later life. *NurseWeek, 16*(25), 21–22.

Callen, B. (2004). Understanding nutritional health in older adults: A pilot study. *Journal of Gerontological Nursing, 30*(1), 36–43.

Caterino, J. M., Emond, J. A., & Camargo, C. A. (2004). Inappropriate medication administration to the acutely ill elderly: A nationwide emergency department study. *Journal of the American Geriatric Society, 52*, 1847–1855.

Center for Climatic Research, University of Delaware. (2004). Impact of heat waves on mortality—Rome, Italy, June–August, 2003. *Morbidity and Mortality Weekly Report, 53*, 369–371.

Centers for Disease Control and Prevention. (2003). Facilitating influenza and pneumococcal vaccination through standing orders programs. *Morbidity and Mortality Weekly Report, 52*, 68–69.

Centers for Disease Control and Prevention. (2004a). *Health United States, 2004 with chartbook on trends in the health of Americans.* Retrieved August 9, 2005, from http:// www.cdc.giv/nchs/data/hus/hus04.pdf

Centers for Disease Control and Prevention. (2004b). Indicators for chronic disease surveillance. *Morbidity and Mortality Weekly Report, 53*(RR-11), 1–114.

Centers for Disease Control and Prevention. (2005a). *CJD (Creutzfeldt-Jakob disease, classic).* Retrieved March 16, 2006, from http:// www.cdc.gov/ncidod/dvrd/cjd/index.htm

Centers for Disease Control and Prevention. (2005b). *Healthy people data*. Retrieved September 5, 2005, from http://wonder.cdc.gov/data2010

Centers for Medicare & Medicaid Services. (2004). Influenza vaccination and self-reported reasons for not receiving influenza vaccination among Medicare beneficiaries > 65 years—United States, 1991–2002. *Morbidity and Mortality Weekly Report, 53*, 1012–1015.

Chang, B. L., Nitta, S., Carter, P., & Markham, Y. K. (2004). Perceived helpfulness of telephone calls: Providing support for caregivers of family members with dementia. *Journal of Gerontological Nursing, 30*(9), 14–21.

Cleveland Clinic. (2005a). *Controlled coughing*. Retrieved March 16, 2006, from http://www.clevelandclinic.org/health/health-info/docs/2400/2413.asp?index=8697

Cleveland Clinic. (2005b). *Diaphragmatic breathing*. Retrieved March 16, 2006, from http://www.clevelandclinic.org/health/health-info/docs/2400/2409.asp?index=9445

Cleveland Clinic. (2005c). *Nutritional guidelines for people with COPD*. Retrieved March 16, 2006, from http://www.clevelandclinic.org/health/health-info/docs/2400/2411.asp?index=9451

Cleveland Clinic. (2005d). *Pursed-lip breathing*. Retrieved March 16, 2006, from http://www.clevelandclinic.org/health/health-info/docs/2400/2408.asp?index=9443

Coeling, H. V., Biordi, D. L., & Theis, S. L. (2003). Negotiating dyadic identity between caregivers and care receivers. *Journal of Nursing Scholarship, 35*, 21–25.

Cooper, K. L., & Kaplan, S. A. (2004). The overactive bladder and incontinence. In R. S. Kirby, C. C. Carson, M. G. Kirby, & R. N. Farah (Eds.), *Men's health* (2nd ed., pp. 417–430). London: Taylor & Francis.

Crews, J. E., & Campbell, V. A. (2004). Vision impairment and hearing loss among community-dwelling older Americans: Implications for health and functioning. *American Journal of Public Health, 94*, 823–829.

Curran, D. R. (2004). Should we discontinue Pap smear screening in women aged > 65 years? *Journal of Family Practice, 53*, 308–309.

Cutler, D. M. (2004). Behavioral health interventions: What works and why? In N. B. Anderson, R. A. Bulatao, & B. Cohen (Eds.), *Critical perspectives on racial and ethnic differences in health in late life* (pp. 643–674). Washington, DC: National Academies Press.

Dash, M. E., Foster, E. B., Smith, D. M., & Phillips, S. L. (2004). Urinary incontinence: The Social Health Maintenance Organization's approach. *Geriatric Nursing, 25*, 81–87.

Davey, A., Janke, M., & Savla, J. (2005). Antecedents of intergenerational support: Families in context and families as context. In M. Silverstein & K. W. Schaie (Eds.), *Annual review of gerontology and geriatrics (Vol. 24), Focus on intergenerational relations across time and space* (pp. 29–54). New York: Springer.

Davis, G. C., Hiemenz, M. L., & White, T. L. (2002). Barriers to managing chronic pain of older adults with arthritis. *Journal of Nursing Scholarship, 34*, 121–126.

Davis, L. L., Burgio, L. D., Buckwalter, K. C., & Weaver, M. A. (2004). Comparison of in-home and telephone-based skill training interventions with caregivers of persons with dementia. *Journal of Mental Health, 10*, 31–44.

Division of Adult and Community Health. (2003a). Hospitalizations for stroke among adults aged >65 years—United States, 2000. *Morbidity and Mortality Weekly Report, 52*, 586–589.

Division of Adult and Community Health. (2003b). Projected prevalence of self-reported arthritis or chronic joint symptoms among persons aged >65 years—United States, 2005–2030. *Morbidity and Mortality Weekly Report, 52*, 489–491.

Division of Adult and Community Health. (2003c). Trends in aging—United States and worldwide. *Morbidity and Mortality Weekly Report, 52*, 101–106.

Division of Adult and Community Health. (2005). Estimated influenza vaccination coverage among adults and children—United States, September 1, 2004–January 31, 2005. *Morbidity and Mortality Weekly Report, 54*, 304–307.

Division of Cancer Prevention and Control, National Center for Chronic Disease Prevention and Health Promotion. (2004). Cancer survivorship—United States, 1971–2001. *Morbidity and Mortality Weekly Report, 53*, 526, 528–529.

Division of Cancer Prevention and Control, National Center for Chronic Disease Prevention and Health Promotion. (2005). Breast cancer screening and socioeconomic status—35 metropolitan areas, 2000 and 2002. *Morbidity and Mortality Weekly Report, 54*, 981–985.

Division of Human Development and Disability. (2002). State-specific prevalence of obesity among adults with disabilities—Eight states and the District of Columbia, 1998–1999. *Morbidity and Mortality Weekly Report, 51*, 805–808.

Division of Nutrition and Physical Activity, National Center for Chronic Disease Prevention and Health Promotion. (2004). Strength training among adults >65 years—United States, 2001. *Morbidity and Mortality Weekly Report, 53*, 25–28.

Division of Surveillance and Informatics. (2003). Non-fatal fall-related traumatic brain injury among older adults—California, 1996–1999. *Morbidity and Mortality Weekly Report, 52*, 276–278.

Division of Unintentional Injury Prevention. (2003). Nonfatal injuries among older adults treated in hospital emergency departments—United States, 2001. *Morbidity and Mortality Weekly Report, 52*, 1019–1022.

Drug Effectiveness Review Project. (2005). *Drug effectiveness review project reports*. Retrieved October 17, 2005, from http://www.ohsu.edu/drugeffectiveness/reports/final.cfm

Dunne, K., Sullivan, K., & Kernohan, G. (2005). Palliative care for patients with cancer: District nurses' experiences. *Journal of Advanced Nursing, 50*, 372–380.

Ebrahim, S., Papacosta, O., Wannamethee, G., & Adamson, J. (2004). Social inequalities and disability in older men: Prospective findings from the British regional heart study. *Social Science & Medicine, 59*, 2109–2120.

Edlund, B. J. (2004). Medication use and misuse. *Journal of Gerontological Nursing, 30*(7), 4.

Edwards, M. (2004). As good as it gets. *AARP Magazine, 47*(6A), 42–49, 90.

Ekwall, A. K., Sivberg, B., & Hallberg, I. R. (2005). Loneliness as a predictor of quality of life among older caregivers. *Journal of Advanced Nursing, 49*, 23–32.

Epidemiology and Surveillance Division. (2004). Influenza and pneumococcal vaccination coverage among persons aged >65 years and persons aged 16–64 years with diabetes or asthma—United States, 2003. *Morbidity and Mortality Weekly Report, 53*, 1007–1012.

Farran, C. J., Loukissa, D., Perraud, S., & Paun, O. (2004). Alzheimer's disease caregiving information and skills. Part II: Family caregiver issues and concerns. *Research in Nursing & Health, 27*, 40–51.

Federal Interagency Forum on Aging-related Statistics. (2004). *Older Americans 2004: Key indicators of well-being*. Washington, DC: Author.

Finfgeld-Connett, D. L. (2004). Treatment of substance misuse in older women: Using a brief intervention model. *Journal of Gerontological Nursing, 30*(8), 30–37.

Finlayson, M., Van Denend, T., & Hudson, E. (2004). Aging with multiple sclerosis. *Journal of Neuroscience Nursing, 36*, 245–251.

Fitzpatrick, A. L., Powe, N. R., Cooper, L. S., Ives, D. G., & Robbins, J. A. (2004). Barriers to health care access and who perceives them. *American Journal of Public Health, 94*, 1788–1794.

Foley, D. J., Heimovitz, H. K., Guralnik, J. M., & Brock, D. B. (2002). Driving life expectancy of persons aged 70 years and older in the United States. *American Journal of Public Health, 92*, 1284–1289.

Fulmer, T. (2002). Elder abuse and neglect assessment. *Try this: Best practices in nursing care to older adults*. New York: Hartford Geriatric Institute for Nursing.

Garand, L., Buckwalter, K. C., & Hall, G. R. (2000). The biological basis of behavioral symptoms in dementia. *Issues in Mental Health Nursing, 21*, 91–107.

Gott, M., Hinchliff, S., & Galena, E. (2004). General practitioner attitudes to discussing sexual health issues with older people. *Social Science & Medicine, 58*, 2093–2103.

Guinn, M. J. (2004). A daughter's journey promoting geriatric self-care: Promoting positive health care interactions. *Geriatric Nursing, 25*, 267–271.

Guralnik, J. M., Alecxih, L., Branch, L. G., & Wiener, J. M. (2002). Medical and long-term care costs when older persons become more dependent. *American Journal of Public Health, 92*, 1244–1245.

Haight, B. K. (2001). Life reviews: Helping Alzheimer's patients reclaim a fading past. *Reflections on Nursing Leadership, 27*(1), 20–22.

Hanks-Bell, M., Halvey, K., & Paice, J. A. (2004). Pain assessment and management in aging. *Online Journal of Issues in Nursing*. Retrieved September 2, 2004, from http://www.nursingworld.org/ojin/topic21/tpc21_6.htm

Harper, S. A., Fukuda, K., Uyeki, T. M., Cox, N. J., & Bridges, C. B. (2005). Prevention and control of influenza: Recommendations of the Advisory Committee on Immunization Practices (ACIP). *Morbidity and Mortality Weekly Report, 54*(RR-8), 1–41.

Heidrick, S. M., & Wells, T. J. (2004). Effects of urinary incontinence: Psychological well-being and distress in older community-dwelling women. *Journal of Gerontological Nursing, 30*(4), 47–54.

Henderson, M. L. (2004). Gerontological advance practice nurses as end-of-life care facilitators. *Geriatric Nursing, 25,* 233–237.

Henley, E. (2004). What the new Medicare prescription drug bill may mean for providers and patients. *Journal of Family Practice, 53,* 389–392.

Henry, M. (2002). Descending into delirium. *American Journal of Nursing, 102*(3), 49–56.

Hoskins, S., Coleman, M., & McNeely, D. (2005). Stress in carers of individuals with dementia and community mental health teams: An uncontrolled evaluation study. *Journal of Advanced Nursing, 50,* 372–380.

Huang, T.-T., & Acton, G. J. (2004). Effectiveness of home visit falls prevention strategy for Taiwanese community-dwelling elders: Randomized trial. *Public Health Nursing, 21,* 247–256.

Huey, F. L. (Ed.). (2001). Global impact of innovations on chronic disease in the genomics era. *The Pfizer Journal* (Global ed.), *11*(2), 1–36.

Hurley, A. C., Gauthier, M. A., Horvath, K. J., Harvey, R., Smith, S. J., Trudeau, S., et al. (2004). Promoting safer home environments for persons with Alzheimer's disease: The home safety/injury model. *Journal of Gerontological Nursing, 30*(6), 43–51.

Imamura, E. (2002). Amy's chat room: Health promotion programmes for community dwelling elderly. *International Journal of Nursing Practice, 8,* 61–64.

Immunization Services Division, National Immunization Program. (2005). Influenza vaccination levels among persons aged > 65 years and among persons aged 18–64 years with high-risk conditions—United States, 2003. *Morbidity and Mortality Weekly Report, 54,* 1045–1049.

International Foundation for Functional Gastrointestinal Disorders. (2003). *Prevalence of bowel incontinence.* Retrieved March 15, 2006, from http://www.aboutincontinence.org/prevalence.html

International Foundation for Functional Gastrointestinal Disorders. (2006a). *Common causes of bowel incontinence.* Retrieved March 15, 2006, from http://www.aboutincontinence.org/causes.html

International Foundation for Functional Gastrointestinal Disorders. (2006b). *Treatment for bowel incontinence.* Retrieved March 15, 2006, from http://www.aboutincontinence.org/treatment.html

Jansson, W., Nordberg, G., & Grafstrom, M. (2001). Patterns of elderly spousal caregiving in dementia care: An observational study. *Journal of Advanced Nursing, 34,* 804–812.

Johnson, B. K. (2004). Sexuality and heart disease: Implications for nursing. *Geriatric Nursing, 25,* 224–226.

Kannus, P., Parkkari, J., Niemi, S., & Palvanen, M. (2005). Fall-induced deaths among elderly people. *American Journal of Public Health, 95,* 422–424.

Kather, T. A. (2005). Colorectal cancer: Guidelines for prevention, screening and treatment. *Advance for Nurses, 20*(5), 15–17.

Kleespies, P. M. (2004). *Life and death decisions: Psychological and ethical considerations in end-of-life care.* Washington, DC: American Psychological Association.

Klein, R., Stoll, K., & Bruce, A. (2004). *Medicaid: Good medicine for state economies, 2004 update.* Retrieved August 30, 2004, from http://www.familiesusa.org

Kolanowski, A. M., Fick, D., Waller, J. L., & Shea, D. (2004). Spouses of persons with dementia: Their healthcare problems, utilization, and costs. *Research in Nursing & Health, 27,* 296–306.

Kwong, E. W.-Y., & Kwan, A. Y.-H. (2004). Stress management methods of the community-dwelling elderly in Hong Kong: Implications for tailoring a stress-reduction program. *Geriatric Nursing, 25,* 102–106.

Laakkonen, M.-L., Pitkala, K. H., Strandberg, T. E., Berglind, S., & Tilvis, R. S. (2004). Living will, resuscitation preferences, and attitudes towards life in an aged population. *Gerontology, 50,* 247–254.

Last Acts. (2002). *Means to a better end.* Retrieved January 29, 2003, from http://www.lastacts.org/files/misc/meansfull.pdf

Lee, S., Colditz, G., Berkman, L., & Kawachi, I. (2003). Caregiving to children and grandchildren and risk of coronary heart disease among women. *American Journal of Public Health, 93,* 1939–1944.

Lee, W. K. M., & Law, K., W.-K. (2004). Retirement planning and retirement satisfaction: The need for a national retirement program and policy in Hong Kong. *Journal of Applied Gerontology, 23,* 212–233.

Leenerts, M. H., Teel, C. S., & Pendleton, M. K. (2002). Building a model of self-care for health promotion in aging. *Journal of Nursing Scholarship, 34,* 355–361.

Levine, C., Hunt, G. G., Halper, D., Hart, A. Y., Lautz, J., & Gould, D. A. (2005). Young adult caregivers: A first look at an unstudied population. *American Journal of Public Health, 95,* 2071–2075.

Lewis, I. D., & McBride, M. (2004). Anticipatory grief and chronicity: Elders and families in racial/ethnic minority groups. *Geriatric Nursing, 25,* 44–47.

Lewis, S. J. (2004, July, Supplement). After menopause: Novel marker helps to identify women at risk for heart disease. *Journal of Family Practice,* S18–S24.

Logue, R. M. (2002). Self-medication and the elderly: How technology can help. *American Journal of Nursing, 102*(7), 51–55.

Loughlin, A. (2004). Depression and social support: Effective treatments for homebound elderly adults. *Journal of Gerontological Nursing, 20*(5), 11–15.

Magnusson, L., & Hanson, E. (2005). Supporting frail older people and their family carers at home using information and communication technology: Cost analysis. *Journal of Advanced Nursing, 51,* 645–657.

Mahan, D. (2004). *Sticker shock: Rising prescription drug prices for seniors.* Retrieved August 30, 2004, from http://www.familiesusa.org

Malavolta, M., Mocchegiani, E., & Bertoni-Freddari, C. (2004). New trends in biomedical aging research. *Gerontology, 50,* 420–424.

Manly, J. J., & Mayeux, R. (2004). Ethnic differences in dementia and Alzheimer's disease. In N. B. Anderson, R. A. Bulatao, & B. Cohen (Eds.), *Critical perspectives on racial and ethnic differences in health in late life* (pp. 95–141). Washington, DC: National Academies Press.

Matesa, J. (2002, November). Barriers to hospice care and some proposed policy solutions. *State Initiatives in End-of-life Care, 17,* 1–8.

Matthews, J. T., Dunbar-Jacob, J., Sereika, S., Schulz, R., & McDowell, B. J. (2004). Preventive health practices: Comparison of family caregivers 50 and older. *Journal of Gerontological Nursing, 30*(2), 46–54.

McGarry, J., & Arthur, A. (2001). Informal caring in late life: A qualitative study of the experiences of older carers. *Journal of Advanced Nursing, 33,* 182–189.

McLeer, S. V. (2004). Mental health services. In H. S. Sultz & K. M. Young, *Health care USA: Understanding its organization and delivery* (4th ed., pp. 335–366). Sudbury, MA: Jones and Bartlett.

Meeks-Sjostrom, D. (2004). A comparison of three measures of elder abuse. *Journal of Nursing Scholarship, 36,* 247–250.

Merrell, J., Kinsella, F., Murphy, F., Philpin, S., & Ali, A. (2005). Support needs of carers of dependent adults from a Bangladeshi community. *Journal of Advanced Nursing, 51,* 549–557.

Miller, C. A. (2004a). Getting older adults through the maze of Medicare prescription drug benefits. *Geriatric Nursing, 25,* 190–191.

Miller, C. A. (2004b). Teaching older adults medication self-care. *Geriatric Nursing, 25,* 318–319.

Minardi, H. A., & Blanchard, M. (2004). Older people with depression: A pilot study. *Journal of Advanced Nursing, 46,* 23–32.

Mitty, E. L. (2001). Ethnicity and end-of-life decision-making. *Reflections in Nursing Leadership, 27*(1), 28–31.

Moeller, J. F., Miller, G. E., & Banthin, J. S. (2004). Looking inside the nation's medicine cabinet: Trends in outpatient drug spending by Medicare beneficiaries, 1997 and 2001; Costly new drugs do have an impact on overall drug spending. *Health Affairs, 23,* 217–225.

Moos, R. H., Brennan, P. L., Schutte, K. K., & Moos, B. S. (2004). High-risk alcohol consumption and late-life alcohol use problems. *American Journal of Public Health, 94,* 1985–1991.

Mouton, C. P., Rodabough, R. J., Rovi, S. L. D., Hunt, J. L., Talamantes, M. A., Brzyski, R. G., et al. (2004). Prevalence and 3-year incidence of abuse among postmenopausal women. *American Journal of Public Health, 94,* 605–612.

Murtaugh, K. N., & Hubert, H. B. (2004). Gender differences in physical disability among an elderly cohort. *American Journal of Public Health, 94,* 1406–1411.

N. A. (2005). Husband fatigue. *The Week, 5*(231), 11.

National Center for Chronic Disease Prevention and Health Promotion. (2002a). *A national public health initiative on diabetes and women's health.* Retrieved October 2, 2002, from http://www.cdc.gov/diabetes/pubs/interim/background.htm

National Center for Chronic Disease Prevention and Health Promotion. (2002b). Prevalence of health-care providers asking older adults about their physical activity levels—United States, 1998. *Morbidity and Mortality Weekly Report, 51,* 412–414.

National Center for Health Statistics. (2005a). Average number of bed days during the preceding 12 months among persons aged >18 years, by age group—United States, 2003. *Morbidity and Mortality Weekly Report, 54,* 803.

National Center for Health Statistics. (2005b). *Health, United States, 2005 with chartbook on trends in the health of Americans.* Retrieved December 23, 2005, from http://www.cdc.gov/nchs/data/hus/hus05.pdf

National Center for Health Statistics. (2005c). Percentage of adults who reported being deaf or having a lot of trouble hearing without a hearing aid, by sex and age group—United States, 2003. *Morbidity and Mortality Weekly Report, 54,* 635.

National Center for Health Statistics. (2005d). Percentage of hospital discharges and days of care, by age group—United States, 2003. *Morbidity and Mortality Weekly Report, 54,* 584.

National Center for Injury Prevention and Control. (2003). Nonfatal physical assault-related injuries among persons aged >60 years treated in hospital emergency departments—United States, 2001. *Morbidity and Mortality Weekly Report, 52,* 812–816.

National Center for Injury Prevention and Control. (2005a). Homicide and suicide rates—National Violent Death Reporting System, six states, 2003. *Morbidity and Mortality Weekly Report, 54,* 377–380.

National Center for Injury Prevention and Control. (2005b). *Older adult drivers: Fact sheet.* Retrieved June 9, 2005, from http://www.cdc.gov/ncipc/factsheets/older.htm

National Center on Birth Defects and Developmental Disabilities. (2005). *Women with disabilities.* Retrieved June 6, 2005, from http://www.cdc.gov/ncbddd/wwomen/default.htm

National Digestive Diseases Information Clearinghouse. (2004). *Fecal incontinence.* Retrieved March 15, 2006, from http://digestive.niddk.nih.gov/ddiseases/pubs/fecalincontinence/

National Heart, Lung, and Blood Institute. (2003). *Chronic obstructive pulmonary disease.* Retrieved March 16, 2006, from http://www.nhbli.nih.gov/public/lung/other/COPD-fact.pdf

National Institute on Aging. (2002). *Alzheimer's disease: Unraveling the mystery.* Washington, DC: U.S. Department of Health and Human Services.

National Institute on Aging. (2004). *Working with your older patient: A clinician's handbook.* Bethesda, MD: Author.

National Institute for Environmental Health Sciences. (2006). *Elderly have higher risk for cardiovascular, respiratory disease from fine particle pollution.* Retrieved March 16, 2006, from http://www.nih.gov/news/pr/mar2006/niehs-08.htm

Naylor, M. (2003). Delirium, depression often overlooked. *American Journal of Nursing, 103*(5), 116.

Neher, J. O. (2004). Clinical commentary. *Journal of Family Practice, 53,* 310.

Newacheck, P. W., & Benjamin, A. E. (2004). Intergenerational equity and public spending; The United States should embrace a new doctrine of fairness to ensure that vulnerable populations are not forced to compete for resources. *Health Affairs, 23,* 142–146.

Okabayashi, H., Liang, J., Krause, N., Akiyama, H., & Sugisawa, H. (2004). Mental health among older adults in Japan: Do sources of social support and negative interaction make a difference? *Social Science & Medicine, 59,* 2259–2270.

Orhon, A. (2002). Elder abuse: Mistreatment of older Americans on the rise. *NurseWeek, 15*(23), 22–23.

Østbye, T., Taylor, D. H. Jr., Yancy, W. S. Jr., & Krause, K. M. (2005). Associations between obesity and receipt of screening mammography, Papanicolaou tests, and influenza vaccination: Results from the Health and Retirement Study (HRS) and the Asset and Health Dynamics Among the Oldest Old (Ahead) study. *American Journal of Public Health, 95,* 1623–1630.

Partnership for Prevention. (2003). *A better Medicare for healthier seniors: Recommendations to modernize Medicare's prevention policies.* Retrieved July 25, 2003, from http://www.prevent.org

Phillips, B. B. (2004). Skip to the loo, my darlin': Urinary incontinence 1850–present. *Geriatric Nursing, 25,* 74–80.

Pinkelman, M. A. (2002). Search for consensus: Prostate. *Community Health Forum, 3*(5), 17–19.

Plese, N. K. (Ed.). (2002). At peace with dying: A healthy approach to the end of life. *The Pfizer Journal, 6*(2), 1–36.

Plese, N. K. (Ed.). (2005a). A profile of caregiving in America (2nd ed.) *The Pfizer Journal, IX*(4), 1–40.

Plese, N. K. (Ed.). (2005b). Global summit on the aging workforce. *The Pfizer Journal, IX*(3), 1–40.

Pricewaterhousecooper's Health Research Institute. (2005). *Acts of charity: Charity care strategies for hospitals in a changing landscape.* Retrieved December 27, 2005, from http://healthcare.pwc.com/cgi-local/hcregister .cgi?link=reg/charitycare.pdf&update=true

Qualls, C. D., Harris, J. L., & Rogers, W. A. (2002). Cognitive-linguistic aging: Considerations for home health care interventions. In W. A. Rogers & A. D. Fisk (Eds.), *Human factors interventions for the health care of older adults* (pp. 47–67). Mahwah, NJ: Lawrence Erlbaum Associates.

Rennard, S. I. (2005). *Patient information: Overview of the management of COPD.* Retrieved March 16, 2006, from http:patients .uptodate.com/print.asp?print=true&file=lung_dis/4567

Resnick, B. (2004). Encouraging exercise in older adults with congestive heart failure. *Geriatric Nursing, 25,* 204–211.

Resnick, B. (2005). Exercise for older adults. *Advance for Nurses, 2*(4), 19–21.

Robbins, R., Rausch, K. J., Garcia, R. I., & Prestwood, K. M. (2004). Multicultural medication

adherence: A comparative study. *Journal of Gerontological Nursing, 30*(7), 25–32.

Robitaille, Y., Laforest, S., Fournier, M., Gauvin, L., Parisien, M., Corriveau, H., et al. (2005). Moving forward in fall prevention: An intervention to improve balance among older adults in real-world settings. *American Journal of Public Health, 95,* 2049–2056.

Rose, M. A. (2004). Planning HIV education programs for older adults: Cultural implications. *Journal of Gerontological Nursing, 30*(3), 34–39.

Rosenfeld, P., & Harrington, C. (2003). Hospital care for the elderly. *American Journal of Nursing, 103*(5), 115.

Safran, D. G., Neuman, T., Schoen, C., Kitchman, M. S., Wilson, I., Cooper, B., et al. (2005). *Prescription drug coverage and seniors: Findings from a 2003 national survey.* Retrieved August 13, 2005, from http://www.cmwf.org/publications/publications_show.htm?doc_id=273944

Samelson, E. J., Zhang, Y., Kiel, D. P., Hannan, M. T., & Felson, D. T. (2002). Effect of birth cohort on risk of hip fracture: Age-specific incidence rates in the Framingham study. *American Journal of Public Health, 92,* 858–862.

Sandison, R., Gray, M., & Reid, D. (2004). Lifestyle factors for promoting bone health in older women. *Journal of Advanced Nursing, 45,* 603–610.

Saxon, S. V., & Etten, M. J. (2002). *Physical change & aging: A guide for the helping professions* (4th ed.). New York: Tiresias Press.

Schlenk, E. A., Dunbar-Jacob, J., & Engberg, S. (2004). Medication non-adherence among older adults: A review of strategies and interventions for improvement. *Journal of Gerontological Nursing, 30*(7), 33–43.

Schneider, J. K., Mercer, G. T., Herning, M., Smith, C. A., & Prysak, M. D. (2004). Promoting exercise behavior in older adults: Using a cognitive behavioral intervention. *Journal of Gerontological Nursing, 30*(4), 45–53.

Seymour, J., Gott, M., Bellamy, G., Ahmedzai, S. H., & Clark, D. (2004). Planning for the end of life: The views of older people about advance care statements. *Social Science & Medicine, 59,* 57–68.

Shepherd, A. J. (2004). An overview of osteoporosis. *Alternative Therapies, 10*(2), 26–33.

Shreffler-Grant, J., Weinert, C., Nichols, E., & Ide, B. (2005). Complementary therapy use among older rural adults. *Public Health Nursing, 22,* 323–331.

Son, G.-R., Therrien, B., & Whall, A. (2002). Implicit memory and familiarity among elders with dementia. *Journal of Nursing Scholarship, 34,* 263–267.

Tabloski, P. A. (2006). *Gerontological nursing.* Upper Saddle River, NJ: Pearson.

Tanner, E. (2004). Chronic illness demands for self-management in older adults. *Geriatric Nursing, 25,* 313–317.

Taylor, D. H. Jr., Hasselblad, V., Henley, S. J., Thun, M. J., & Sloan, F. A. (2002). Benefits of smoking cessation for longevity. *American Journal of Public Health, 92,* 990–996.

Teunissen, T. A. M., de Jonge, A., van Weel, C., & Lagro-Janssen, A. L. M. (2004). Treating urinary incontinence in the elderly—Conservative measures that work: A systematic review. *Journal of Family Practice, 53,* 25–32.

Turcu, A., Toubin, S., Mourey, F., D'Athis, P., Manckoundia, P., & Pfitzenmeyer, P. (2004). Falls and depression in older people. *Gerontology, 50,* 303–308.

U.S. Census Bureau. (2004a). *Health insurance coverage: 2003.* Retrieved September 30, 2004, from http://www.census.gov

U.S. Census Bureau. (2004b). *Poverty: 2003 highlights.* Retrieved September 30, 2004, from http://www.census.gov

U.S. Census Bureau. (2005). *Statistical abstract of the United States, 2004–2005.* Retrieved May 5, 2005, from http://www.census.gov/prod/2004pubs/04statab

U.S. Department of Health and Human Services. (2000). *Healthy people 2010* (Conference edition, in two volumes). Washington, DC: Author.

U.S. Preventive Services Task Force. (2005a). *The guide to clinical preventive services, 2005.* Retrieved August 13, 2005, from http://www.ahrq.gov/clinic/pocketguide.htm

U.S. Preventive Services Task Force. (2005b). *Screening for abdominal aortic aneurysm.* Retrieved August 13, 2005, from http://www.ahrq.gov/clinic/uspstf/uspsaneu.htm

Validation Training Institute. (2003). *What is validation?* Retrieved March 16, 2006, from http://www.vfvalidation.org/whatis.html

Vellone, E., Sansoni, J., & Cohen, M. Z. (2002). The experience of Italians caring for family members with Alzheimer's disease. *Journal of Nursing Scholarship, 34,* 323–329.

Vivarai-Dresler, G., & Bakker, D. A. (2004). Blood pressure monitoring: Older adults' perceptions. *Journal of Gerontological Nursing, 30*(1), 44–52.

Vogel, C. (2003). Dementia: Prompt detection, family education make the difference. *NurseWeek, 16*(8), 21–22.

Wang, H.-H. (2001). A comparison of two models of health-promoting lifestyle in rural elderly Taiwanese women. *Public Health Nursing, 18,* 204–211.

Weeks, S. K., McGann, P. E., Michaels, T. K., & Penninx, B. W. J. H. (2003). Comparing various short-form geriatric depression scales leads to the GDS-5/15. *Journal of Nursing Scholarship, 35,* 133–137.

Wells, Y., Foreman, P., Gething, L., & Petralia, W. (2004). Nurses' attitudes toward aging and older adults: Examining attitudes and practices among health services providers in Australia. *Journal of Gerontological Nursing, 30*(9), 5–13.

Wiebe, C. (2004). Drug import programs defy federal warnings, reap benefits. *Medscape Business of Medicine, 5*(2). Retrieved October 13, 2005, from http://www.medscape.com/viewarticle/490299

Williams, A., & Jester, R. (2005). Delayed surgical fixation of fractured hips in older people: Impact on mortality. *Journal of Advanced Nursing, 52,* 63–69.

Williams, J. R. (2004). Gerontological nurse practitioner care guidelines: Sleep management in elderly patients. *Geriatric Nursing, 25,* 310–312.

Williams, K., Kemper, S., & Hummert, M. L. (2004). Enhancing communication with older adults: Overcoming elderspeak. *Journal of Gerontological Nursing, 30*(10), 17–25.

Williams, M. E. (2005). *Physical diagnosis in elderly people.* Retrieved April 24, 2005, from http://www.medscape.com/viewprogram/3955_pnt

Wooten, J., & Galavis, J. (2005). Polypharmacy: Keeping the elderly safe. *RN, 68*(8), 44–50.

World Health Organization. (2004). *The world health report 2004.* Geneva, Switzerland: Author.

World Health Organization. (2005). *World health report 2005: Make every mother and child count.* Retrieved December 16, 2005, from http://www.who.int/why/2005/annexesen.pdf

Yan, E. C.-W., & Tang, C. S.-K. (2004). Elder abuse by caregivers: A study of prevalence and risk factors in Hong Kong Chinese families. *Journal of Family Violence, 19,* 269–277.

Yoon, S.-J. L, & Horne, C. (2001). Herbal products and conventional medicines used by community-residing older women. *Journal of Advanced Nursing, 33,* 51–59.

Yoon, S. L., & Horne, C. (2004). Perceived health promotion practices by older women: Use of herbal products. *Journal of Gerontological Nursing, 30*(7), 9–15.

You, L., Deans, C., Liu, K., Zhang, M. F., & Zhang, J. (2004). Rising awareness of fall risk among Chinese older adults: Use of the home fall hazards assessment tool. *Journal of Gerontological Nursing, 30*(6), 35–42.

Yuan, Z., Dawson, N., Cooper, G. S., Einstadter, S., Cebul, R., & Rimm, A. A. (2001). Effects of alcohol-related disease on hip fracture and mortality: A retrospective cohort study of hospitalized Medicare beneficiaries. *American Journal of Public Health, 91,* 1089–1093.

Zerwekh, J. V. (2006). *Nursing care at the end of life: Palliative care for patients and families.* Philadelphia: F. A. Davis.

Zhan, L. (2004). Caring for family members with Alzheimer's disease. *Journal of Gerontological Nursing, 30*(8), 19–29.

Zhan, L., & Chen, J. (2004). Medication practices among Chinese American older adults: A study of cultural influences. *Journal of Gerontological Nursing, 30*(4), 24–33.

Meeting the Needs of Poor and Homeless Populations

Advocacy in Action

Safe at Home

Homeless women and children face a variety of challenges in their lives and do not need to experience any further risks to their health. However, students working in a group of homes for homeless women and their children noted a number of safety hazards that put the children, in particular, at risk of injury. Each of the homes had been a single-family dwelling but now housed three or four homeless women and many young children.

Most of the women were attempting to escape abusive situations and often did not have the knowledge or energy to engage in childproofing the homes. In addition, the staff was not always aware of structural safety hazards present in the homes. The students decided that safety was a significant issue that they could address. They began by assessing the safety hazards in the seven homes. All the homes had fenced play areas for the children, but in some of them the surface below the play areas was hard and in others play equipment was in poor repair and presented several safety hazards. Inside the homes, there were a number of other safety hazards. The women frequently left medications and sharp utensils within easy reach of small children. Cleansers and other toxic materials were in easy reach, and there were no outlet covers or latches on the cabinet doors. Most of the mothers had little knowledge of home safety or potential hazards.

Based on their assessment, the students undertook a number of initiatives. They created a home safety training manual for each house and conducted safety education classes for the mothers living there. In addition, they obtained donations of outlet covers and cabinet latches from local merchants that they installed in each house. They also alerted the agency responsible for the homes regarding the play area and equipment hazards, and the administrator was able to get a local construction company to redesign the outdoor areas, put in safe play surfaces, and construct safe play equipment. With the safety training manual, agency staff were able to orient subsequent residents to safety issues in the homes, and the project took on a life of its own.

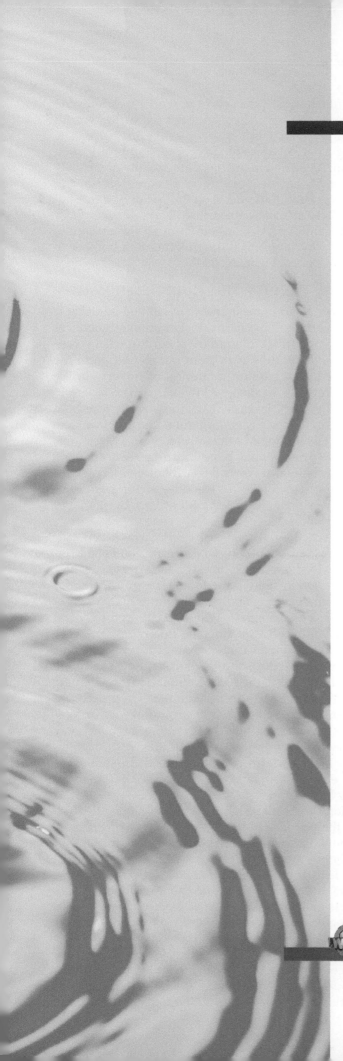

Meeting the Needs of Poor and Homeless Populations

CHAPTER OBJECTIVES

After reading this chapter, you should be able to:

1. Analyze the effects of factors contributing to poverty and homelessness.
2. Identify biophysical, psychological, physical environmental, sociocultural, behavioral, and health system factors that influence the health of poor and homeless clients.
3. Describe approaches to primary prevention of homelessness and analyze related roles of community health nurses with respect to each.
4. Identify major areas of emphasis in primary prevention of health problems in poor and homeless clients.
5. Identify areas in which secondary preventive interventions may be required in the care of poor and homeless individuals and analyze the role of the community health nurse in these interventions.
6. Identify strategies for tertiary prevention of poverty and homelessness at the aggregate level.
7. Describe considerations in implementing care for poor and homeless individuals.
8. Identify the primary focus of evaluation for care of poor and homeless clients.

KEY TERMS

criminalization
deindustrialization
deinstitutionalization
gentrification
homeless individual
means-tested income transfers
noninstitutionalization
poverty
safe havens
structural unemployment
worst-case housing

 MediaLink
http://www.prenhall.com/clark

Additional interactive resources for this chapter can be found on the Companion Website. Click on Chapter 20 and "Begin" to select the activities for this chapter.

As we have seen in several previous chapters, sociocultural factors play a significant role in determining the health status of population groups. The health-related effects and community health nursing roles with respect to two interrelated sociocultural factors, poverty and homelessness, are explored in detail in this chapter.

OVERVIEW OF POVERTY AND HOMELESSNESS

In 1948, the United Nations General Assembly adopted the Universal Declaration of Human Rights, which stated that "everyone has the right to a standard of living adequate for the health and well-being of himself and his family, including food, clothing, housing, and medical care social services, and to the right to security in the event of unemployment, sickness, disability, widowhood, old age, or other lack of livelihood in circumstances beyond his control" (cited in Thiele, 2002, p. 712). The following year, in the United States, the Housing Act of 1949 proposed "the realization as soon as feasible of the goal of a decent home and suitable living environment for every American family" (cited in Freeman, 2002, p. 709). To further the objectives of these two pieces of legislation, the World Health Organization developed six *Health Principles of Housing* as follows. Healthful housing:

- protects against communicable diseases through access to a safe water supply, sanitary disposal of excreta and solid wastes, drainage of surface water, support for personal and domestic hygiene, safe food protection, and structural safeguards against disease transmission
- protects against injury, chronic disease, and poisoning by means of safe construction materials, structural safety, ventilation and light, and absence of exposure to hazardous conditions or substances
- reduces psychological and social stress
- provides an improved housing environment
- supports informed use of housing
- protects populations at risk (Thiele, 2002)

The responsibility of governments with respect to housing were further delineated in the core principles of housing justice emphasized by the National Coalition for the Homeless (2005n). These principles include the right of every person to basic economic rights, including housing; the responsibility of society to meet housing needs; the need for economic and social support for adequate housing; the right of homeless individuals to services and programs provided to housed individuals; the need for tailored services and programs to meet the needs of people without adequate housing; and the right to equal access to housing regardless of one's life circumstances. The final principle of the Coalition is that provision of universal access to adequate housing is a measure of an effective society.

Unfortunately, many of the world's societies do not achieve these principles of housing justice. Worldwide, more than 1 billion people live in inadequate housing in urban areas alone (Population Information Program, 2003), and many more are literally or virtually homeless. Adequate housing is a community health concern because of its effects on the health of the population. These effects occur in three ways: through poor physical conditions of housing, through the absence of affordable housing, and through location of housing in unhealthy places (Freeman, 2002).

Defining Poverty and Homelessness

Both poverty and homelessness are defined in multiple ways. **Poverty** is "having insufficient money, goods, or means of support" (Wilton, 2004, p. 26), but what is considered *sufficient* may vary from one definition to the next. The most common definition of poverty in the United States is an income lower than the federally identified poverty level. In 2005, the poverty threshold for a family of four was an annual income less than $19,350 (Center for Medicaid and State Operations, 2005). The "near poor" have incomes 100% to 199% above the federal poverty level (National Center for Health Statistics, 2003). In Canada, poverty is determined by *low-income cut-offs* identified by Statistics Canada (Wilton, 2004).

Poverty may also be defined in terms of the percent of one's income spent on essential goods and services (e.g., food, shelter, clothing) or one's income relative to the median income in the local area. In Canada, for example, the poor generally spend more than 56.2% of their income on essentials (Wilton, 2004). In the context of the U.S. Rural Rental Housing Loan Program, very low income is defined as an income 50% below the area median income (AMI), and low-income households are below 50% to 80% of the AMI (National Coalition for the Homeless, 2005f). Measurable definitions of poverty are important because they often determine clients' eligibility for assistance programs. For example, eligibility may be restricted to individuals or families with incomes at or below the defined poverty level. In some programs, eligibility may be set at 100% or 150% above poverty level.

Homelessness also has multiple definitions, depending on the purpose of the definition. One of the most commonly used definitions is that posed by the Stewart B. McKinney Homeless Assistance Act of 1987, the first federal legislation in the United States dealing with the problem of homelessness. In the McKinney Act, a **homeless individual** is defined as a person who "lacks a fixed, regular, and adequate nighttime residence; and . . . has a primary residence that is: (a) a supervised publicly or privately operated shelter designed to provide temporary accommodations . . . (b) an institution that provides a temporary residence for individuals intended to be institutionalized, or (c) a public or private place not

*T*he World Health Organization Regional Office for Europe has described homelessness as "a complex concept embracing states of rooflessness, houselessness, living in insecure accommodation, or living in inadequate accommodation" (Wright & Tompkins, 2005, p. 2). The *roofless* include people without shelter, newly arrived immigrants, and those displaced by disaster or violence. Those who are *houseless* are living in temporary shelter, but also include those who are released from prisons, hospitals, or foster homes with nowhere to go. Those *living in insecure accommodation* include those doubled up with friends and family, as well as those who are in the process of being evicted and "squatters" who take up residence in areas not designed for human habitation (e.g., warehouses and city parks). Those who are *living in inadequate accommodation* include people living in overcrowded or substandard housing. Having a home is defined as "having an adequate dwelling (or space) over which a person and his/her family can exercise exclusive possession, being able to maintain privacy and enjoy social relations, and having a legal title to occupy" (p. 2).

Compare the WHO definition of homelessness to that used in the McKinney Act in the United States. What are the implications for determining the extent of homelessness? For determining eligibility for services designed to address the needs of homeless populations? How does the definition of having a home relate to the criminalization of homelessness seen in many jurisdictions in the United States?

designed for, or ordinarily used as, a regular sleeping accommodation for human beings" (National Coalition for the Homeless, 2005t, p. 1). Being homeless has also been defined as "having spent more than seven consecutive nights in a shelter or other non-dwelling" (Swigart & Kolb, 2004, p. 162). Unfortunately, these definitions fail to recognize the large segment of the population who are virtually homeless but are living doubled and tripled up with friends or family or who are living in substandard housing (National Coalition for the Homeless, 2005s). In various studies, anywhere from 46% to 82% of homeless families had been living with others just prior to becoming homeless, and a typical family may spend as long as 4 years doubled up with friends or family members (Bolland & McCallum, 2002).

A more inclusive definition that does include these populations as well as others (e.g., those living in hotels) is provided in the definition of homeless children and youth in the McKinney-Vento Act dealing with the education of homeless children and youth. In this legislation, homeless children and youth are

(a) individuals who lack a fixed, regular, and adequate nighttime residence . . . and (b) include (i) children and youth who are sharing the housing of other persons due to loss of housing, economic hardship, or a similar reason; are living in motels, hotels, trailer parks, or camping grounds due to lack of alternative adequate accommodations; are living in emergency or transitional shelters; are abandoned in hospitals; or are awaiting foster care placement; (ii) children and youth who have

a primary nighttime residence that is a public or private place not designed for or ordinarily used as a regular sleeping accommodation for human beings . . . (iii) children and youth who are living in cars, parks, public spaces, abandoned buildings, substandard housing, bus or train stations, or similar settings, and (iv) migratory children who qualify as homeless for purposes of this subtitle because the children are living in circumstances described in clauses (i) through (iii). (National Coalition for the Homeless, 2005t)

The Magnitude of Poverty and Homelessness

There are no exact figures on the number of poor or homeless persons in the United States. In 2003, 12.5% of all persons in the United States had incomes below poverty level, an increase from 12.1% in 2002. This amounts to 35.9 million people (U.S. Census Bureau, 2005). From 1982 to 1998, the income of the wealthiest 1% of the American population increased by 42%, whereas that for the poorest 40% decreased by 76% (Wise, 2004). Despite these figures, the median per capita income is highest in the Americas, at $15,850 per year. The poorest region is Africa, where the per capita income is only $560. Fewer than 5% of the population of the European Region lives in poverty, compared to 39% in the African Region. An estimated 70% of the world's extremely poor population is women (World Health Organization [WHO], 2003, 2005).

The relationship between poverty and homelessness is well established and is best conveyed by the following statement: "Being poor can mean that one is an illness, an accident, or a paycheck away from homelessness" (Bringing America Home, 2005e, p. 1). As with poverty, the exact number of homeless persons is unknown and, in fact, varies from one day to the next. The best estimate is that approximately 3.5 million people, including 1.35 million children, are homeless in the United States in any given year. These figures include approximately 1% of the total U.S. population (National Coalition for the Homeless, 2005o) and 6.3% of those in poverty (Milby, Schumacher, Wallace, Freedman, & Vuchinich, 2005). Approximately one tenth of these people are chronically homeless (Caton et al., 2005). The number of homeless people may be largely underestimated due to the failure to include those who are homeless for short periods of time, those who are housed with others, or those who are just invisible to officials (National Coalition for the Homeless, 2005s; Sherman & Redlener, 2003, p. 1).

Worldwide, 20 to 40 million urban families are homeless and many others live in temporary structures. Each year several million of the world's families are forcibly evicted from the places where they are living (Population Information Program, 2003). U.S. homelessness rates tripled between 1987 and 1997, and even though the number of shelter beds doubled in many locations and tripled in others, the need for shelter remains largely unmet (National Coalition for the Homeless, 2005o). In 2004, requests for shelter in 27 U.S. cities increased by 7%, and 32% of requests were denied due to lack of resources (National Coalition for the Homeless, 2005k).

An estimated 6.5% of all adults in the United States, or 12 million people, have been literally homeless at some time in their lives (Anderson & Rayens, 2004), and on any given night 500,000 to 700,000 persons may be homeless (Swigart & Kolb, 2004). Who are these homeless individuals? In 2003, 39% of the homeless were children under 18 years of age (National Coalition for the Homeless, 2005t). Approximately 42% of these children were under 6 years of age, and 20% were over 11 years of age. Half of these children have been homeless more than once, and 23% have been homeless three or more times (Clement, 2003). About 5% of the homeless are *unaccompanied youth*, "individuals under the age of eighteen who lack parental, foster, or institutional care" (National Coalition for the Homeless, 2005, p. 1). Between 500,000 and 1 million young people run away from home each year, and 200,000 may be on the streets at any one time (Clement, 2003).

Families are the fastest-growing segment of the homeless population, accounting for 40% of the urban homeless population in 2004 and a larger proportion of the homeless in rural areas (National Coalition for the Homeless, 2005k). The number of families represented among the urban homeless increased by 5% in only 2 years, and in rural areas, single mothers with children make up the bulk of the homeless population (Bringing America Home, 2005b). As noted by the National Coalition for the Homeless, "Homelessness is a devastating experience for families. It disrupts virtually every aspect of family life, damaging the physical and emotional health of family members, interfering with children's education and development, and frequently resulting in separation of family members" (2005k, p. 1). Members

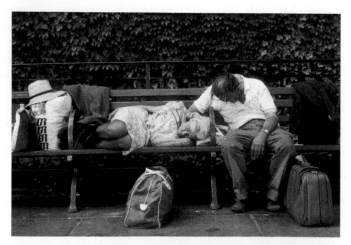

Due to overcrowding in shelters, many homeless individuals have no choice but to sleep outside. (© Andrew Holbrooke/The Image Works)

of ethnic minority groups are more likely to experience poverty and homelessness in urban areas than is the Caucasian population. Overall, African Americans comprise 49% of the homeless population, 35% are Caucasian, 13% Hispanic, 2% Native American, and 1% Asian. In a study in Philadelphia, 20% of African American women had been homeless sometime in the prior 7 years, compared to 4.8% of Hispanic women, 1.2% of Caucasian women, and 0.9% of Asian women (Webb, Culhane, Metraux, Robbins, & Culhane, 2003). In rural areas, on the other hand, homeless individuals and families are more likely to be Caucasian (National Coalition for the Homeless, 2005t). Homelessness in minority populations has been found to be more often due to external socioeconomic factors (e.g., poverty and unemployment) than to internal factors such as substance abuse (Cooke, 2004).

Another rapidly increasing segment of the homeless population is the elderly. For example, there was a 60% increase in the number of people over 55 years of age in Massachusetts shelters from 1999 to 2002. There is some debate regarding the age at which a homeless person should be considered elderly. Generally, however, 50 years of age is used as a cut-off because homeless people tend to age faster than the general population and a 50-year-old homeless individual may have a health status similar to that of a 70-year-old in the general population (National Coalition for the Homeless, 2005m). The increase in homelessness among the elderly is due, in large part, to the loss of affordable housing in the context of fixed incomes.

Older householders have approximately one chance in three of experiencing *worst-case housing*. **Worst-case housing** is defined as having an income below 50% of the area median income, being involuntarily displaced from housing, paying more than half of one's income for rent and utilities, or living in substandard housing (National Coalition for the Homeless, 2005k). Only 37% of very-low-income elderly receive federal housing assistance, and current Supplemental Security Income (SSI) benefits (an additional Social Security benefit for low-income elderly individuals) fall well below poverty level, and pay less than half of the fair market rent (FMR) in even the most generous states (National Coalition for the Homeless, 2005m).

Older homeless individuals are also less likely than others to request shelter due to fears of victimization. In one study, half of the older homeless persons responding had been robbed and one fourth had been assaulted in the previous year. Older homeless persons, like most elderly people, also tend to have more health problems than their younger counterparts and are less likely to be aware of eligibility for benefits and more likely to need assistance in navigating the social services system (National Coalition for the Homeless, 2005m).

U.S. veterans are another group that experience homelessness, accounting for roughly 23% of the total homeless population and 33% of homeless men.

According to Veterans Administration (VA) estimates, as many as 200,000 veterans may be homeless on any given night, and 529,000 to 840,000 veterans are homeless at some time during the year (National Coalition for Homeless Veterans, n.d.). Veterans have been found to be as much as three times more likely to become homeless than the general population (Nyamathi et al., 2004). Somewhat surprisingly, homelessness among veterans has not been linked to combat experience, but is associated with high rates of mental illness and addictive disorders. Approximately half of homeless veterans experience problems with substance abuse, and an estimated 45% experience mental illness (National Coalition for Homeless Veterans, n.d.). Homeless female veterans have been found to be even more likely than male veterans to have serious psychiatric disorders and less likely to be employed or to have addictive disorders (National Coalition for the Homeless, 2005l). Although the Veterans Administration provides services to more than 100,000 homeless veterans each year, at least 80% of the homeless veteran population is not served by the VA. A portion of this population is served by the more than 200 community-based veterans organizations across the country (National Coalition for Homeless Veterans, n.d.).

Epidemiologic Factors Affecting the Health of Poor and Homeless Populations

The epidemiology of poverty and homelessness has two aspects, factors that contribute to these conditions and factors that influence their effects on the health status of poor and homeless populations. Here we will examine both aspects in light of considerations in each of the dimensions of health.

Biophysical Considerations

Biophysical factors, in conjunction with factors in other dimensions, may lead to poverty and homelessness. Conversely, poverty and homelessness have serious consequences for biophysical health that vary with age and prior health status.

Certain health conditions may contribute to poverty and homelessness due to limited ability to work (Nielsen, Juon, & Ensminger, 2004). For example, people with HIV/AIDS are at greater risk for homelessness than the general population for a number of reasons. Hospitalization and excessive fatigue may interrupt employment, leading to loss of income and consequent inability to pay for housing. They may also experience discrimination and job loss due to their condition. In one study conducted in several cities, 44% to 50% of housed clients with HIV/AIDS feared becoming homeless due to inability to afford housing. In another study, 40% of 12,000 people with HIV/AIDS surveyed had been homeless at least once (National Coalition for the Homeless, 2005j).

Homeless individuals, particularly homeless youth, may also be at greater risk for HIV infection as a result of sexual abuse and exploitation and the practice of engaging in sex for money (Robertson et al., 2004). The median prevalence of HIV/AIDS in the homeless population is three times that in the general population, but may be as high as 62% in some subpopulations of the homeless. Homeless individuals with HIV/AIDS also tend to be sicker and have higher mortality rates than those with housing because of the additional stress of being homeless (National Coalition for the Homeless, 2005j). Homelessness, particularly among those with HIV/AIDS, also increases the risk of tuberculosis (TB), due to crowded conditions in shelters, and homeless individuals with TB usually have more advanced disease than their housed counterparts (National Coalition for the Homeless, 2005j).

Poverty has long been linked to ill health. One measure of this link is the number of days of activity limitation experienced due to illness. From 1993 to 2001, 15% of Americans with annual incomes under $15,000 experienced 14 or more days of activity limitation, compared to only 6.2% of those with incomes over $50,000 (Zahran et al., 2005).

The health effects of poverty and homelessness are exacerbated for both the young and the elderly. For example, homeless children are twice as likely as other children to report fair or poor health and four times more likely to experience developmental delays (Bringing America Home, 2005d). In addition, homeless children are two to six times more likely than other children to have asthma and twice as likely to experience lead poisoning. They also have a higher incidence of dental problems, poor nutrition, anemia, ear infection, upper respiratory infection and bronchitis, diarrhea, skin conditions, accidental injuries, obesity, and failure to thrive (Clement, 2003; Sherman & Redlener, 2003). Homeless children are also less likely to be up to date on immunizations. For example, in one study, only 11% of sheltered adolescents were adequately immunized (Ensign, 2001). Homeless adolescents often experience sexually transmitted diseases (STDs) and pregnancy. Approximately 80% of homeless youth are sexually active before 15 years of age. They have incidence rates for HIV infection two to ten times higher than other teenagers and are also at risk for hepatitis B. Other health problems common in this

EVIDENCE-BASED PRACTICE

Characteristics of homeless populations and the factors contributing to their homelessness vary from one geographic locale to the next. Solutions to the problem of homelessness must be based on causes specific to the local area. How might you go about determining the extent and causes of homelessness in your own area? Who comprises the homeless population in your area and what are their health needs? What needs for primary, secondary, and tertiary prevention are evident in your local homeless population?

population include skin conditions, injuries, dental problems, and poor nutrition (Clement, 2003).

Health problems common among homeless adults include asthma, bronchitis, hypertension, heart disease, peptic ulcer, cancer, arthritis, diabetes, and STDs (Wilson, 2004). Other frequently noted problems include malnutrition and TB and other respiratory diseases, due to the lack of housing and overcrowding in shelters (Krieger & Higgins, 2002). Homeless individuals tend to experience higher mortality from most causes than does the housed population (Wilde, Albanese, Rennells, & Bullock, 2004). Additional problems include frostbite, leg ulcers, liver disease, peripheral vascular disease, hepatitis C, vision problems, skin conditions, and trauma due to accidental injury and assault (Kushel, Perry, Bangsberg, Clark, & Moss, 2002; National Coalition for the Homeless, 2005h; Swigart & Kolb, 2004). As we can see from this list of common conditions, homeless persons often suffer multiple acute and chronic conditions that require long-term treatment and monitoring that is difficult in circumstances of homelessness (National Coalition for the Homeless, 2005h). Inadequate diet and lack of access to medications and health care supplies make disease management difficult. In addition, survival stress experienced by many homeless persons may lead them to put health needs at a lower priority than basic survival needs (Archambault, 2002).

The elderly are at particular risk of health problems stemming from homelessness. All of the usual problems of the elderly are intensified by homelessness. The homeless elderly are particularly susceptible to the effects of communicable diseases, exposure, burns, and trauma due to alcohol use, physical or mental impairment, or assault. The elderly homeless population is also more likely than younger groups to experience chronic disability due to physical, mental, or emotional impairment.

Psychological Considerations

Psychological factors can lead to homelessness when people are unable to cope with the demands of daily life and have limited support systems. Family dynamics in the family of origin have been linked to homelessness in adulthood. In one study, for example, homeless women were less likely to have good support networks, were less likely to call on existing networks for assistance, and had networks that were less functional than stably housed women. Women who were unable to engage in reciprocal relationships or who reported conflictive relationships in childhood were at greater risk of homelessness. The authors noted the "significance of families of origin and learning how to develop and utilize support systems in preventing or reducing homelessness" and attributed increased vulnerability to homelessness as adults to the absence or inhibited development of abilities to interact effectively with support systems (Anderson & Rayens, 2004).

Mental illness is another psychological factor that contributes to homelessness. Estimates of the extent of psychiatric illness in the homeless population vary, but best estimates suggest that 20% to 25% of the homeless population experiences severe mental illness (National Coalition for the Homeless, 2005r), and 45% of homeless veterans have psychiatric diagnoses (Nyamathi et al., 2004). Some authors note that these figures only take into account homeless individuals with serious diagnoses and fail to account for many other mental health problems experienced by this population (Archambault, 2002). Others caution that the prevalence of mental illness in a specific homeless population changes over time and that intervention strategies need to address these changes (North, Eyrich, Pollio, & Spitznagel, 2004).

Mental illness interferes with one's ability to perform instrumental activities of daily living that permit one to remain adequately housed. In one study, 86% of the homeless individuals surveyed had a history of drug or alcohol problems or mental illness, and 30% experienced all three at some point in their lives (Wilde et al., 2004). Homeless clients with psychiatric illness are often noncompliant with therapeutic recommendations, exhibit more symptoms, and have higher rates of hospitalization for mental illness than housed persons with mental health problems (Caton et al., 2000).

Many authors cite the move to deinstitutionalize the mentally ill in the 1950s and 1960s as the cause of increasing homelessness among this population (Bohrer & Faulkner, 2004; McLeer, 2004). **Deinstitutionalization** was the process of discharging large numbers of mentally ill persons from mental institutions in an attempt to enable them to live in the least restrictive environment possible. This move was prompted by recognition of the appalling conditions prevalent in many institutions for the mentally ill. Although the intent of deinstitutionalization was laudable, the results were not. Unfortunately, there was no concurrent move to provide the community services needed for the mentally ill to live in noninstitutional settings, leaving them to fend for themselves. Other authors, however, point out that the increase in homeless mentally ill persons did not actually occur until the 1980s, when income and housing assistance programs for this population were withdrawn (National Coalition for the Homeless, 2005r). Loss of these socioeconomic supports prevented many mentally ill clients, prohibited from working by their disabilities, from being able to pay rent and resulted in their homelessness. In addition, the stigma of mental illness, combined with the stigma of homelessness, makes it more difficult for these individuals to obtain needed services (Bohrer & Faulkner, 2004).

Some homeless persons without preexisting mental illness exhibit psychological problems as a result of their homelessness. For example, data indicate that one third of homeless women have attempted suicide, compared to only one fourth of housed women (National Coalition for the Homeless, 2005k). Similarly, in one study, more than half of homeless adolescents had considered suicide (Clement, 2003). Homeless youth have also been found to have high rates of depression and conduct disorder, and rates of post-traumatic stress disorder (PTSD) are three times higher in this population than among adolescents in general (National Coalition for the Homeless, 2005p). Younger children's mental health is also affected by homelessness, and homeless children are more likely than their housed age mates to experience anxiety, depression, and withdrawal (Bringing America Home, 2005d). In addition, homelessness has been linked to child behavior problems, and fear of homelessness may lead to mental health problems in children (Krieger & Higgins, 2002).

Mental illness may also affect one's ability to escape homelessness. Homeless mentally ill individuals have been found to be homeless for longer periods of time than other homeless persons and to have less family contact, more barriers to employment, and more contact with the criminal justice system (National Coalition for the Homeless, 2005r). Conversely, good mental health, as evidenced in effective coping skills, has been linked to shorter episodes of homelessness (Caton et al., 2005).

Physical Environmental Considerations

Physical environmental factors also contribute to the effects of homelessness on health. Exposure to cold, even in the mildest climates, can lead to hypothermia (Clement, 2003). This is particularly true when people are lying on concrete or are clothed in wet garments. Overcrowding and poor sanitary conditions in shelters contribute to the spread of communicable diseases among a population that is already debilitated by exposure and poor nutritional status. As noted earlier, TB is rapidly spread in overcrowded shelter environments (Division of Applied Public Health Training, 2003).

Unsafe physical environments also present health hazards for young children. In addition to the potential for physical injury, the restrictions placed by parents on children's activities in unsafe surroundings may result in developmental delays.

Rural environments also pose physical environmental hazards for the poor and homeless due to the lack of available shelters and lack of access to assistance services. Rural poor and homeless individuals are more likely than members of the urban homeless population to live in a car, camper, or severely deteriorated housing (National Coalition for the Homeless, 2005s).

Sociocultural Considerations

Sociocultural dimension factors play a major role in the development of poverty and homelessness and in their effects on health. Lack of affordable housing, inadequate social support and welfare reform, mobility, and employment are some of the societal conditions that contribute to conditions of poverty and homelessness.

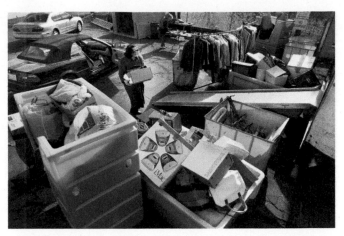

Thrift stores help the poor and the homeless to stretch their resources, but still may not meet all their needs. (Chip Somodevilla/Getty)

Other considerations to be addressed in this dimension include school attendance for homeless children and youth and considerations related to criminal justice, civil rights, and violence.

LACK OF AFFORDABLE HOUSING In addition to poverty, lack of affordable housing is the primary cause of homelessness in the United States. From 1973 to 1993, more than 2 million low-rental housing units disappeared from the housing market. Some were abandoned due to poor condition, others were demolished in the process of gentrification, and still others became unaffordable due to increases in rents. During the same period the number of households needing low-income housing increased significantly. From 1995 to 1997, the number of housing units renting for less than $300 per month declined by 19%, and between 1991 and 1995, the median rent for low-income housing increased by 21% (Bringing America Home, 2005b). Currently there is a gap of 4.4 million units between the available housing supply and the need for low-rent housing (National Coalition for the Homeless, 2005k), and it is estimated that an increase of 250,000 low-rent units would be needed each year for the next 20 years to meet the demand (Bringing America Home, 2005b).

Part of the loss of affordable housing stems from **gentrification**, which is defined as the displacement of low-income housing by higher-income space use such as luxury apartments, condominiums, or office buildings. Another aspect of the problem is the loss of many

BUILDING OUR KNOWLEDGE BASE

*L*ack of affordable housing is one of the primary factors contributing to homelessness in many areas of the United States. What strategies would you use to determine the availability of low-income housing in your area? How do housing costs compare to local wages for different subgroups in the community?

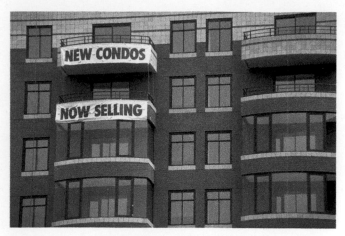

Single-room-occupancy hotels (SROs) that once provided low-cost shelter in many inner-city neighborhoods are being replaced by high-rent condominiums and luxury apartments. (© Rachel Epstein/The Image Works)

single-room occupancy (SRO) units in inner city areas. From 1970 to the mid-1980s, more than 1 million SROs were lost, many to the gentrification process in city center areas in large metropolitan settings. During this period, New York City lost an estimated 87% of downtown SRO units, Chicago lost all of its SROs, Los Angeles lost half, and San Francisco lost 43% (National Coalition for the Homeless, 2005a).

In rural areas homelessness is often precipitated by the occurrence of major structural or physical problems that make houses unsafe for human habitation. Approximately 30% of rural households in the United States, or 6.2 million households, have at least one major problem with housing. Housing availability in rural areas is also complicated by long distances to workplaces, lack of transportation, and insecure tenancy due to changes in local real estate markets (e.g., trailer park displacement by high-income single-family dwellings). Interestingly, many rural areas that are experiencing economic growth have the worst levels of low-income housing availability. When industry moves into an area, property values increase and so do rents, pricing out low-income residents (National Coalition for the Homeless, 2005s).

Worldwide, millions of people cannot afford housing that meets regulatory code standards. In addition, regulatory constraints control land acquisition and construction and do not foster development of low-income housing. In many parts of the world, it would take low-income families 15 to 30 years to be able to afford legal housing by saving 30% to 50% of their annual income (Population Information Program, 2003). Unfortunately, many people's incomes do not cover the basic necessities of life, much less allow for this level of savings.

POVERTY, SOCIAL SUPPORT, AND WELFARE REFORM The percentage of poor people in the U.S. population increased from 11.3% in 2000 to 12.1% in 2002, and the actual number of poor people increased by 4.3 million.

Increases in poverty stem from both declining wages and changes in public assistance programs. Since the 1980s income growth has not kept pace with rising housing costs. Family and individual incomes have declined while housing costs increased (National Coalition for the Homeless, 2005e; 2005o).

The American economy is increasingly divided into a highly paid skilled labor sector and a low-paid service sector (Freeman, 2002). In 1967, someone earning minimum wage could expect to support a family of three above poverty level. From 1981 to the 1990s, the federal minimum wage remained at $3.15 per hour, then increased in 1996 to $5.15 per hour. No increase in the minimum wage has been legislated at the federal level in the intervening years. Legislation in some states has increased the mandated minimum wage slightly beyond the federal minimum. Because of high rates of inflation, the real purchasing power of the minimum wage has decreased by 26% since 1979, and a full-time year-round employee receiving a federally defined minimum wage actually receives $1,778 less a year than the identified poverty level for a family of two. In no state, even those with the most generous minimum wage legislation, could one afford the fair market rent for a two-bedroom apartment. In fact, at the median state minimum wage, someone would need to work 87 hours per week to afford such an apartment at a cost of 30% of their monthly income, the federal definition of affordable housing (National Coalition for the Homeless, 2005e).

Many people, however, pay far more than 30% of their income for housing costs. In fact, 4.9 million households experience worst-case housing, paying more than 50% of their income for housing costs and having an income below 50% of the median for their geographic area. It is estimated that a minimum wage of $14.66 per hour would be required to enable a family to afford a two-bedroom home. This amount is nearly three times the current federal minimum wage and twice the minimum wage of any state (Bringing America Home, 2005e).

Changes in government programs to assist the poor have contributed to increased poverty and homelessness in two ways. First, the level of assistance provided has not kept pace with the rate of inflation. Consequently, individuals and families receiving aid fall deeper into poverty. Second, budgetary cutbacks have actually reduced benefits in some instances and stiffened eligibility requirements so that fewer of the working poor are eligible for aid. At the same time, taxes paid by the poor have increased. Some authors have noted a shift from welfare to "workfare" programs in the United States as well as in the United Kingdom and Canada (Wilton, 2004).

In 1996, the U.S. Congress passed the Personal Responsibility and Work Reconciliation Act, replacing the Aid to Families with Dependent Children (AFDC) program with the Temporary Aid to Needy Families (TANF) program, placing lifetime limits on receipt of

ETHICAL AWARENESS

You are visiting a formerly homeless client, a single mother with three children under 8 years of age. She has been in subsidized housing for only 3 months. She is now working, and you discover that she is making about $50 more than the maximum that allows her to qualify for her housing subsidy. You know that there is a long list of people who are waiting to obtain subsidized housing, many of whom are in worse straits than this mother. Will you report her increased income to the housing authorities? Why or why not?

benefits, and requiring recipients to be employed within 2 years of receiving benefits. The change also divorced Medicaid benefits from cash assistance programs. The intent of the legislation was to move recipients off the welfare rolls and to obtain gainful employment for them. TANF benefits and food stamps together, however, do not exceed the poverty level income in any state (National Coalition for the Homeless, 2005k). From 2000 to 2003, the number of poor children increased by 11%, yet the number of people receiving TANF benefits decreased by 9% (National Coalition for the Homeless, 2005k). Unfortunately, although many TANF recipients are finding employment, it is usually in low-paying jobs without benefits or sick leave, making it difficult for homeless women with children to provide adequately for their children. The federal legislation did not mandate support for childcare for working mothers, and although some states provide this assistance, many do not, making it even more difficult for low-income women to adequately care for dependent children.

Women on welfare are also more likely to have physical health problems than other women, and in 1997, as a result of welfare reforms, 675,000 people (including 400,000 children) lost access to federally funded health insurance (National Coalition for the Homeless, 2005h). In some studies, as many as 20% of

women previously on AFDC had chronic disabilities that limited their ability to work (Nielsen et al., 2004). Current and former welfare recipients have lower health status than the general population on several indicators, including glycosylated hemoglobin, blood pressure, body mass index, physical function, and smoking (Kaplan et al., 2005). Neither the health status nor the employability of many former AFDC recipients was considered in the design of welfare reforms.

Other federal programs that provided low-rent housing or housing subsidies to low-income individuals and families have also been cut. The U.S. federal government has ceased to build affordable housing and has actually demolished many older structures, replacing previous federal housing with housing vouchers intended to bridge the difference between an individual's or family's income and the cost of private rental (so called "section 8") housing. The point has been made, however, that housing vouchers may not be of much assistance in areas where low-income housing is scarce (Freeman, 2002). The average wait for section 8 housing is 24 months, but may be as long as 8 to 10 years in some areas (Sherman & Redlener, 2003).

Only about a third of poor renter households actually receive housing subsidies, and the availability of assistance is declining. For example, in 1976, 400,000 section 8 vouchers were authorized, but that number was reduced to 34,000 in 2003 (Bringing America Home, 2005b). Overall, federal housing support declined by 49% from 1980 to 2003 (National Coalition for the Homeless, 2005k). In addition, U.S. housing policies benefit the wealthy through mortgage interest tax deductions, reducing tax revenues that could help subsidize housing for the poor. It is estimated that the federal government loses $4 in income tax revenues for every $1 spent on housing assistance for the poor and homeless (Bringing America Home, 2005b). Federal housing assistance programs are summarized in Table 1♦.

TABLE 1	Federal Housing Assistance Programs	
Program	Focus	Eligibility/Requirements
Section 811. Supportive Housing for Persons with Disabilities Program	• Small group homes, independent living projects, multifamily housing developments	• Very-low-income persons with disabilities over 18 years of age • Families with at least one disabled member
Section 202. Supportive Housing for the Elderly Program	• Construction, rehabilitation, or acquisition of structures to serve as supportive housing • Provision of support activities • Rental assistance to cover difference between costs and income	• Very-low-income persons age 62 years and older
Section 8. Housing Choice Voucher Program	• Rental assistance through a voucher system that permits renters access to privately owned housing	• Very-low-income families, elderly and disabled individuals • Income cannot exceed 50% of median income of area

Continued on next page

TABLE 1	Federal Housing Assistance Programs *(continued)*	
		• Renters pay 30% of monthly income for rent and utilities
Section 8. Single-Room Occupancy	• Rehabilitation of existing structures to provide SRO units • Rental assistance to meet difference between cost and 30% of income • Rental assistance provided for 10-year period • May involve provision of some support services	• Very-low-income homeless individuals • Renters pay approximately 30% of income for rent • Rent must be equal to or less than 75% of HUD-established fair market rent (FMR) for an efficiency/studio unit
HOPE VI	• Destruction and replacement of public housing units or dramatic rehabilitation of existing units • Integration of low-income renters in middle-income areas • Provision of support services	• Intensive screening • Agreement to counseling and employment services
Public Housing	• Provision of rental housing to low-income families and individuals	• Low-income family, elderly, or disabled individual • U.S. citizen or eligible immigrant • Renters pay highest of (a) 30% of income, (b) 10% of monthly gross income, (c) shelter allowance, (d) locally determined minimum up to $50
Home Investment Partnerships Program	• Funding grants to states or communities to build, buy, or rehabilitate housing units for rental or ownership • Provision of rental assistance for occupants	• Local jurisdictions must contribute 25% match for funds • Income below 80% of area median
Section 502. Rural Home Ownership Direct Loan Program	• Loans to build, repair, renovate, or relocate houses (including mobile/manufactured homes) • Assistance with site purchase and water and sewage disposal arrangements	• Low- and very-low-income rural families without adequate housing • Able to afford mortgage payments, taxes, and insurance • 40% of funds must be used to serve families with incomes less than 50% of area median income
Section 515. Rural Rental Housing Loans	• Competitive mortgage loans to provide affordable rental housing • Provision of funds to buy and improve land and water and waste disposal systems	• Very-low-, low-, and moderate-income families, elderly, and disabled individuals • Renters pay higher of 30% of income or basic rent
Section 514/516. Farm Labor Housing Loans and Grants	• Loans and grants to buy, improve, or repair housing for farm laborers and those involved in aquaculture or on-farm processing	• U.S. citizens or permanent legal residents (temporary laborers, even if legally admitted, are not eligible) • Retired or disabled farm laborers living in such housing may remain there after retirement or disability

Data from: National Coalition for the Homeless. (2005). Federal housing assistance programs. Retrieved November 29, 2005, from http://www.nationalhomeless.org/publications/facts

MOBILITY Residential instability and population mobility are additional sociocultural factors that contribute to poverty and homelessness and to the lack of available social support systems. With the increasing mobility of the population, extended family members are often less available to help with material assistance. Extended family support may be hampered by international mobility as well as movement within states and nations.

CULTURAL COMPETENCE

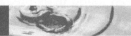

*H*omelessness is much less prevalent among some cultural groups than others (e.g., Muslims). Why do you think this might be the case? What other cultural groups do you think might exhibit similar protective factors for homelessness? How would you go about determining whether your assumption is correct?

Some homeless families and individuals may move to another location in an attempt to find work or housing. Approximately 70% of homeless families remain in the same general area, but the other 30% move (Clement, 2003). Loss of affordable housing may also mean moving to an area where shelter is available or moving from one shelter setting to another. As we will see later, this mobility poses difficulties in educating homeless children and youth.

A history of residential instability and mobility in childhood has also been linked to adult homelessness. Residential stability in childhood has been associated with both physical and mental health in middle adulthood. It has been hypothesized that residential stability permits the development of social capital and the ability to make social network connections that protect against homelessness later in life (Bures, 2003).

EMPLOYMENT Unemployment and underemployment are other major social factors contributing to homelessness. Although many people remain employed, there has been a shift in the job market from relatively well-paid manufacturing jobs to lower-paid employment in service industries (e.g., janitorial work). This phenomenon is referred to as **structural unemployment** or **deindustrialization** because it arises from changes in the nation's economic and occupational structure, such as the shifts from heavy to light industry and from manufacturing to technological occupations (Hirsch, Kett, & Trefil, 2002). In structural unemployment, jobs may be available, but those who are unemployed do not have the skills needed to qualify for them (Unemployment types, 2006). The emergence of high-technology occupations requires new sets of skills that many displaced workers do not have. Such changes in the structure of the job market have resulted in a situation in which 8.7 million people were unemployed in 2003 (U.S. Census Bureau, 2005).

The percentage of homeless people who are jobless varies from group to group. Overall, 42% of the homeless are employed, but many homeless individuals work at low-paying jobs that do not provide sufficient income to meet basic survival needs. An estimated 46% of jobs with the most growth from 1994 to 2005 provide incomes of less than $16,000 a year (Bringing America Home, 2005e). Many poor and homeless individuals are underemployed, a measure of those who are unemployed plus those who desire full-time work, but can only find part-time employment. Using this measure, in 2004, 9.9% of the U.S. population was underemployed, compared to an unemployment rate of 5.5%. In addition to declining real wages noted earlier, job security and stability have also declined, and displaced workers may have difficulty finding another job. Even when they do find work, however, many take jobs that pay an average of 13% less than former salaries. These workers also often find themselves in jobs that do not provide the benefits available from previous employment (National Coalition for the Homeless, 2005e).

Finding employment is difficult for most homeless individuals. Those with mental illness find it hard to maintain a job, if they can get one, because of their instability. Homeless single women with children, who account for almost half of homeless families, have problems of childcare while they work. In one study, for example, 30% of former welfare recipients reported having to leave work due to caregiving responsibilities (Kneipp, Castleman, & Gailor, 2004).

Even homeless persons with employable skills in areas where jobs are available may have difficulty negotiating the employment process. Lack of transportation may make it difficult to go to an interview or to get to work when a job is found. In addition, job application and interviews take time, which may prevent the individual from securing food or shelter for the night when these are obtained only after long waits in line in competition with many other homeless persons. Moreover, the homeless person may also find that he or she is penalized for working by reduction or even loss of assistance benefits and publicly financed health care coverage. Homeless individuals who cannot find regular work may engage in day labor or "shadow work." Shadow work may involve selling junk, personal possessions, or plasma; begging or panhandling; scavenging for food, salable goods, or money; and theft, all of which may carry criminal penalties in some jurisdictions (National Coalition for the Homeless, 2005q).

SCHOOL ATTENDANCE School attendance and its effects on school performance are other considerations affecting poor and homeless populations. In 2000, more than 930,000 children in kindergarten through 12th grade were homeless (Bringing America Home, 2005c). Frequent moves by homeless families result in frequent changes of school. Approximately 60% of U.S. children make an unscheduled school change between grades 1 and 12 (Kogut, 2004), often as a result of residential instability. It is estimated that every change results in the loss of 3 to 6 months of education. This affects school performance, and 23% of homeless children have repeated one or more grades (National Coalition for the Homeless, 2005d). In addition, homeless children and youth are four times more likely than their housed age mates to be below the 10th percentile in vocabulary and reading skills (Clement, 2003).

As noted by the National Coalition for the Homeless (2005d, p. 3), "School is one of the few stable, secure places in the lives of homeless children and youth—a place where they can acquire the skills needed to help them escape poverty." Unfortunately, the stability of the school environment is complicated by residency requirements, delay in the transfer of records, lack of transportation, and, often, lack of immunization records. Additional problems lie in getting children and youth assessed for special education needs, providing counseling, and promoting participation in before- and after-school activities. Unaccompanied youth also face problems with guardianship and liability. Approximately 87% of homeless children and youth are enrolled in school, but only 77% attend on a regular basis (National Coalition for the Homeless, 2005d).

The McKinney Act of 1987 attempted to fund states to provide educational services to homeless children and youth. The McKinney-Vento Act further requires school districts to maintain children in their prior schools whenever possible, to provide transportation as needed, and to provide immediate enrollment when a child moves to a new school regardless of prior receipt of official documents. Unfortunately, funds to provide these services are generally lacking. In 1990, Congress authorized $50 million for Education for Homeless Children and Youth (EHCY) programs, but the funds were never appropriated (National Coalition for the Homeless, 2005d). The 2003 EHCY budget was funded at $55 million, $15 million less than the amount authorized. The two McKinney Acts are also intended to fund preschool services for homeless preschoolers, yet only 15% of homeless preschool-age children were enrolled in preschool programs in 2000 (Bringing America Home, 2005c), partly because of long waiting times (30 days to 12 months) for public preschool programs (National Coalition for the Homeless, 2005d). School may be the only place that many poor children receive any health care. Difficulties with school attendance not only impair educational performance, but may also detract from the health status of these children.

CRIMINAL JUSTICE, CIVIL RIGHTS, AND VIOLENCE Homelessness and lack of basic necessities to support life may lead to crime, as well as prostitution, to obtain money. More often, however, homeless individuals are arrested for actions that, if conducted in private, would be perfectly acceptable. The homeless are overrepresented in jail, and recently released prisoners are at high risk of homelessness due to disruption of family and community ties. Mentally ill inmates have an even more difficult time reintegrating into society and have an even higher risk of homelessness (Kushel, Hahn, Evans, Bangsberg, & Moss, 2005). Approximately 54% of homeless men have a history of incarceration at some time in their lives (Cooke, 2004). A history of arrest has also

been found to be predictive of longer periods of homelessness than those experienced by persons without criminal records (Caton et al., 2005).

Many cities criminalize activities of homeless persons in an effort to render them invisible to the general public through incarceration "under the guise of assumed threats to public safety" (National Coalition for the Homeless, 2005q, p. 3). **Criminalization** is defined as "the process of legislating penalties for the performance of life-sustaining functions in public" (National Coalition for the Homeless, 2005q, p. 4). As noted by one author, "Homeless people are in a double bind. For them socially legitimated space does not exist, and so they are denied access to public space and public activity by laws of a capitalist society that is anchored in private property and privacy" (Mitchell, 2003, p. 135). This concept is further highlighted in statements by the National Coalition for the Homeless (2005q) that "because people without homes have no option but to perform necessary functions in public, they are vulnerable to judgment, harassment, and arrest for committing 'nuisance' violations in public" (p. 4) and that "cities have turned to the criminal justice system for housing, treatment, and even as a means of 'disappearing' homeless people" (p. 9).

Earlier, we saw that the number of available shelter beds is insufficient to meet the need in many jurisdictions. Another barrier to shelter that keeps people on the street and vulnerable to arrest for *nuisance* crimes is the cost of shelter, which may be as high as $5 to $10 per night and thus beyond the means of the most destitute homeless (National Coalition for the Homeless, 2005q). Fines imposed for *illegal* activities further deplete the money available to homeless individuals for obtaining housing. In addition, mental health and drug courts may also reserve shelter beds for sentencing purposes, further restricting the availability of shelter for many homeless individuals (Bringing America Home, 2005f).

In surveys conducted throughout the nation, 80% of communities have laws against camping or sleeping in public areas, yet 100% of these communities lack sufficient shelter beds to meet local needs. Police often conduct sweeps of areas where homeless people congregate prior to major political, entertainment, or sports events, and homeless people are banned outright from some high-income residential and tourist areas. In many places, public parks have been designated as "family" parks, making them off-limits for people without children. Similarly, bars have been placed in the center of public benches to prevent people from lying down on them. Increased policing of gentrified areas and tourist centers effectively removes the homeless from the sight of the more affluent members of society (Bringing America Home, 2005f).

Existing laws are selectively enforced, with homeless people, particularly members of ethnic minority groups, more often being arrested for nuisance activities than housed individuals (Bringing America Home,

2005f). The criminalization of activities by the homeless is costly to society and uses money that could be better spent in more positive initiatives to end homelessness. In fact, the cost of jailing a homeless offender, excluding the cost of police activity, is estimated to range from $40 to $140 per day. This is in excess of the cost of providing housing and other services, estimated at $30 per day (National Coalition for the Homeless, 2005q). The cost of criminalization is also higher than the cost of creating new affordable housing. In addition to the societal cost, criminalization also increases barriers to housing and other services for people who now have criminal records (Bringing America Home, 2005f).

Discrimination in terms of civil rights violations is not the only form of discrimination encountered by homeless individuals and families. In some cases, discrimination in housing markets may actually cause homelessness. Despite legislation to the contrary, Black individuals and families, elderly poor, people with HIV/AIDS, and those with psychiatric disorders frequently encounter discrimination in their efforts to obtain housing (Northridge, Stover, Rosenthal, & Sherard, 2003). In addition, exclusionary zoning ordinances prohibit construction of multifamily units or high-density housing in many high-income neighborhoods. Requirements for significant acreage upon which to build further restrict development of affordable housing and increase the price of what housing is available (Freeman, 2002).

Discrimination against the poor and homeless, at its extreme, results in violence and victimization. The National Coalition for the Homeless (2005g) identifies three types of perpetrators of *hate crimes*: mission offenders, scapegoat offenders, and thrill seekers. Mission offenders perceive themselves to be on a mission to cleanse the world of certain types of undesirable people. Scapegoat offenders engage in violence in response to feelings of frustration with circumstances (e.g., unemployment) that they attribute to members of a particular group. Thrill seekers act violently to derive pleasure from hurting others. The Coalition noted that most violence against homeless persons is committed by thrill seekers; however, they also state that the frequency of violence against the homeless rises with increased police action against this group and with negative city responses or portrayals of the homeless as responsible for societal ills.

Think Advocacy

The Bringing America Home Act (Bringing America Home, 2005a) is an ambitious piece of legislation aimed at addressing the multiple factors that contribute to homelessness in the United States. Access the Web site at http://www.bringingamerica-home.org to see what organizations have endorsed this legislation. What organizations in your area might endorse the Act? How might you organize a campaign to support this piece of legislation?

From 1999 to 2004, a total of 386 violent acts against homeless individuals, resulting in 156 deaths, were reported. Victims ranged in age from 4 months to 74 years, and the perpetrators were as young as 11 years and as old as 65. In 2004 alone, 105 events were reported and 25 deaths occurred, with perpetrators ranging from 12 to 45 years of age (National Coalition for the Homeless, 2005g).

Violence may also be a cause of homelessness. For example, studies of homeless women indicate that 25% to 50% of them were abused in the year prior to becoming homeless. In one study, 46% of the women had remained in an abusive situation because of lack of other options. Loss of cash assistance programs may further limit the options for escape available to abused women and children (National Coalition for the Homeless, 2005c). Homeless youth may also be prior victims of abuse. Approximately 46% of runaway youth have been physically abused and 17% have been sexually abused (National Coalition for the Homeless, 2005p). Homeless youth are also at greater risk for violence and victimization on the street than adults. For example, in one study, 85% of homeless youth had witnessed a stabbing or shooting (Clement, 2003).

Behavioral Considerations

Behavioral considerations that are particularly relevant to the poor and homeless populations include diet and nutrition, rest, substance abuse, and sexual activity. Inadequate nutrition among poor and homeless individuals is a lifestyle factor leading to ill health. As housing and heating costs increase for poor families, food expenditures tend to decrease. In higher-income families, on the other hand, exceptionally cold weather and increased heating costs tend to be associated with increased food expenditures (Bhattacharya, DeLeire, Haider, & Currie, 2003). One million U.S. households are considered food insecure, and 3 million people experience hunger (Wehler et al., 2004).

The homeless, even those housed in shelters, rarely have access to kitchen facilities. Some shelters do provide meals, but they are rarely adequate to meet the nutritional needs of those served. This is particularly true in the case of homeless children, who frequently exhibit anemia or serious growth failure, and who go hungry twice as often as housed children (Bringing America Home, 2005d). In one survey, 20% of homeless individuals reported one or fewer meals a day; 39% reported hunger and the inability to afford food; and 40% had gone without food for one or more days (Clement, 2003). The homeless may also have difficulty meeting special dietary needs posed by chronic illness and pregnancy.

Homeless individuals may also have difficulty obtaining adequate rest. Because of increased crime and victimization at night, many homeless individuals may attempt to sleep in the daytime when they are less vulnerable to attack. This further limits their ability to obtain many services that are offered only during the day. The inability to rest frequently places homeless individuals at greater risk for a variety of health problems and worsens existing health conditions. For example, the inability to lie down to rest may lead to venous stasis and contribute to leg and foot ulcers. These adverse effects on circulation are made worse if the homeless individual smokes. Smoking also intensifies the effects of respiratory infections contracted from others in crowded shelters.

Substance abuse is a behavioral factor that may contribute to homelessness when the abuser is unable, because of his or her addiction, to meet, or even care about, needs for shelter. Substance abuse may also lead to expenditure of money for alcohol or drugs that could be used for shelter. On the other hand, homelessness may lead to use and abuse of alcohol and drugs as a form of escape, or alcohol or drugs may be used to relieve symptoms of psychiatric illness. The precise connection between homelessness and substance abuse, however, is unclear. Competition for scarce housing resources may put those with drug and alcohol abuse problems at a disadvantage relative to other homeless individuals. Findings of studies showing a consistent link between addiction and homelessness have been called into question because of the preponderance of long-term shelter users and single homeless men in these studies (National Coalition for the Homeless, 2005a).

Changes in disability benefits have also made individuals with addictive disorders more vulnerable to homelessness. The Clinton administration eliminated eligibility for SSI and Social Security Disability Insurance (SSDI) for people whose disability is related to substance abuse (National Coalition for the Homeless, 2005a). In one study, 3% of homeless individuals had recently lost SSI or SSDI benefits, leaving them unable to support prior rents.

Nonheterosexual sexual orientation may be a precursor to homelessness, particularly among young people. In one study, for example, 35% of homeless youth reported homosexual or bisexual orientation as their reason for leaving home (Rew, Fouladi, & Yockey, 2002). Sex trading, or the exchange of sex for money or food, is a lifestyle that may arise as a result of homelessness. Sex trading is particularly prevalent among adolescent runaways who find no other way to earn enough money to support themselves (Clement, 2003). Homelessness has also been linked to sex trading among men who have sex with men (MSM) (Newman, Rhodes, & Weiss, 2004). Sex trading and injection drug use among some members of the homeless population place this group at risk for communicable diseases such as HIV infection and hepatitis B and C. Homelessness and poverty may also affect other health-related behaviors. For example, women with a history of adverse socioeconomic

circumstances at some point in their lives have been shown to be less likely to use hormone replacement therapy (Lawlor, Smith, & Ebrahim, 2004). Poverty and homelessness may also make it more difficult for people to engage in health-promoting and illness-preventing activities. We have already seen that homelessness is associated with decreased immunization levels among children. On a more positive note, some research has indicated that homeless individuals, particularly women, are open to healthy lifestyle behaviors when they are able to engage in them. For example, homeless women have been found to engage in behaviors related to physical activity, diet, and stress management (Wilson, 2004).

Health System Considerations

Health system factors may contribute to homelessness or limit access to care for poor and homeless persons. For example, medical bills for catastrophic illness, particularly for those who do not have health insurance, may catapult individuals and families into homelessness. As we saw earlier, thousands of people lost insurance coverage in 1997 as a result of changes in welfare benefits; another 725,000 individuals who were laid off lost employment-based health insurance (National Coalition for the Homeless, 2005k). In 2003, 16.5% of the U.S. population under 65 years of age had no health insurance (National Center for Health Statistics, 2005). Catastrophic illness in this population could easily lead to depletion of any existing savings, inability to pay rent, and eventually homelessness.

Noninstitutionalization of the mentally ill is another health system factor that may contribute to homelessness. **Noninstitutionalization** refers to a lack of hospitalization of persons with mental problems who are in need of care. Often, particularly in urban areas, people with mental illness are not hospitalized until they have deteriorated to the point where they are a danger to themselves or others. Such tolerance of deviant behavior prevents mentally ill individuals from obtaining help when they need it and when they could most easily benefit from it. In other situations, long waits for treatment may prevent individuals with mental illness or substance abuse disorders from obtaining help in a timely fashion and may lead to subsequent homelessness as they become less and less able to cope with life. Even when treatment becomes available, homeless individuals with no contact address cannot be reached and may be dropped from long waiting lists (National Coalition for the Homeless, 2005a).

More often than causing homelessness, however, health care system factors make it more difficult for homeless individuals to obtain health care and to prevent or resolve health problems. Financial costs are one barrier to health care for the homeless. Approximately 55% of the homeless population lacks health insurance (Wilde et al., 2004). Lacking regular health care providers, homeless individuals and families have rates of emergency department (ED) use three times those of the general population. For example, 40% of homeless individuals in one study made one or more ED visits in the previous year, and 8% had made three or more visits (Kushel et al., 2002). Many homeless individuals do not receive any care. Ten percent of homeless parents indicated that their children needed health care but did not receive it due to costs (Clement, 2003). Similarly, 13% of sheltered adolescents delayed getting recommended care due to costs (Ensign, 2001). Homeless veterans, on the other hand, may be slightly more likely to have a regular source of health care and receive needed care (Nyamathi et al., 2004). Some assistance is provided to help homeless individuals and families obtain needed health care. In 1987, the McKinney Act authorized creation of the Health Care for the Homeless (HCH) program. The program, which was reauthorized in 1996 under the Health Centers Consolidation Act and in 2002 under the Health Care Safety Net Amendments Act, provides grants to community-based organizations to support primary care services for homeless individuals (National Coalition for the Homeless, 2005h, 2005i). Some homeless individuals, particularly children, may also be eligible for Medicaid; however, the National Women's Law Center (2004) has noted that even eligible persons may not enroll in the Medicaid program because of the complexity of the enrollment process.

Cost is not the only barrier to health care access. Other problems include lack of transportation, long waits for service (which may mean missing a meal at the soup kitchen or being unable to obtain shelter for the night), fragmentation of services due to lack of case management, and billing practices that result in attaching the wages of those who earn next to nothing. Lack of childcare for other children may also prevent homeless parents from obtaining care for themselves or their children. Provider barriers include insensitivity to the needs and circumstances of the homeless and unwillingness to provide care to those with no means of payment.

Personal barriers posed by homeless persons themselves include priority placed on survival over health needs, denial of illness, fears of loss of personal control, lack of money, and embarrassment over personal appearance and hygiene. Homeless individuals and families may also lack the expertise or the energy to complete the processes involved in registration or application for services.

Lack of preventive care is a common problem among this population. Few pregnant homeless women receive prenatal care. These women and their offspring are at higher risk for complications of pregnancy than is the general population. Homeless women are also less likely to receive preventive services. Preventive care is also lacking for young children.

Think Advocacy

Wilde, Albanese, Rennells, and Bullock (2004) described the development of a nursing clinic for homeless men by nursing faculty and students. Based on the success of the clinic, shelter staff are more knowledgeable regarding the health needs of the homeless population and better able to meet those needs. How might you and your classmates establish such a service to serve the local homeless population? What services would be needed? Which of these services could be provided by nurses? By other health care and social service professionals? How might you go about obtaining these other services?

Compliance with treatment recommendations may also be difficult. Homeless clients may be unable to afford prescribed medications or may not have a watch to time doses correctly. They may not have access to water to take oral medications, and syringes for insulin may be lost or stolen. Other difficulties include retaining potency in medications exposed to frequent temperature changes and obtaining prescription refills. Treatment for HIV/AIDS is particularly difficulty among the homeless due to the complexity of most treatment regimens (National Coalition for the Homeless, 2005j).

Mental health services for poor and homeless populations are also lacking. Some observers have noted a mismatch between traditional community mental health services and the needs of the homeless population. Comprehensive services are seldom offered at one location, and mental health services seldom address the social factors contributing to homelessness.

COMMUNITY HEALTH NURSING AND CARE OF POOR AND HOMELESS POPULATIONS

Community health nurses may encounter homeless clients in a number of venues. They may work in or with shelters for homeless people. Or they may encounter virtually homeless people during home visits to other clients with whom homeless individuals may be staying. Community health nurses may also encounter homeless clients who seek to obtain services from other agencies where nurses are employed. Finally, homeless clients may be referred to community health nurses by other agencies and providers.

Homeless individuals may be reluctant to admit to their homelessness for a variety of reasons. They may feel embarrassed about their condition or may want to forestall intrusion into what they may feel is their own affair. Community health nurses should be alert to indicators of possible homelessness in clients they encounter. For example, a community health

Advocacy in Action

Interpreting for the Homeless

As an outreach nurse with Health Care for the Homeless in Phoenix, Arizona, I was constantly advocating for the homeless clients I served. Many individuals who are homeless have histories of mental illness, substance abuse, and physical abuse. They often do not trust the health care system and have generally had less than satisfying encounters with health care providers who could only identify the negative effects of their lifestyle rather than attempt to understand how to deliver culturally appropriate care to this vulnerable population.

As an outreach nurse, I was responsible for locating homeless individuals who were at risk, engaging them in services, and coordinating their health care. The locating wasn't difficult, but engaging and coordinating care proved to be. As clients came to trust me, I was able to schedule them for medical appointments and assured them that I would provide transportation and, more importantly, accompany them to appointments when possible.

Homeless people can be uncomfortable with meeting new people and having to sit in a waiting room full of people who may not appreciate their presence. They are concerned that the appointment may affect their ability to work that day. Picking up cans and panhandling do not allow for sick time. Many of my clients lived outside and did not have access to clean clothes or showers. I was prepared for the attitudes of the public, but not the attitude of the providers. The providers were quick to identify clients' negative health behaviors regardless of the reason they were seeking treatment. Rather than provide positive reinforcement for making and keeping an appointment, providers admonished clients for not coming in sooner. There was no consideration for their lifestyle in developing treatment plans. Clients who lived on the street would be told to go home, elevate the broken extremity, put ice on it, and call their orthopedic surgeon—none of which is possible for people living under a bridge or in a shelter.

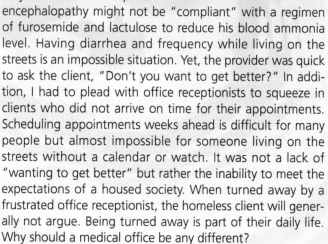

Countless times I acted as an "interpreter" for my clients. I had to explain why someone with hepatic encephalopathy might not be "compliant" with a regimen of furosemide and lactulose to reduce his blood ammonia level. Having diarrhea and frequency while living on the streets is an impossible situation. Yet, the provider was quick to ask the client, "Don't you want to get better?" In addition, I had to plead with office receptionists to squeeze in clients who did not arrive on time for their appointments. Scheduling appointments weeks ahead is difficult for many people but almost impossible for someone living on the streets without a calendar or watch. It was not a lack of "wanting to get better" but rather the inability to meet the expectations of a housed society. When turned away by a frustrated office receptionist, the homeless client will generally not argue. Being turned away is part of their daily life. Why should a medical office be any different?

I am an advocate for a marginalized population that is unable to demand the medical care it deserves. I explain to providers how best to meet the needs of people who are homeless. I assist clients in navigating a health care system that has little understanding of the unique characteristics of people who are homeless. As an assistant clinical professor at ASU College of Nursing, I am educating new client advocates. During the senior year in community health nursing, I supervise students at a local shelter where they provide care to over 400 homeless residents. As a result of this clinical experience, the population welcomes over 60 new advocates each year.

Kay Jarrell, MS, RN
Clinical Assistant Professor
Arizona State University College of Nursing

nurse may note that a client has not taken a shower or washed his or her clothes in some time. Or the client may be hesitant when asked for a home address or may give the address of a known homeless shelter. Clients who report living with other family members or friends may also be virtually homeless. When faced with these indicators, the community health nurse can tactfully explore if the client is indeed homeless and if assistance is desired.

In other instances, clues may be more subtle. For example, in a hearing related to a college academic integrity violation related to plagiarism, the student explained his purchase of a paper from an Internet source as a result of not being able to work in his dorm room because his roommate was using drugs and he was afraid to be associated with him. When a community health nurse faculty member, who happened to be a member of the hearing committee, asked where the student was staying if he was not living in the dorm, he reported that he was living in one of the student lounges on campus. In addition to dealing with the academic integrity violation, the committee took immediate steps to obtain adequate housing for the student. However, his homeless plight would not have been identified if the community health nurse had not caught the cue buried in his defense of plagiarism.

Assessing the Health of Poor and Homeless Populations

The first step in the care of poor and homeless segments of the population is assessing their health status and identifying the factors that influence their health. The community health nurse examines factors that contribute to homelessness in the population as well as the effects of homelessness on health. The focused assessment below provides some questions that can be used in assessing the health of the homeless population. The assessment tool included in Appendix I on the Companion Website can be used to assess the health of homeless clients.

Assessment data for poor and homeless populations may be somewhat more difficult to obtain than data about other, more easily observed populations.

Community health nurses working with homeless individuals or groups of homeless persons would be particularly alert for commonly encountered health problems. In addition, they would assess individual clients for the presence of any other chronic or communicable diseases, as well as for high prevalence rates for these conditions in the homeless population. Information regarding prevalent conditions can be sought from health professionals and agencies that care for homeless people. Some data on the age, gender, and ethnic composition of the homeless population may be available from shelter sites and social service agencies. Local churches may also have a sense of the number and types of homeless people served. Local government agencies may also have data on the extent of the homeless population and its composition.

FOCUSED ASSESSMENT

Assessing the Homeless Population

Biophysical Considerations

- What is the age composition of the homeless population? The ethnic and gender composition?
- What developmental effects has homelessness had? What acute and chronic health problems are prevalent? What is the prevalence of pregnancy?
- What is the immunization status of the homeless population (particularly children)?

Psychological Considerations

- What is the extent of mental illness in the homeless population? What is the extent of depression, anxiety, and suicide?
- What stresses are experienced by this population? How does the homeless population cope with stress?
- What are individual and group responses to being homeless? To seeking help?

Physical Environmental Considerations

- What are the effects of climatic conditions on the homeless population?
- Where do homeless individuals in the community seek shelter? How adequate are shelter facilities? What hygiene facilities are available to homeless persons?
- Do environmental conditions pose other health hazards for homeless individuals (e.g., flooding under bridges used for shelter)?

Sociocultural Considerations

- What is the community attitude to homelessness? To homeless individuals?
- What is the extent of family support available to the homeless individual? What is the extent of community support available to the homeless population?
- To what extent does family violence contribute to homelessness in the community?
- What effects do education, economic, and employment factors have on homelessness in the community? What proportion of the eligible homeless population is receiving financial assistance? What proportion of the homeless is employed? In what kind of work?

- What childcare resources are available to homeless women with children?
- What education programs are available for homeless children?
- What transportation resources are available to the homeless population?
- What is the availability of low-cost housing in the community? What is the availability of shelter for homeless persons? For individuals with special needs?
- What proportion of the homeless population consists of families? What proportion of homeless families are headed by women?
- What is the extent of crime victimization among homeless individuals?

Behavioral Considerations

- What food resources are available in the community for homeless individuals? What nutritional deficits do homeless individuals exhibit? What is the nutritional value of food available to homeless individuals and families?
- What is the extent of drug and alcohol abuse in the homeless population?
- What is the prevalence of smoking in the homeless population?
- Are there facilities available in the community for homeless individuals to rest during the day? What health effects does lack of rest have on the homeless individual?
- What is the extent of prescription medication use among the homeless population? Do homeless individuals have access to resources to help with medication expenses?
- What is the extent of sex trading and unsafe sexual activity in the population?

Health System Considerations

- What health care services are available to homeless persons in the community? To what extent are these services integrated with other services needed by the homeless population? What is the availability of mental health services for homeless individuals? Drug and alcohol treatment services? To what extent are preventive health services available to and utilized by the homeless population?
- Where do homeless persons usually obtain health care? What are the attitudes of health care providers toward homeless individuals?
- How is health care for homeless persons financed?

Information on the prevalence of specific conditions and immunization status can be obtained in surveys of the homeless population. Surveys of homeless individuals will need to be conducted in places where they congregate. For example, a community health nurse might survey individuals living in a shelter or those who take advantage of community meal programs. Because of the time needed to complete surveys, the lack of resources available to them (e.g., pens or pencils for completing written surveys), and varied levels of education among the homeless population, surveys will be most effective if conducted verbally in the context of other services. For example, the nurse might survey clients as they wait in line at a local soup kitchen or approach them for a few minutes of their time after they finish a meal. Privacy is often lacking in the lives of homeless individuals, and community health nurses should refrain from asking for highly personal information in public settings. Homeless individuals with substance abuse problems may also be wary of admitting these and other illicit behaviors (e.g., theft of food) unless assured of confidentiality. Community health nurses should endeavor to ask survey questions in language appropriate to the client's understanding and in ways that do not imply value judgments. Homeless individuals themselves may be involved in the development of survey tools that address their perceived needs in a sensitive and culturally appropriate manner. Community health nurses can also advocate for the involvement of homeless individuals in data collection and analysis and payment for temporary employment in these activities.

Surveys can also be a mechanism for collecting information on the extent of mental illness and the level of coping skills in the population. Psychiatric treatment facilities may also have data on the number of homeless individuals served and the types of diagnoses seen.

Environmental conditions and their effects on the homeless are often best assessed through observation. What is the local weather and how does it affect the homeless population? The adequacy of shelter facilities can be observed by visits to existing shelters. Other places where homeless people congregate can also be observed. At the same time, observations in public places can provide some information on the attitude of others toward obviously homeless individuals as well as on the extent of police activities related to the homeless. Local police records can also provide information on arrests for nuisance crimes.

The extent of family violence as a precursor to homelessness can best be determined by surveys of homeless individuals, particularly women and youth. Police and other protective services agencies are another source of information on family violence. These agencies may also provide information on the availability of shelters for victims of abuse. Shelter personnel can likewise be a source of information on the homeless population.

Educational and employment information can be obtained in a similar manner. Local social service agencies or employment offices may have information on places where homeless individuals may go to seek day labor. Observation and questioning of people in these locations can provide information on the kinds of jobs available and wages paid, as well as potential job hazards faced by the homeless population. Perusal of the local newspaper can also provide a sense of the job opportunities that may be available to homeless individuals. General community employment and economic data may be available from local chambers of commerce or government employment offices. Census data also include this information but may be outdated, depending on the recency of data collection.

Social service agencies and telephone books are potential sources of data regarding childcare availability. In addition, the community health nurse can contact local childcare providers to determine the availability of care for children in low-income families. Similarly, school districts can provide information on the availability of public preschool programs. School districts can also provide information on the number of homeless children enrolled in local schools, as well as the services available to meet their needs.

Information on shelter availability would most likely be obtained from social service agencies, local churches, or local government offices. These organizations may also have information regarding food resources and other services available to poor and homeless populations. Information on specific nutritive intake, however, is best obtained by observation in shelters or surveys of homeless individuals. Surveys could also be used to determine the extent of health-related behaviors such as smoking, alcohol and drug use, and sex trading, as well as the use of prescription medications. Crime victimization data would be available from local police departments.

General information on the availability of health services can be obtained from telephone directories, and specific agencies can be contacted to determine the type and extent of services provided to homeless individuals. Emergency departments, in particular, may have information on the frequency with which homeless individuals use ED services as a substitute for primary care. Local officials and health care agencies can also be contacted to determine how health care services for poor and homeless individuals are funded.

Diagnostic Reasoning and Care of Poor and Homeless Populations

Based on the assessment of the health status of poor and homeless clients and factors contributing to that status, nursing diagnoses may be derived at any of several levels. At the individual client level, the community health nurse may make diagnoses related to the existence of homelessness. As discussed before, the diagnostic statement includes underlying factors if identifiable, for example, "homelessness due to inability to pay for shelter" or "homelessness due to mental illness and inability to care for self."

Other kinds of diagnoses made at the individual or family level might relate to specific health problems resulting from or intensified by homelessness. As an example, the nurse might make a diagnosis of "stasis ulcers due to excessive walking and standing and inability to lie down at night" or "malnutrition due to inability to afford food and lack of access to cooking facilities."

Nursing diagnoses may also be made at the group or community level. For example, the community health nurse may diagnose a significant problem of homelessness in the community. Such diagnoses might be stated as "an increase in the homeless population due to recent closure of major community employer" or "an increase in the number of homeless families due to unemployment and reductions in public assistance programs." Diagnoses may also be made at the aggregate level relative to specific problems engendered by homelessness, for example, "increased prevalence of tuberculosis due to malnutrition and crowding in shelters for the homeless" or "increased incidence of anemia among homeless children due to poor nutrition."

Planning and Implementing Health Care for Poor and Homeless Populations

Planning to meet the needs of homeless clients should focus on long-term as well as short-term solutions to problems. Planning should also reflect the factors contributing to the needs of the homeless in a particular locale. For example, if most of the homelessness in one community is due to unemployment, long-term interventions would most likely be directed toward improving employment opportunities in the area or increasing the employability of those involved. If, on the other hand, a significant portion of homelessness in the area is due to mental illness and inability to care for self, attention would be given to providing supportive services for the mentally ill.

Planning should address the underlying factors contributing to homelessness as well as its health consequences. For example, providing shelter on a nightly basis may decrease the risk of exposure to cold for homeless persons but does nothing to relieve homelessness. In planning to meet the health needs of homeless clients, community health nurses may work independently or in conjunction with other health care and social service providers. When planning to address factors contributing to homelessness, however, the community health nurse frequently is part of a group of government officials and concerned citizens who have assumed responsibility for dealing with the overall problem of homelessness. The principles of coalition building will be helpful to community health nurses working with others to address problems of homelessness and poverty in the community.

Efforts to alleviate homelessness and its consequences may take place at the primary, secondary, or tertiary level of prevention. Community health nurses may be involved in activities at any or all three levels. As is true in caring for any client, planning care for a homeless client or population begins with prioritizing health needs. In many instances, the first priority would be obtaining shelter, a secondary preventive measure. Other health needs could then be addressed in terms of their priority. For each of the health care needs identified for the homeless client or population, the community health nurse would develop specific outcome objectives and design interventions at the primary, secondary, or tertiary level of prevention. Planning efforts should be a joint function of the community health nurse, homeless clients, who best know their situation and the kinds of interventions that are likely to be successful in that situation, and other concerned individuals.

Primary Prevention

Primary prevention may be directed at either preventing homelessness or preventing its health consequences. Primary prevention can occur at the individual or family level or at community levels. Community health nurses can help prevent individuals and families from becoming homeless by assisting them to eliminate factors that may contribute to homelessness. For example, if a family is threatened with eviction because of a parent's unemployment, the nurse can assist family members to obtain emergency rent funds from local social service agencies. The nurse can also encourage the family to apply for ongoing financial aid programs or assist the parent to find work.

As noted earlier, some people become homeless because of underlying psychiatric illness and an inability to deal with the requirements for maintaining shelter. Severely disturbed people may just wander away from home and take up residence on the streets. Homelessness in this group can be prevented by referrals for psychiatric therapy and counseling. Case management in the transition from hospital or prison to community may help to prevent homelessness in mentally ill or inmate populations. Nurses may also provide support services to families caring for mentally ill members to prevent these persons from becoming part of the homeless population. Placement in a sheltered home might also be an approach to preventing homelessness in the mentally disturbed person when family members either cannot or do not wish to care for the client. In addition, the community health nurse can monitor the effectiveness of therapy and watch for signs of increasing agitation or disorientation that may precede wandering. The nurse can also assist the disturbed person by giving concrete direction in such tasks as paying rent.

Runaway children and teenagers are another segment of the homeless population for whom homelessness may be prevented through primary preventive interventions. Efforts of community health nurses to promote effective communication in families and enhance parenting skills may prevent young people from feeling a need to run away. Similarly, efforts to prevent or deal with child abuse may prevent runaways.

Primary prevention at the community level to reduce the incidence of poverty and homelessness requires major changes in societal structure and thinking. Some suggested avenues for intervention include federal support for low-cost housing, increases in the minimum wage, and access to supportive services for the mentally and physically disabled to allow them to function effectively in society. Another suggestion aimed at reducing the incidence of poverty in families with children to prevent their homelessness is to provide childcare assistance and paid parental occupational leaves as needed.

Creating employment opportunities and programs to train people in employable skills is another possible primary preventive measure for both poverty and homelessness. Current public job training programs, however, have been criticized for their failure to facilitate job placement for those who complete the programs. Job training programs directed specifically toward the local job market have been suggested as more appropriate approaches to unemployment. Another societal intervention could be to provide a guaranteed annual income to all citizens. Such an approach is exemplified in part by social insurance programs such as Social Security and unemployment insurance that are not restricted to the poor but available to all eligible participants. Other social programs that may help to prevent homelessness include legal assistance to prevent evictions as well as increased housing subsidies (Caton et al., 2000). Changes in housing codes and tax laws to prevent loss of welfare benefits or allowing tax credits in shared housing situations may also be helpful. There is also a need for "discharge planning" for housing assistance for people displaced by building condemnation or renovation or release from prisons and other institutions.

Community health nursing involvement in such activities occurs primarily through advocacy and political action. As advocates, community health nurses can make policy makers aware of the needs of the homeless and can contribute to efforts to plan programs that prevent homelessness. Nurses can also engage in political activities to influence policies that help to eliminate these conditions. Comprehensive legislation was introduced before the U.S. Congress in November 2005 as part of the Bringing America Home Act (H.R. 4347). At that time, the bill was assigned to the House Ways and Means Committee. In March 2006, it was referred to the Subcommittee on Health, where it remains at this writing (Library of Congress, 2006). This legislation is a broad-based initiative acknowledging housing as a basic right for all and making provisions for a living wage, universal health care, dramatic services expansion for homeless individuals, and protection for temporary workers similar to that enjoyed by full-time employees. The Act also addresses civil rights protection for the homeless and the construction of new housing or rehabilitation of existing low-income housing (Bringing America Home, 2005a; National Coalition for the Homeless, 2005b). Community health nurses can be actively involved in promoting passage of this and similar legislation.

Community health nurses can also work to promote adoption of sound housing policies. Criteria for such policies include the creation of a social contract for decent housing funded at the federal level, redistribution of federally funded housing benefits (e.g., giving priority to localities with the greatest need), federal funding at levels needed to assure housing access, and policies that are sensitive to local housing market conditions (e.g., increasing subsidies in high-cost communities or building more housing in areas where housing is scarce) (Freeman, 2002).

Primary prevention may also be undertaken with respect to specific health problems experienced by homeless persons. Here, community health nurses may work with individuals, families, or groups of people. For example, community health nurses working with homeless substance abusers might advocate a program providing clean syringes to injection drug users. Failing that, the nurse might provide a simple bleach solution for injection equipment to minimize the risk of blood-borne diseases such as hepatitis and AIDS. Similarly, nurses may provide assistance to families with budgeting and meal planning to provide nutritious meals on limited incomes.

Community-based avenues for preventing homelessness among the mentally ill include providing access to services within the community that enable these persons to care for themselves adequately without institutionalization. Efforts may also be needed to ensure hospitalization for those persons who cannot be adequately maintained in the community. Treatment for substance abuse and secure places for convalescence after hospital discharge might also serve to prevent homelessness in this subgroup.

Also at the group level, nurses may engage in primary prevention for specific problems by encouraging community groups to provide shelters for homeless individuals. Nurses may also provide basic health care for the homeless, focusing particularly on primary preventive measures such as influenza vaccine and routine immunizations for children. For example, immunization services may be provided in nontraditional settings such as soup kitchens, shelters, and so on (Postema & Breiman, 2000). Adequate ventilation, reduced crowding, and use of ultraviolet lights in shelters may also help to prevent the spread of communicable disease.

Another area for primary prevention of the health consequences of homelessness is adequate nutrition. Community health nurses can advocate for food programs for the needy, including the homeless. They can also serve as consultants to existing food programs to ensure that meals are nutritionally adequate to meet the needs of the population served. Community health nursing activities in this area may also include attempts to arrange diets for homeless clients with special needs (e.g., assisting a diabetic client to select foods from those prepared in a shelter that approximate a diabetic diet as closely as possible).

Community health nurses can also work with other concerned citizens to initiate programs to provide adequate clothing and shoes for homeless clients. Efforts may also be needed to arrange for the homeless to bathe and wash their clothing. In some cities, day shelters that do not provide sleeping accommodations often provide homeless individuals an opportunity to shower and wash their clothing. These shelters may also provide a clean change of clothing on a periodic basis.

Another aggregate approach to preventing specific health problems among the homeless is providing universal access to health care through national health insurance or similar programs at the state level. Nurses can promote such programs through political activity and advocacy and may also be involved in implementing them by providing direct services to the homeless.

Secondary Prevention

Secondary prevention is designed to alleviate existing homelessness and its health effects. Community health nurses working with homeless individuals must first address their priority concerns for shelter and basic necessities before other health needs can be addressed (Drennan & Joseph, 2005). At the individual level, secondary interventions may include referral for financial assistance via "means-tested income transfers." **Means-tested income transfers** involve the distribution of cash or noncash assistance to individuals and families on the basis of income. As noted earlier, such programs frequently serve only the poorest of the poor and may necessitate loss of all resources before eligibility can be confirmed. Community health nurses may need to function as advocates to assist clients through the bureaucratic process frequently involved. This is particularly true for elderly clients and those with mental health problems. At the community level, nurses can advocate a review of eligibility criteria for means-tested income transfer programs so that a greater proportion of the homeless population is served.

Shelter is an immediate need for homeless individuals. The community health nurse can assist the homeless client to locate temporary shelter. This may be accomplished by means of referrals to existing shelters. If the nurse is not aware of homeless shelters provided in the community, he or she can contact a local YMCA or YWCA, a Salvation Army service center, or local churches for information on shelter availability. When organized shelter facilities are not available, the nurse may try contacting local houses of worship to see if members of religious congregations can provide shelter for a homeless person on a short-term basis. In making a referral for emergency shelter, the community health nurse would consider the needs of the particular client. Ideally, for example, the elderly and women and children would be referred to shelters where they are protected from victimization. Similarly, homeless persons with chronic health problems should be referred to shelters where health services are available and their conditions can be monitored on an ongoing basis.

At the aggregate level, community health nurses can work with government officials and other concerned citizens to develop shelter programs for homeless individuals or families. Avenues that might be pursued include school gymnasiums, churches, and public buildings. Many cities have used these and other buildings as temporary nighttime shelters for the homeless during cold weather. Plans might also be developed for more adequate shelters that provide other services as well as a place to sleep.

For homeless persons with significant mental health problems, it may be necessary to create specialized shelters called **safe havens**, which are secure, stable places of residence that place few demands on those receiving help. Many mentally ill homeless individuals are not able to deal with the behavioral restrictions and other policies imposed by many typical homeless shelters. They need a place with limited restrictions that offers the same bed each night, a place to stay during the day, and a place to store their belongings. Because of the special needs of this segment of the homeless population, safe havens do not limit the length of stay for those served. Safe havens then become a stage in clients' progressive movement toward permanent housing in which they can learn to trust and relearn skills needed to maintain a permanent residence while unlearning the distrust required for survival on the streets.

Homeless persons with mental illness also require services tailored to meet their needs. Several authors note that the constant search for shelter, food, and other necessities interferes with treatment for mental illness and substance abuse problems. It is therefore helpful to combine treatment services with shelter and other services needed by the mentally ill and substance-abusing segments of the homeless population (Milby et al., 2005). Although this population has been characterized as generally noncompliant with treatment recommendations, pilot projects that involve outreach, available—but not mandatory—group therapy, and case management services have been shown to be effective in ensuring housing stability in this population (Shern et al., 2000). The provision of abstinence-only shelter for substance abusers is somewhat controversial. On one hand, abstinence-contingent shelter has been found to be useful in promoting treatment (Milby et al., 2005). On the other hand, the National Coalition for the Homeless (2005a) has noted that complete abstinence may not be a realistic goal for this population and that programs are needed that recognize and address the probability of relapse. Provision of housing assistance seems to be the key factor in helping this and other segments of the homeless population to remain housed. One study in New York, for example, demonstrated that 80% of those who received subsidized housing remained housed irrespective of the presence of mental and social disorders. Conversely, only 18% of those who did not receive housing subsidies were able to maintain a stable residence (National Coalition for the Homeless, 2005k).

Shelters are an emergency resource, not a solution to the problem of homelessness. Community health nurses should help homeless clients find ways to meet long-term shelter needs. For individual clients, this may mean referrals for employment assistance or other services to eliminate factors that resulted in homelessness. At the community level, nurses can participate in planning long-term solutions to the problems of homelessness. Unfortunately, such planning has not often been the focus of community attempts to deal with the problem. Community health nurses can advocate and participate in planning efforts to provide low-cost housing, employment assistance, job training, and other services needed to resolve community problems of homelessness. Initiating these planning activities may require political activity on the part of the community health nurse.

Planning for long-term resolution of the problem of homelessness for runaways involves a different set of strategies. The community health nurse can explore with the youngster his or her reasons for running away from home. Nursing interventions are then directed toward modifying factors that led the child to run away. For example, if the child was abused, the nurse can institute measures to prevent further abuse if the youngster returns to the home, or foster home placement can be arranged. If problems stem from poor family communication, the nurse can make a referral for family counseling or other therapeutic services. The nurse can also serve as a liaison between the child and his or her family, negotiating for changes that make the child's return possible.

Particular care should be taken to involve the child in planning interventions to resolve his or her situation. A child returned to his or her family unwillingly will probably run away again. In addition, such actions on the part of the community health nurse may also destroy

any faith the child may have had in health care providers as a source of assistance.

At the aggregate level, community health nurses should alert community policy makers to the need for coordinated services for the homeless offered in a single location to meet the health and social needs of homeless clients (Rosenbaum & Zuvekas, 2000). They should also make sure that planning groups in which they participate plan services to address the needs of the homeless for housing, food, clothing, employment, childcare services for working parents, and adequate preventive and therapeutic health care services. Planning should also include avenues for outreach and follow-up services, particularly for the homeless who may be lost to service. Such comprehensive programs require changes in health care and social systems that may necessitate legislation and public policy formation that can be guided by nursing input.

Community health nurses can also provide curative services for a variety of health problems experienced by the homeless. For example, they may make referrals for food supplement programs or provide treatment for skin conditions or parasitic infestations. They will also be actively involved in educating clients for self-care. Homeless clients may have difficulty with simple aspects of treatment regimens. For example, if the homeless client does not have access to a clock or watch, it may be difficult to take medications as directed. Nurses can suggest the use of medications that can be taken in conjunction with set activities, such as on arising or at bedtime.

The special needs of homeless children and older persons require particular attention. One suggestion is age-segregated shelters or services specifically designed for older persons and families with children to prevent their victimization by other subgroups within the homeless population. Special attention also needs to be given to meeting the nutritional needs of these vulnerable groups as well as those of pregnant women.

Tertiary Prevention

Tertiary prevention may be aimed at preventing a recurrence of poverty and homelessness for individuals, families, or groups of people affected. Conversely, the emphasis may be placed on preventing the recurrence of health and social problems that result from conditions of poverty and homelessness.

Community health nursing involvement in tertiary prevention may entail political activity to ensure the provision of services to relieve poverty and homelessness on a long-term basis. This means involvement by nurses in efforts to raise minimum wages or to design programs to educate the homeless for employment in today's society. Advocacy and political activity may also be needed to ensure the adequacy of community services for the mentally ill to allow them to care for themselves or to support their families as caregivers.

At the individual or family level, community health nurses may be involved in referral for employment assistance or for educational programs that allow homeless clients to eliminate the underlying factors involved in their homelessness. Moreover, nurses might assist clients to budget their incomes more effectively or engage in cooperative buying efforts to limit family expenses. Community health nurses may also be actively involved in monitoring the status of mentally ill clients in the home and in assisting families of these clients to obtain respite care and other supportive services needed to prevent the mentally ill client from returning to a state of homelessness. In such cases, nurses also monitor medication use and encourage clients to receive counseling and other rehabilitative services.

Another avenue for tertiary prevention that may be employed at either the individual or group level is advocacy to prevent the criminalization of normal activities of life for homeless people. The National Coalition for the Homeless (2005q) has developed several recommendations that community health nurses and other advocates of homeless populations can implement. These include:

- Monitoring and documenting local arrests, fines, and harassment of homeless persons
- Empowering and organizing the homeless to advocate for themselves
- Providing legal advocacy for homeless individuals and advocating legislation to prevent criminalization
- Controlling and monitoring the activities of private security guards
- Mustering public and professional support for the Bringing America Home Act

Evaluating Care for Poor and Homeless Populations

Evaluating the effects of nursing interventions with poor and homeless clients can take place at two levels: the individual level and the population level. At the individual level, evaluation of the effectiveness of interventions reflects the client care objectives developed by the nurse and client in planning care. For example, if an objective for a homeless family was to provide them with an income sufficient to meet survival needs, the nurse and family would determine whether this objective has been achieved. Does the family now have sufficient income to provide adequate housing, appropriate nutrition, and other needs? If the objective was to find employment for the mother or father, has this been accomplished?

Evaluation of aggregate-level interventions must also be undertaken. For example, nurses and other concerned individuals will want to determine whether shelter programs are sufficient to meet the needs of the homeless population. Evaluation of tertiary prevention programs focuses on the extent to which interventions prevent people from returning to poverty and again becoming homeless. Are job training programs effective in increasing the income of participants above the poverty level? Criticism of current welfare programs seems to indicate that such programs do not effectively relieve the problems of the poor and homeless. If current programs are not effectively alleviating the problem, other solutions must be sought; community health nurses must be actively involved in developing those solutions.

The Working Group on Homeless Health Outcomes (1996) of the Bureau of Primary Health Care suggested that evaluation of programs for the homeless address both systems-level and client-level outcomes. Systems-level outcomes to be considered include ease of access to programs; the comprehensiveness of services offered; continuity of care, including appropriate referrals, follow-up, and case management; the degree to which an integrated set of services is provided; cost-effectiveness; focus on prevention; and client involvement in the design and implementation of services. Client-level outcomes include client involvement in and commitment to treatment, improved health status, improved functional status, effective disease self-management, improved quality of life, client choice of providers, and client satisfaction.

An additional focus for evaluation is the achievement of those national health objectives that relate to low-income individuals and families. The current status of some of these objectives is presented on page 570. Targets for achievement of other national objectives among the poor and near poor have also been developed, and the degree of success in achieving these targets can be assessed by visiting the *Healthy People 2010◆* data Web site at http://wonder.cdc.gov/data2010. As we can see from the data, none of the objectives have reached the targets and little progress has been made with respect to most of them. Two of the objectives are actually moving away from the target, indicating that considerable work yet remains to protect the health of the poor, and particularly the homeless, population.

Poverty and homelessness are growing problems in the United States and throughout the world, and community health nurses may encounter poor and homeless individuals and families in a variety of settings. Community health nurses can provide direct health care services to these clients. They may also be actively involved in identifying and planning to deal with factors that contribute to poverty and homelessness.

HEALTHY PEOPLE 2010
Goals for Population Health◆

OBJECTIVE	BASELINE	MOST RECENT DATA	TARGET
■ 1-1. Increase the proportion of poor people with health insurance	65%	69%	100%
■ 1-4. Increase the proportion of poor people with a regular source of health care	79%	80%	96%
■ 1-6. Reduce the proportion of poor families with difficulty or delay in getting care	17%	NDA	7%
■ 8-22. Increase the proportion of poor families living in pre-1950s housing that has been tested for the presence of lead-based paint	18%	22%	50%
■ 8-23. Reduce the proportion of occupied housing units that are substandard	6.2%	NDA	3%
■ 11-1. Increase the proportion of poor households that have access to the Internet at home	NDA	NDA	80%
■ 14-24. Increase receipt of all immunizations among poor children	70%	68%	80%#
■ 19-4. Reduce growth retardation in low-income children	8%	8%	5%
■ 19-18. Increase food security and reduce hunger	69%	NDA	94%
■ 28-4. Reduce blindness and visual impairment in poor children and adolescents	34%	35%	20%#

NDA—No data available

 # Objective moving away from target

Data from: Centers for Disease Control and Prevention (2005). Healthy people data. Retrieved September 5, 2005, from http://wonder.cdc.gov/data2010

Case Study

A Homeless Family

Crystal is a 16-year-old girl with a 3-month-old baby boy. She has been referred for community health nursing services by her teacher at a special program for adolescents with children. In this program, the girls attend school while childcare services are provided for the children. During the day, the girls participate in the care of their infants and learn about childcare as well as the usual high school subject material. Crystal has been referred because she has not been coming to school and her teacher is concerned. The school does not have a home address or phone number for Crystal, but the teacher gives you the phone number of Crystal's grandmother. After several attempts, you finally contact the grandmother, who agrees to give Crystal a message to get in touch with you. The grandmother says that Crystal does not live with her and that she sees her only occasionally.

The following week you receive a call from Crystal. She is reluctant to give you an address but agrees to come to the health department with the baby. When she arrives, she tells you that she has not been going to school because the baby was ill and cannot return to the childcare center without a doctor's note that the baby is well. Crystal says she cannot afford to see a doctor. She has no health insurance and no money for health care. She began the application process for Medicaid but never followed through because it was "too much hassle." She lives with her mother and stepfather in a camper shell at a construction site where her stepfather is temporarily employed. She refuses to give you the location of this construction site, saying that they will probably move to a new site soon. Crystal says her parents provide her with food and formula for the baby, who appears clean and well nourished. The baby has not begun his immunizations, again because of lack of funds for health services.

Crystal says she is in good health but has not had a postpartum checkup. Although not currently sexually active, she has a steady boyfriend and is contemplating sexual intimacy with him. She asks about various types of contraceptives.

The father of her baby is no longer in the area and is not aware that Crystal had a baby. Crystal's own father is also removed from the picture and Crystal does not know where he is. When asked about her grandmother, Crystal says that they do not get along well and that her grandmother hardly speaks to her since she got pregnant.

Crystal is anxious to complete high school and enroll in a program to become a beautician. She tried recently to get a part-time job in a fast-food restaurant, but was told they wanted someone with experience. She socializes somewhat with the girls at school and goes with several of them to take their babies to the park and similar outings.

1. What health problems are evident in this situation? What are the biophysical, psychological, physical environmental, sociocultural, behavioral, and health system factors influencing these problems?
2. What primary prevention measures would you undertake with Crystal and her son?
3. What secondary prevention measures would be warranted to deal with existing health problems? Describe specific actions you would take to resolve these problems.
4. What could be done in terms of tertiary prevention to prevent further consequences or recurrence of health problems in this situation?
5. How would you evaluate the effectiveness of your interventions with Crystal? Describe the specific evaluative criteria you would use and how you would obtain the evaluative data needed.

Test Your Understanding

1. What are some of the biophysical, psychological, physical environmental, sociocultural, behavioral, and health system considerations that contribute to poverty and homelessness or affect the health of poor or homeless people?

2. Describe at least three approaches to primary prevention of homelessness. How might community health nurses be involved in each approach?

3. What are the major areas of emphasis in primary prevention of health problems among homeless clients?

4. What are three areas in which secondary preventive activities may be appropriate in the care of poor and homeless

clients? What kinds of secondary preventive measures might a community health nurse employ in these areas?

5. Identify at least two strategies for tertiary prevention of homelessness at the aggregate level. How might community health nurses be involved in implementing these strategies?

6. What is the primary focus in evaluating care for homeless clients? Is this focus the same for evaluating care for individuals and families and care for groups of homeless people?

EXPLORE MediaLink

http://www.prenhall.com/clark
Resources for this chapter can be found on the Companion Website

Audio Glossary
Appendix I: Adult Health Assessment and
   Intervention Guide
Exam Review Questions

Case Study: Promoting the Health of the
   Homeless
MediaLink Application: Lenny Kravitz on
   Poverty (video)

Media Links
Challenge Your Knowledge
Update *Healthy People 2010*
Advocacy Interviews

References

Anderson, D. G., & Rayens, M. K. (2004). Factors influencing homelessness in women. *Public Health Nursing, 21,* 12–23.

Archambault, D. (2002). The health needs of homeless men. *Community Health Forum, 3*(5), 37–39.

Bhattacharya, J., DeLeire, T., Haider, S., & Currie, J. (2003). Heat or eat? Cold-weather shocks and nutrition in poor American families. *American Journal of Public Health, 93,* 1149–1154.

Bohrer, G. J., & Faulkner, P. (2004, October 4). Beyond standardized care for the homeless mentally ill. *NurseWeek,* pp. 31–33.

Bolland, J. M., & McCallum, D. M. (2002). Touched by homelessness: An examination of hospitality for the down and out. *American Journal of Public Health, 92,* 116–118.

Bringing America Home. (2005a). *Bringing America home: The campaign.* Retrieved November 29, 2005, from http://www.bringingamericahome.org

Bringing America Home. (2005b). *People need affordable housing.* Retrieved November 29, 2005, from http://www.bringingamericahome.org

Bringing America Home. (2005c). *People need education.* Retrieved November 29, 2005, from http://www.bringingamericahome.org

Bringing America Home. (2005d). *People need health care.* Retrieved November 29, 2005, from http://www.bringingamericahome.org

Bringing America Home. (2005e). *People need livable incomes.* Retrieved November 29, 2005, from http://www.bringingamericahome.org

Bringing America Home. (2005f). *People need their civil rights protected.* Retrieved November 29, 2005, from http://www.bringingamericahome.org

Bures, R. M. (2003). Childhood residential stability and health at midlife. *American Journal of Public Health, 93,* 1144–1148.

Caton, C. L. M., Dominguez, B., Schanzer, B., Hasin, D. S., Shrout, P. E., Felix, A., et al. (2005). Risk factors for long-term homelessness: Findings from a longitudinal study of first-time homeless single adults. *American Journal of Public Health, 95,* 1753–1759.

Caton, C. L. M., Hasin, D., Shrout, P. E., Opler, L. A., Hirschfield, S., Dominguez, B., et al. (2000). Risk factors for homelessness among indigent urban adults with no history of psychotic illness: A case-control study. *American Journal of Public Health, 90,* 258–263.

Center for Medicaid and State Operations. (2005). Medicaid at a glance, 2005. Retrieved December 21, 2005, from http://www.cms.hhs.gov/Medicaideligibility/downloads/MedGlance05.pdf

Centers for Disease Control and Prevention. (2005). *Healthy people data.* Retrieved September 5, 2005, from http://wonder.cdc.gov/data2010

Clement, M. S. (2003). *Children at health risk.* Malden, MA: Blackwell.

Cooke, C. L. (2004). Joblessness and homelessness as precursors of health problems in formerly incarcerated African American men. *Journal of Nursing Scholarship, 36,* 155–160.

Division of Applied Public Health Training, Epidemiology Program Office. (2003). Tuberculosis outbreak in a homeless population—Portland, Maine, 2002–2003. *Morbidity and Mortality Weekly Report, 52,* 1184–1185.

Drennan, V. M., & Joseph, J. (2005). Health visiting and refugee families: Issues in professional practice. *Journal of Advanced Nursing, 49,* 155–163.

Ensign, J. (2001). The health of shelter-based foster youth. *Public Health Nursing, 18,* 19–23.

Freeman, L. (2002). America's affordable housing crisis: A contract unfulfilled. *American Journal of Public Health, 92,* 709–712.

Hirsh, E. D., Jr., Kett, J. F., & Trefil, J. (Eds.), (2002). Structural unemployment. In *The new dictionary of cultural literacy* (3rd ed.). Retrieved March 19, 2006, from http://www.bartleby.com/59/18/structuralun.html

Kaplan, G. A., Siefert, K., Ranjit, N., Raghunathan, T. E., Young, E. A., Tran, D., et al. (2005). The health of poor women under welfare reform. *American Journal of Public Health, 95,* 1252–1258.

Kneipp, S. M., Castleman, J. B., & Gailor, N. (2004). Informal caregiving burden: An overlooked aspect of the lives and health of women transitioning from welfare to employment? *Public Health Nursing, 21*, 24–31.

Kogut, B. H. (2004). Why adult literacy matters. *Phi Kappa Phi Forum, 84*(2), 26–28.

Krieger, J., & Higgins, D. L. (2002). Housing and health: Time again for public health action. *American Journal of Public Health, 92*, 758–768.

Kushel, M. B., Hahn, J. A., Evans, J. L., Bangsberg, D. R., & Moss, A. R. (2005). Revolving doors: Imprisonment among the homeless and marginally housed population. *American Journal of Public Health, 95*, 1747–1752.

Kushel, M. B., Perry, S., Bangsberg, D., Clark, R., & Moss, A. R. (2002). Emergency department use among the homeless and marginally housed: Results from a community-based study. *American Journal of Public Health, 92*, 778–784.

Lawlor, D. A., Smith, G. D., & Ebrahim, S. (2004). Socioeconomic position and hormone replacement therapy use: Explaining the discrepancy in evidence from observational and randomized controlled studies. *American Journal of Public Health, 94*, 2149–2154.

Library of Congress. *H.R. 4347*. Retrieved March 19, 2006, from http://thomas.loc.gov/cgi-bin/bdquery/z?d109:h4347

McLeer, S. V. (2004). Mental health services. In H. S. Sultz & K. M. Young (Eds.), *Health care USA: Understanding its organization and delivery* (4th ed., pp. 335–366). Sudbury, MA: Jones and Bartlett.

Milby, J. B., Schumacher, J. E., Wallace, D., Freedman, M. D., & Vuchinich, R. E. (2005). To house or not to house: The effects of providing housing to homeless substance abusers in treatment. *American Journal of Public Health, 95*, 1259–1265.

Mitchell, D. (2003). *The right to the city: Social justice and the fight for public space*. New York: Guilford Press.

National Center for Health Statistics. (2003). *Health United States, 2003: Chartbook on trends in the health of Americans*. Washington, DC: Author.

National Center for Health Statistics. (2005). Percentage of persons aged <65 years without health insurance, by age group and number of uninsured months—United States, 2003. *Morbidity and Mortality Weekly Report, 54*, 385.

National Coalition for Homeless Veterans. (n.d.). *Facts and media: Background and statistics*. Retrieved March 19, 2006, from http://www.nchv.org/background.cfm

National Coalition for the Homeless. (2005a). *Addiction disorders and homelessness*. Retrieved November 29, 2005, from http://www.nationalhomeless.org/publications/facts

National Coalition for the Homeless. (2005b). *Bill to end homelessness in America introduced in Congress*. Retrieved November 29, 2005, from http://www.nationalhomeless.org/publications/facts

National Coalition for the Homeless. (2005c). *Domestic violence and homelessness*. Retrieved November 29, 2005, from http://www.nationalhomeless.org/publications/facts

National Coalition for the Homeless. (2005d). *Education of homelessness children and youth*. Retrieved November 29, 2005, from http://www.nationalhomeless.org/publications/facts

National Coalition for the Homeless. (2005e). *Employment and homelessness*. Retrieved November 29, 2005, from http://www.nationalhomeless.org/publications/facts

National Coalition for the Homeless. (2005f). *Federal housing assistance programs*. Retrieved November 29, 2005, from http://www.nationalhomeless.org/publications/facts

National Coalition for the Homeless. (2005g). *Hate, violence, and death on Main Street, USA, June 2005*. Retrieved November 29, 2005, from http://www.nationalhomeless.org/publications/facts

National Coalition for the Homeless. (2005h). *Health care and homelessness*. Retrieved November 29, 2005, from http://www.nationalhomeless.org/publications/facts

National Coalition for the Homeless. (2005i). *Health care for the homelessness program*. Retrieved November 29, 2005, from http://www.nationalhomeless.org/publications/facts

National Coalition for the Homeless. (2005j). *HIV/AIDS and homelessness*. Retrieved November 29, 2005, from http://www.nationalhomeless.org/publications/facts

National Coalition for the Homeless. (2005k). *Homeless families with children*. Retrieved November 29, 2005, from http://www.nationalhomeless.org/publications/facts

National Coalition for the Homeless. (2005l). *Homeless veterans*. Retrieved November 29, 2005, from http://www.nationalhomeless.org/publications/facts

National Coalition for the Homeless. (2005m). *Homelessness among elderly persons*. Retrieved November 29, 2005, from http://www.nationalhomeless.org/publications/facts

National Coalition for the Homeless. (2005n). *Housing justice*. Retrieved November 29, 2005, from http://www.nationalhomeless.org/publications/facts

National Coalition for the Homeless. (2005o). *How many people experience homelessness?* Retrieved November 29, 2005, from http://www.nationalhomeless.org/publications/facts

National Coalition for the Homeless. (2005p). *Homeless youth*. Retrieved November 29, 2005, from http://www.nationalhomeless.org/publications/facts

National Coalition for the Homeless. (2005q). *Illegal to be homeless, 2004 report*. Retrieved November 29, 2005, from http://www.nationalhomeless.org/publications/facts

National Coalition for the Homeless. (2005r). *Mental illness and homelessness*. Retrieved November 29, 2005, from http://www.nationalhomeless.org/publications/facts

National Coalition for the Homeless. (2005s). *Rural homelessness*. Retrieved November 29, 2005, from http://www.nationalhomeless.org/publications/facts

National Coalition for the Homeless. (2005t). *Who is homeless?* Retrieved November 29, 2005, from http://www.nationalhomeless.org/publications/facts

National Women's Law Center. (2004). *Making the grade on women's health*. Retrieved August 13, 2005, from http://www.nwlc.org/pdf/HR04findings_and_titlepage.pdf

Newman, P. A., Rhodes, F., & Weiss, R. (2004). Correlates of sex trading among drug-using men who have sex with men. *American Journal of Public Health, 94*, 1998–2003.

Nielsen, M. J., Juon, H.-S., & Ensminger, M. (2004). Preventing long-term welfare receipt: The theoretical relationship between health and poverty over the early life course. *Social Science & Medicine, 58*, 2285–2301.

North, C. S., Eyrich, K. M., Pollio, D. E., & Spitznagel, E. L. (2004). Are rates of psychiatric disorders in the homeless population changing? *American Journal of Public Health, 94*, 103–108.

Northridge, M. E., Stover, G. N., Rosenthal, J. E., & Sherard, D. (2003). Environmental equity and health: Understanding complexity and moving forward. *American Journal of Public Health, 93*, 209–214.

Nyamathi, A., Sands, H., Pattatucci-Aragon, A., Berg, J., Leake, B., Hahn, J. E., et al. (2004). Perception of health status by homeless US veterans. *Family and Community Health, 27*(1), 65–74.

Population Information Program, Center for Communication Programs. (2003). *Population reports: Meeting the urban challenge*. Retrieved July 25, 2003, from http://www.jhucpp.org

Postema, A. S., & Breiman, R. F. (2000). Adult immunization programs in nontraditional settings: Quality standards and guidance for program evaluation. *Morbidity and Mortality Weekly Report, 49*(RR-1), 1–13.

Rew, L., Fouladi, R. T., & Yockey, R. D. (2002). Sexual health practices of homeless youth. *Journal of Nursing Scholarship, 34*, 139–145.

Robertson, M. J., Clark, R. A., Charlebois, E. D., Tulsky, J., Long, H. L., Bangsberg, D. R., et al. (2004). HIV seroprevalence among homeless and marginally housed adults in San Francisco. *American Journal of Public Health, 94*, 1207–1217.

Rosenbaum, S., & Zuvekas, A. (2000). Health care use by homeless persons: Implications for public policy. *Health Services Research, 34*, 1303–1304.

Sherman, P., & Redlener, I. (2003). Homeless women and their children in the 21st century. In H. M. Wallace, G. Green, & K. J. Jaros (Eds.), *Health and welfare for families in the 21st century* (2nd ed., pp. 469–480). Sudbury, MA: Jones and Bartlett.

Shern, D. L., Tsemberis, S., Anthony, W., Lovell, A. M., Richmond, L., Felton, C., et al. (2000). Serving street-dwelling individuals with psychiatric disabilities: Outcomes of a psychiatric rehabilitation clinical trial. *American Journal of Public Health, 90*, 1873–1878.

Swigart, V., & Kolb, R. (2004). Homeless persons' decisions to accept or reject public health disease-detection services. *Public Health Nursing, 21*, 162–170.

Thiele, B. (2002). The human right to adequate housing: A tool for promoting and protecting individual and community health. *American Journal of Public Health, 92*, 712–715.

Unemployment types. (2006). *Wikipedia*. Retrieved March 19, 2006, from http://

en.wikipedia.org/wiki/Unemployment_types

U.S. Census Bureau. (2005). *Statistical abstract of the United States: 2004–2005.* Retrieved August 16, 2005, from http://www.census.gov/prod/2004pubs/04statab

Webb, D. A., Culhane, J., Metraux, S., Robbins, J. M., & Culhane, D. (2003). Prevalence of episodic homelessness among adult child-bearing women in Philadelphia, PA. *American Journal of Public Health, 93,* 1895–1896.

Wehler, C., Weinreb, L. F., Huntington, N., Scott, R., Hosmer, D., Fletcher, K., et al. (2004). Risk and protective factors for adult and child hunger among low-income housed and homeless female-headed households. *American Journal of Public Health, 94,* 109–115.

Wilde, M. H., Albanese, E. P., Rennells, R., & Bullock, Q. (2004). Development of a student nurses' clinic for homeless men. *Public Health Nursing, 21,* 354–360.

Wilson, M. (2004). Health-promoting behaviors of sheltered homeless women. *Family and Community Health, 28*(1), 51–63.

Wilton, R. (2004). Putting policy into practice? Poverty and people with serious mental illness. *Social Science & Medicine, 58,* 25–39.

Wise, P. (2004). The transformation of child health in the United States; Social disparities in child health persist despite dramatic improvements in child health overall. *Health Affairs, 23,* 9–25.

Working Group on Homeless Health Outcomes, Bureau of Primary Health Care. (1996). *Meeting proceedings.* Rockville, MD: Health Resources and Services Administration.

World Health Organization. (2003). *Right to water.* Geneva, Switzerland: Author.

World Health Organization. (2005). *World health statistics 2005.* Retrieved September 21, 2005, from http://www.who.int/health-info/statistics/whostat2005en1.pdf

Wright, N. M. J., & Tompkins, C. N. E. (2005). *How can health care systems effectively deal with the major health care needs of homeless people?* Retrieved December 12, 2005, from http://www.euro.who.int/HEN/Syntheses/homeless/ 20050124_11

Zahran, H. S., Kobau, R., Moriarty, D. G., Zack, M. M., Holt, J., & Donehoo, R. (2005). Health-related quality of life surveillance—United States 1993–2002. *Morbidity and Mortality Weekly Report, 54*(SS-4), 1–35.

Care of Clients in Official and Voluntary Health Agencies

CHAPTER OBJECTIVES

After reading this chapter, you should be able to:

1. Discuss the legal and regulatory parameters of nursing in official health agencies.
2. Describe the core functions and essential services of local health departments.
3. Discuss educational preparation for nursing in official health agencies.
4. Analyze the core competencies of the public health workforce as they relate to nursing in official health agencies.
5. Analyze community nursing diagnoses as they relate to nursing in official health agencies.
6. Analyze the role of the community health nurse in carrying out the core functions and essential services in local health departments.
7. Define faith community nursing.
8. Describe the philosophy of nursing in a faith-based community.
9. Describe the scope and standards of nursing in a faith-based community.
10. Differentiate among models for nursing in a faith-based community.
11. Describe the roles and functions of community health nurses in a faith-based community.

KEY TERMS

faith community
faith community nurses
health ministry
parish nursing
public health nurse (PHN)
whole person health

MediaLink

http://www.prenhall.com/clark

Additional interactive resources for this chapter can be found on the Companion Website. Click on Chapter 22 and "Begin" to select the activities for this chapter.

From Chapter 22 of *Community Health Nursing: Advocacy for Population Health*, 5/e. Mary Jo Clark. Copyright © 2011 by Pearson Education. Published by Prentice Hall. All rights reserved.

Advocacy in Action

Connie's Dilemma

Connie, a 40-year-old recovering drug abuser, called me one day with a request. She and her fiancé, also a recovering drug abuser and the father of her baby, had been looking for a Narcotics Anonymous meeting and had been unable to find one they could attend at a convenient time for both of them. She asked if I, as parish nurse, would approach the Parish Council and present her request to start up a Narcotics Anonymous meeting on Saturday evenings in the parish hall.

Realizing that Connie could not make the request herself and remain anonymous, I agreed to do so. However, I also realized that because of a past experience with the Youth Group, when some teens had used the parish hall for meetings that included the use of marijuana, the Parish Council would be reluctant to grant permission. After investigating the experience of other churches that provided space, exploring the liability of the parish, and testing out the request among several members of the Parish Council, I presented Connie's request. In making the presentation, I emphasized the mission of the parish, which was to "raise the dead in spirit," provided the testimony of other pastors of churches that had Narc Anon meetings, and addressed the issue of the parish's liability. Connie's request was granted unanimously. The first Narc Anon meeting was held within a month, with 10 persons in attendance. Six months later, the number had grown to 40. Now, 8 years later, the Narc Anon meetings continue with an average attendance of 80 members. Truly, the spirits of those Narcotics Anonymous members have been raised.

Judith Mouch, MSN, MA
University of Detroit Mercy

Community health nursing focuses on the health of population groups, and that this focus, rather than the practice setting, is the core of community health nursing. The U.S. health care delivery system is composed of official and voluntary health agencies, both of which provide settings for the practice of community health nursing. In this chapter, we will explore exemplars of official and voluntary health agencies, the local health department and faith-based organizations, as settings for community health nursing practice. Local and state health departments and federal public health agencies are the official government agencies responsible for the overall health of the population. However, they are assisted in performing this responsibility by a wide variety of private-sector, nonprofit voluntary agencies and organizations. Faith communities that choose to engage in health-related ministries are a relatively new type of voluntary organization that engages in community health nursing activities.

COMMUNITY HEALTH NURSING IN AN OFFICIAL AGENCY: THE LOCAL HEALTH DEPARTMENT

Many community health nurses are employed in official health agencies, often at the local health department level. Although community health roles and functions in local health departments may vary somewhat from one jurisdiction to another, there are usually many similarities encountered in practice in these settings. In this chapter, we will examine some of those commonalities as well as some of the differences between the community health nursing role in official agencies and in voluntary organizations as exemplified by a faith-based health ministry.

Community health nursing in the United States originated in voluntary activities by nurses who were known as "public health nurses" because of their focus on the health of populations as well as of the individuals and families who comprised that population. The title *public health nurse*, or PHN, however, is now most commonly reserved for nurses who engage in public health practice within official public health agencies. This use of the title *public health nurse* is also true in other places, such as the United Kingdom (Carr & Davidson, 2004) and Ontario, Canada (Fliesser, Schofield, & Yandreski, 2003). Not all nurses who work in official public health agencies are public health nurses. Public health nurses generally have a specifically defined role related to the health of the whole population even though they may provide services to individuals and families within the population. For example, some local health departments employ public health nurses and another category of

nurses who may be called registered general nurses or clinic nurses, who may be responsible for the care of specific individuals. In Ireland, for example, public health nurses have a population focus with an emphasis on health promotion, and registered general nurses are responsible for secondary and tertiary prevention with individual clients (Clarke, 2004). Similar differentiation among nursing staff occurs in some health departments in the United States as well. For these reasons, we will use the term *public health nurse* in this chapter when referring to those community health nurses working in official health agencies whose focus of practice is the health of the entire population.

Legal and Regulatory Parameters of Public Health Nursing

Official health agencies are the only setting where community health nurses work in which many of their activities are derived from federal or state legislative mandates or local ordinances. Official agencies are charged by the particular level of government with protecting the health of the public, and public health nurses working in these agencies are actively involved in carrying out that mandate. For example, one of the functions of official public health agencies is to protect the public from communicable diseases. Under this mandate, public health nurses may investigate reports of communicable diseases. For instance, a public health nurse might conduct a follow-up interview of a community resident for whom a primary care provider has made a diagnosis of hepatitis A. In addition to obtaining information on the possible source of the client's infection and educating the client and family members to prevent the spread of disease, the public health nurse may be responsible for assuring that a close contact who prepares food in a local restaurant is removed from work until he or she has received hepatitis A vaccine and/or immune globulin and is determined

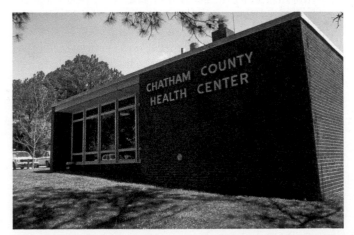

Public health nurses most often practice in official health agencies such as county health departments. (Billy E. Barnes/PhotoEdit)

to be free of disease. Similarly, public health nurses may be responsible for assuring that a chronic typhoid carrier does not work as a food handler or even provide food to groups of people (e.g., church members) on a volunteer basis.

Public health nurses are also charged with making sure that other health-related regulations are adhered to. For example, in the event of an influenza pandemic, quarantine measures may be instituted, and public health nurses may be responsible for assuring that those affected abide by quarantine restrictions. Similarly, clients with communicable tuberculosis (TB) who refuse treatment may be placed on home isolation under a judicial order. In this instance, it is often the public health nurse who makes sure that the client remains in his or her home and that only persons who have received chemoprophylaxis for TB are allowed to visit the home. Although clients must consent to treatment by public health nurses or official agencies, because of the legal mandate to protect the health of the public, failure to accept treatment for a communicable disease can result in restrictions of liberty when the appropriate court proceedings are implemented.

Public Health Functions and Essential Services in Local Health Departments

Local health department jurisdictions may include a city, a county, or a group of counties. For example, public health services for most of Los Angeles County are provided by the county department of health, but Pasadena and Long Beach, two cities within the county, have their own independent health departments. In some largely rural areas, on the other hand, one health department may provide services in several counties.

Many of the functions and activities of local health departments are mandated by state law or local ordinances. In addition to legislated functions, local health departments have primary responsibility for performance of the core functions and essential services of public health at the local level. The core functions of public health are assessment, policy development, and assurance. These core functions were identified by the Institute of Medicine in its 1988 report, *The Future of Public Health*.

In 1994, in the context of health care reform legislation proposed by then President Clinton, a Public Health Functions Steering Committee was formed to develop a consensus on the essential elements of population-based health services. The committee was composed of representatives of the American Public Health Association (APHA), the Association of Schools of Public Health, the Association of State and Territorial Health Officials, the Environmental Council of the States, the Institute of Medicine, the National Association of County and City Health Officials, the National Association of State Alcohol and Drug Abuse Directors, the National Association of State

Mental Health Program Directors, the Public Health Foundation, and the U.S. Public Health Service. The committee identified the basic obligations of official health agencies and a set of essential services required to fulfill those obligations and accomplish the core functions of public health. The obligations identified included:

- Preventing epidemics and the spread of disease
- Protecting the public against environmental hazards
- Preventing injuries
- Promoting healthy behaviors and mental health
- Responding to disasters and aiding communities to recover from their effects
- Assuring the quality and accessibility of health services in the area (American Public Health Association, n.d.)

In meeting these obligations, official health agencies are responsible for the performance of certain essential services (National Public Health Performance Standards Program, n.d.). The core functions of public health and related essential services are presented in Table 1◆. The role of the public health nurse in providing these essential services is addressed later in this chapter.

Many local health departments have begun to redesign services to better address the core functions and essential services. Until recently, services were determined, in large part, by funding sources rather than the needs of the public (Avila & Smith, 2003). For example, Los Angeles County Department of Health Services has restructured its services around the essential services. The intent of the program is to protect and improve the health of the entire population while continuing to function as a safety net agency, providing services for those with no other source of care (Fielding, Luck, & Tye, 2003).

Some local health departments have used the 10 essential services to derive a system of indicators to assess the effectiveness of system performance. These indicators can be grouped as structural, process, and outcome indicators. Structural indicators address the infrastructure of the system and assess areas such as the adequacy of personnel to meet the needs of the population. Process indicators examine the ways in which services are provided, efficiency, and use of resources. Outcome indicators may address either intermediate or ultimate program outcomes. An example of an intermediate outcome might be increased immunization rates, whereas a related ultimate outcome might be decreased incidence of vaccine-preventable diseases (Derose, Asch, Fielding, & Schuster, 2003).

At the national level, the 10 essential public health services have been used to develop National Public Health Performance Standards for services provided by national, state, and local health systems (National Public Health Performance Standards Program, 2001). The performance standards include specific indicators related to each of the essential services. Local health departments may perform essential services themselves or

TABLE 1	Core Functions and Related Public Health Services
Core Function	**Essential Services**
Assessment	• Monitor health status to identify community health problems.
	• Diagnose and investigate health problems and health hazards in the community.
Policy development	• Inform, educate, and empower people regarding health issues.
	• Mobilize community partnerships to identify and solve health problems.
	• Develop policies and plans that support individual and community health efforts.
Assurance	• Enforce laws and regulations that protect health and ensure safety.
	• Link people to needed health care services and assure the provision of health care when otherwise unavailable.
	• Assure a competent public health and personal health workforce.
	• Evaluate effectiveness, accessibility, and quality of personal and population-based health services.
	• Research for new insights and innovative solutions to health problems.

Data from: National Public Health Performance Standards Program. (n.d.). The essential public health services. Retrieved January 16, 2006, from http://www.cdc.gov/od/nphpsp/EssentialPHServices.htm

assure that they are performed by some group or agency in the local jurisdiction (Beaulieu & Schutchfield, 2002).

Public Health Personnel

Community health nurses working in official public health agencies collaborate with a variety of people from other health-related and non-health-related disciplines. The Public Health Functions Project of the U.S. Department of Health and Human Services has recommended several specific occupational categories for public health practice. The breadth of disciplines represented will depend on the size of the public health agency, but community health nurses may encounter some or all of the disciplines included in Table 2◆. As noted earlier, local health departments may also employ nurses who are not public health nurses to provide care to individual clients and families that is not population-based. These nurses were not included in the occupational categories identified by the Public Health Functions project because their focus is not on the health of the overall population. For example, registered nurses, vocational nurses, or assistive personnel may work in STD clinics or in family planning, prenatal, or well-child clinics, providing services to specific clients in need of them. Health departments may also employ nurse practitioners to provide primary care services. Public health nurses may provide direct services within clinics, but they also have a broader practice mandate for addressing the overall health of the population. Public health nurses may also be responsible for supervising the practice of other nursing personnel.

Lay outreach workers or community health workers (CHWs) and volunteers are other categories of personnel that may be supervised by public health nurses. Community health workers may be used in outreach, screening and case finding, and health education activities. They may also assist with translation services for professional staff. Volunteers serve many of the same functions as CHWs except they are not paid personnel. For example, either CHWs or community volunteers may participate in house-to-house screening for lead exposure or to identify uninsured residents, providing them with referrals to services as needed.

In addition to supervising the activities of other nursing personnel, CHWs, and volunteers, public health nurses collaborate with other members of the public health team as well as other segments of society (e.g., residents, teachers, protective services personnel, government officials) to accomplish the core functions of public health. For example, a public health nurse might collaborate with teachers, school administrators, and health department substance abuse counselors and health educators to design a program to prevent substance use and abuse by local high school students. Local police and businesspeople who sell alcoholic beverages might also be involved in the collaborative effort. As another example, the nurse might refer a family with a rodent infestation to an environmental specialist for assistance or refer clients in need of specific services to a public health dentist or physician.

Public Health Nursing in a Local Health Department

Public health nurses are responsible for a large proportion of the essential services provided by local health departments. In the remainder of our discussion of the public health nursing role in the local official health agency, we will explore educational preparation for public health nursing, the use of nursing diagnoses in public health nursing, public health nursing as it relates to the core functions and essential services of public health agencies, and specific public health nursing roles in a local health department.

TABLE 2	Frequently Encountered Public Health Personnel
Occupational Category	**Description**
Alcohol/substance abuse counselor	Assesses and treats persons with alcohol or drug dependency problems; may engage in prevention programs
Biostatistician	Analyzes and interprets community health data
Epidemiologist	Investigates the determinants and distribution of disease, disability, and other health outcomes and develops means for prevention and control
Environmental engineer	Applies engineering principles to control, eliminate, ameliorate, and/or prevent environmental health hazards (assisted by environmental engineering technicians or technologists)
Environmental scientist/specialist	Applies biological, chemical, and public health principles to control, eliminate, ameliorate, and/or prevent environmental health hazards (assisted by environmental science technicians or technologists)
Health educator	Designs, organizes, implements, communicates advice on, and evaluates the effect of educational programs and strategies to support and modify health-related behaviors of individuals, families, organizations, and communities
Health information system specialist	Develops and maintains computer data and information systems
Health services manager/administrator	Plans, organizes, directs, controls, and/or coordinates health services, education, or policy
Mental health/substance abuse social worker	Provides services for persons having mental, emotional, or substance abuse problems
Mental health counselor	Emphasizes prevention and works with individuals and groups to promote optimal mental health; may help individuals deal with existing mental health problems
Occupational safety and health specialist	Collects data on workplace environments and exposures, implements and evaluates programs to limit chemical, physical, biological, and ergonomic risks to workers
Psychologist/mental health provider	Diagnoses and treats mental disorders by using individual, child, family, and group therapies
Public health social worker	Identifies, plans, develops, implements, and/or evaluates programs to address the social and interpersonal needs of populations
Public health attorney/ hearing officer	Advises on legal issues in enforcement of health regulations; may prosecute violation of public health regulations
Public health dentist	Provides preventive and curative dental services (assisted by public health dental workers such as dental hygienists and assistants)
Public health laboratory scientist	Develops, coordinates, and provides laboratory services; may provide oversight for regulation of laboratory practices and procedures (assisted by public health laboratory technicians or technologists)
Public health nurse	Provides nursing services to population groups, individuals, and families
Public health pharmacist	Develops and implements public policy for pharmaceuticals; may dispense pharmaceutical preparations
Public health physician	Provides preventive and curative physical health services
Public health policy analyst	Analyzes needs and plans for development of health programs, facilities, and resources; analyzes and evaluates the implications of alternative policies
Public health veterinarian	Provides preventive and curative services related to animals and control of animal diseases transmissible to people
Public health/public relations/ information/health communications/media specialist	Assists in the development and implementation of programs to communicate health-related messages

Data from: Public Health Functions Project. (2000). The public health workforce: An agenda for the 21st century. *Retrieved May 19, 2001, from http://web.health.gov/phfunctions*

Preparation for Public Health Nursing

When Florence Nightingale initiated the concept of public health nursing, she made it clear that this area of specialty practice required educational preparation beyond basic nursing preparation (Buhler-Wilkerson, 2001; McDonald, 2000). A similar need for postgraduate preparation for public health nursing was perceived in the United States.

Today, in some jurisdictions (e.g., California), **public health nurse (PHN)** is a legal term that designates a registered nurse who meets specific educational requirements for state certification for aggregate-level practice (including a minimum of a baccalaureate degree in nursing) (Board of Registered Nursing, 2004). Required educational preparation for PHN certification in California includes content in physical, mental, and developmental assessment; surveillance and epidemiology related to chronic and communicable diseases; health promotion and disease prevention; multicultural health care; research methodology and statistics; health education; and population-based practice. Other content requirements include legal and health care financing issues, family violence, case management, and emergency preparedness and response. In addition, public health nurses must complete a supervised clinical learning experience in public settings working with individuals, families, and communities (State of California, n.d.). Nurses with public health nurse certification in California are not restricted to employment in official public health agencies, nor do all nurses working in public health agencies have state PHN certification, as noted earlier.

Educational preparation beyond basic nursing education is required for public health nursing in other countries as well. For example, in Ireland, public health nurses must have educational preparation in general nursing, midwifery, and public health nursing and must be registered in all three areas (Clarke, 2004). Irish public health nurses must also have a minimum of 2 years of clinical nursing practice (Hanafin, Houston, & Cowley, 2002). Similarly, public health nursing practice in Finland requires a year of advanced studies in health promotion beyond the required 3 years of general nursing education (Jakonen, Tossavainen, Tupala, & Turunen, 2002). In Japan, public health nurses hold a different license from other nurses that is based on additional educational preparation and passing a national specialty examination (Yamashita, Miyaki, & Akimoto, 2005). Advanced educational preparation is also required for public health nursing in the United Kingdom (Nursing & Midwifery Council, 2004) and Manitoba, Canada (Manitoba Health, 1998).

Standards and Competencies for Public Health Nursing

Public health nurses working in local health departments should conform to the general standards and principles of community/public health nursing. The standards reflect the use of the nursing process in population-based practice and are related to assessment of community health problems; diagnosis and priority setting; outcomes identification; planning, implementation, and coordination of programs and ser-vices. The standards also address the nurse's role in health education and health promotion, consultation, regulatory activities, and population health status evaluation. Additional areas of professional performance addressed by the standards include quality of practice, education, professional practice evaluation, collegiality and professional relationships, collaboration, ethics, research, resource

utilization, leadership, and advocacy on the part of community health nurses (American Nurses Association, 2007). Similar sets of standards for public and community health nursing practices have been created in other countries such as the United Kingdom (Nursing & Midwifery Council, 2004) and Canada (Community Health Nurses Association of Canada, 2003). These sets of standards have a more distinct population focus than U.S. standards and may be obtained at http://www. nmc-uk.org/AFrameDisplay.aspx?DocumentID=234 and http://www.communityhealthnursescanada.org/Standards/STandards%20Practice%20jun04.pdf, respectively.

To carry out the core functions of public health and provide the essential public health services, public health personnel, including nurses, must possess a basic set of skills. Requisite skills include research and analytic skills to collect, analyze, and interpret community health data; communication skills related to presentation, advocacy, and leadership; policy development and program planning skills; and skills derived from the basic public health sciences such as biostatistics and epidemiology. Additional skills required of those employed in public health agencies include cultural skills related to cultural competence and cultural sensitivity; financial planning and management skills such as contract negotiation and financial and organizational management skills; and skills in teaching (Public Health Functions Project, 2000). These basic competencies have been adapted to public health nursing in the Public Health Nursing Competencies developed by the Quad Council of Public Health Nursing Organizations (2004).

Organizational Structures for Public Health Nursing

In addition to the overall redesign of health care delivery programs, some local health departments are returning public health nursing to the primary public health mission— improving the health of the entire population, with health department nurses providing primary care only as safety net agencies. For example, the Los Angeles County Department of Health Services has redesigned the public health nurse role in the agency, identifying two categories of public health nurses: district nurses and specialty program nurses. District nurses are so called because each nurse is responsible for addressing the health needs of all who reside in his or her district or assigned geographic area. District nurses are generalists educated to address a wide range of health needs across the age spectrum. Specialty program nurses, on the other hand, have special preparation in particular program areas such as tuberculosis control, maternal–child health, sexually transmitted disease control, and so on (Avila & Smith, 2003).

The intent in redesigning the public health nursing role was to accomplish three objectives:

• Movement away from a categorical focus on specific diseases and conditions to a more holistic approach

- Provision of consultation services to the community (either individuals or groups) with respect to health issues
- Participation as a service planning area team member addressing the broad spectrum of needs in the area

To this end, the district nurses have begun to conduct annual community assessments of their districts based on the 10 leading health indicators developed for the *Healthy People 2010*◆ objectives and other local health needs.

These assessments are intended to identify community assets as well as problems and provide the foundation for area health care planning (Avila & Smith, 2003). Community assessment by nurses in official public health agencies might be conducted in light of the focused assessment provided below. A complete tool to guide community assessment is included in Appendix G on the Companion Website and in the *Community Assessment Reference Guide* 🗒 designed to accompany this text.

FOCUSED ASSESSMENT

Assessing Communities Using the Leading Health Indicators

Physical Activity

- What is the extent of physical activity in the community?
- What are community attitudes toward physical activity?
- What opportunities for physical activity are available for various age groups in the population?
- To what extent does the prevalence of physical disability or illness among community members influence physical activity?
- What physical environmental, socioeconomic, or cultural factors discourage physical activity in the community?
- What health effects related to lack of physical activity are prevalent in the community?

Overweight and Obesity

- What is the prevalence of overweight/obesity in the community?
- What cultural and socioeconomic factors contribute to overweight/obesity in the community?
- What resources exist for dealing with problems of overweight and obesity in the community?
- What health effects related to overweight and obesity are prevalent in the community?

Tobacco Use

- What is the extent of tobacco use in the community?
- Is tobacco advertising targeted to specific subsegments of the community?
- What legislative and regulatory factors influence tobacco use and sales in the community?
- What is the availability of tobacco use cessation assistance for people who want to quit?
- What health effects related to tobacco use are prevalent in the community?

Substance Abuse

- What is the extent of substance abuse in the community?
- In what subsegments of the population is substance abuse typically found?
- What substances are typically abused? By which subsegments of the population?
- What psychological, cultural, and socioeconomic factors influence substance abuse in the community?
- What is the availability of substance abuse treatment in the community?
- What harm-reduction strategies, if any, are in use in the community?
- What health effects related to substance abuse are prevalent in the community?

Responsible Sexual Behavior

- What is the extent of unprotected sexual activity in the community?
- What is the incidence of unwanted pregnancy in the community?
- What are the incidence and prevalence of sexually transmitted diseases (STDs) in the community?
- What is the extent of sexual activity by adolescents in the community?
- To what extent do members of the community engage in sexual activity with multiple sexual partners?
- To what extent is sexual activity by community members influenced by drug and alcohol use?
- What health services are available in the community to address pregnancy and STDs?

Mental Health

- What is the extent of mental illness in the community?
- What types of mental illness are prevalent?
- What are community attitudes toward mental health problems?
- What health services are available in the community to address mental health problems? How accessible are they to members of the population?

Injury and Violence

- What is the incidence of unintentional injury in the community? What types of injuries typically occur? What are the factors that influence the occurrence of unintentional injuries?
- What is the incidence of intentional injury resulting from violence? What types of violence are particularly prevalent in the community?
- What is the prevalence of disability as a result of accidental or intentional injury?
- What is the community attitude toward violence? What strategies are employed in the community to prevent violence?
- What services are available to address the needs of victims of intentional or unintentional injury?
- What services are available to address the needs of perpetrators of violence?

Environmental Quality

- What environmental pollutants are present in the community? What is the source of pollutants?
- What legal and regulatory factors influence environmental quality in the community?
- What health effects related to poor environmental quality are prevalent in the community?
- What other effects, if any, does the physical environment have on community health (e.g., opportunities for physical activity, safety concerns)?

Continued on next page

Immunization

- What are community immunization levels?
- What are community attitudes toward and levels of knowledge about immunizations?
- What socioeconomic or cultural factors impede immunizations?
- How available and accessible are immunization services to community members?
- What are the incidence and prevalence of immunizable diseases in the community?

Access to Care

- What proportion of the population is covered by health insurance?
- What proportion of the population has a regular source of health care?

- What is the extent of nonemergent care provided in local emergency departments?
- What proportion of the population receives preventive health services?
- To what extent do members of the population forgo health care for economic or other reasons (e.g., lack of knowledge, transportation to services, etc.)?

Other Indicators

- What other health problems are prevalent in the community (e.g., heart disease, hypertension, cancer, diabetes)?
- To what extent are these problems controlled in affected members of the community?
- What preventive activities are undertaken in the community with respect to these problems?

In the Irish public health nursing service and the British National Health System, distinctions are made between public health nurses, who have a population focus to their practice, and community health nurses, who provide more services on an individual client/family level. District nurses in Sweden are similar to those in Los Angeles County, and a similar approach is used in Finland, where public health nursing services may be based on sectoral or population-based models or a combination of both. Sectoral practice reflects a focus on a particular age group or health problem, similar to that of specialty program nurses in Los Angeles County, whereas population-based practice is similar to district nursing practice, described above (Jakonen et al., 2002). Some countries and U.S. health departments have separated services provided to specific population groups. Other countries, such as Australia, have begun to reunite functions under a generalist public health nurse role (Hanafin et al., 2002). Public health nurses working in specific jurisdictions need to become familiar with the organizational structure of public health nursing services and identify their particular role within that structure.

Nursing Diagnoses, Intervention Outcomes, and Public Health Nursing

As indicated throughout this text, community health nurses engage in the diagnostic reasoning process to develop community nursing diagnoses that are designed to direct intervention to achieve specific designated outcomes. One study of field records in one county health department found that 65 nursing diagnoses among those developed by the North American Nursing Diagnosis Association (NANDA) and 128 nursing interventions identified in the Nursing Interventions Classification (NIC) were used by public health nurses (Rivera & Parris, 2002).

Similarly, six population-based community nursing outcomes developed as part of the Nursing Outcomes Classification (NOC) have been tested for their applicability to nursing practice by public health nurses in official health agencies. The six diagnoses were (a) community competence, (b) community health status, (c) community health: immunity, (d) community risk control: chronic disease, (e) community risk control: communicable disease, and (f) community risk control: lead exposure. All of the outcomes were rated by practicing public health nurses as important and all of the outcome indicators were found to be important in assessing the achievement of outcomes. In addition, 45% of the indicators were felt to be capable of being influenced by nursing interventions, suggesting that community-level diagnoses may be useful in identifying and improving the health status of population groups (Head et al., 2004).

Public Health Nursing and Public Health Functions and Services

The efforts of public health nurses in local health departments are directed toward the accomplishment of the core public health functions and provision of the essential services outlined earlier. These efforts may be undertaken with individual clients and families as well as with population groups. With respect to the core function of assessment, for example, the public health nurse in a local health department may assess the health status of populations, target groups, families, or individuals. Similarly, he or she may recommend policy and program development to meet the needs of entire populations or subgroups of individuals and families within the population. The policy development function may also involve activities to develop standards of practice and criteria for service delivery. Finally, in relation to the assurance function, public health nurses may provide direct services to individuals and families, or evaluate the quality and effectiveness of health care services. Public health nursing roles and functions may also be examined in relation to the essential services provided by public health agencies as depicted in Table 3◆.

TABLE 3	Essential Public Health Services and Related Community Health Nursing Functions
Essential Service	**Community Health Nurse Function**
Monitor health status to identify community health problems.	• Conduct community assessments. • Collect data to monitor status of identified community health problems.
Diagnose and investigate health problems and health hazards in the community.	• Identify community assets and needs. • Identify factors contributing to community health problems. • Identify community health hazards and alert appropriate authorities.
Inform, educate, and empower people regarding health issues.	• Plan and implement health education programs. • Develop and disseminate health-related messages to the public. • Assist with community organization and empowerment.
Mobilize community partnerships to identify and solve health problems.	• Identify key community members. • Assist community members to articulate needs and plan to address them. • Identify potential coalition members to address particular health issues.
Develop policies and plans that support individual and community health efforts.	• Participate in community health program planning based on identified needs. • Advocate for relevant and culturally sensitive health care programs. • Advocate for involvement of community members in health program planning, implementation, and evaluation.
Enforce laws and regulations that protect health and ensure safety.	• Identify violations of health-related regulations and inform appropriate authorities. • Educate the public regarding health-related regulations.
Link people to needed health care services and assure the provision of health care when otherwise unavailable.	• Make referrals for health care services as needed. • Provide direct health care services as appropriate.
Assure a competent public health and personal health workforce.	• Assist in the education of community health nurses and other health care professionals.
Evaluate effectiveness, accessibility, and quality of personal and population-based health services.	• Participate in the planning and conduct of program evaluations to determine effectiveness, accessibility, and quality of services. • Use evaluative data to improve health care delivery.
Research for new insights and innovative solutions to health problems.	• Identify relevant research questions and participate in designing and conducting studies to answer them. • Test innovative practice models and delivery systems.

Several of the national health objectives for 2010 address the infrastructure and functions of local public health agencies (Centers for Disease Control and Prevention [CDC], 2005). These objectives can be viewed on the *Healthy People 2010*◆ Web site at http://wonder.cdc.gov/data2010. The targets for selected objectives are presented on the next page. Public health nurses may be actively involved in the accomplishment of these objectives. For example, public health nurses are the health care professionals most likely to develop and implement culturally and linguistically appropriate health promotion and disease prevention programs related to many of the health problems addressed in the objectives. Similarly, public health nurses may help to inform information systems personnel of the types of data needed in geographic information systems or assist local health authorities to develop health improvement plans that address state and national priorities.

Public Health Nursing Roles in a Local Health Department

Public health nurses working in local health departments also perform community health nursing roles. The extent to which they engage in any one particular role, however, will depend on the focus and organizational structure of the particular health department. By virtue of their population health focus, public health nurses engage in all of the population-oriented roles. For example, community health nurses engage in the case-finding role in the context of other responsibilities. For example, a public health nurse working in a family planning clinic or making a home visit for child health may identify a woman who shows signs of intimate partner violence or notice a visitor to the home who has symptoms of tuberculosis. Similarly, public health nurses perform the leadership role in assisting community members to take action regarding a community health problem such as adolescent pregnancy or a high incidence of bicycle accidents among school-aged children. One population-oriented role that public health nurses may or may not be actively involved in is the researcher role. Even if public health nurses are not actively involved in conducting research, they will endeavor to incorporate research findings into their practice.

Delivery-oriented roles are performed by public health nurses primarily in the context of population-based delivery systems. For example, public health nurses may help develop systems that coordinate care for groups of clients with specific kinds of health problems

HEALTHY PEOPLE 2010
Goals for Population Health

OBJECTIVE	BASELINE	TARGET
7-11. Increase the number of health departments that provide access to culturally and linguistically competent health promotion and disease prevention programs related to:		
c. Cancer	30%	50%
g. Educational and community-based programs	33%	50%
h. Environmental health	22%	50%
i. Family planning	42%	50%
m. Heart disease and stroke	28%	50%
n. HIV	45%	50%
o. Immunizations and infectious diseases	48%	50%
q. Maternal and child health	47%	50%
r. Mental health	18%	50%
s. Nutrition and overweight	44%	50%
t. Occupational safety and health	13%	50%
u. Oral health	25%	50%
v. Physical activity and fitness	21%	50%
y. Sexually transmitted diseases	41%	50%
z. Substance abuse	26%	50%
aa. Tobacco use	24%	50%
23-3. Increase the proportion of local health data systems that use geocoding to promote use of geographic information systems	45%	90%
23-12. Increase the proportion of local jurisdictions that have a health improvement plan linked with their state plan	32%	80%

Data from: Centers for Disease Control and Prevention. (2005). Healthy people data. Retrieved September 6, 2005, from http://wonder/cdc.gov/data2010

Think Advocacy

Esperanza Gutierrez is a public health nurse working for the Jackson County Health Department. She is responsible for a low-income area in which many Latino clients live. Many of her clients live in apartment complexes owned by a few absentee Caucasian landlords. On several of her visits, Esperanza has noticed that the apartments are in need of repair and many are lacking smoke detectors, although they are required in rental units by state law. Others have bars on the windows that would prevent escape in case of fire. Her clients tell her that they have spoken to their landlords about repairs, but have received no response or are told to call a repairman and pay for the repairs themselves. Many of her clients speak no English and are afraid to report the safety hazards to the local housing authority for fear they will be evicted in retaliation. There are not enough rental units to meet the housing demand in the area, and apartments are often rented within a day of vacancy.

- What factors are influencing this situation?
- What action might Esperanza take to remedy the situation?
- What other segments of the county government might she involve in her efforts? What other community agencies might she involve? How might she go about obtaining their involvement?
- How might residents of the apartment complexes become involved?

requiring assistance from several health and social service sectors (e.g., those with HIV infection or pregnant adolescents). Similarly, public health nurses engage in collaboration with a wide variety of others in developing services and programs to meet the needs of population groups. They may also collaborate with others and coordinate care for individual and family clients. In the liaison role, public health nurses may serve as liaisons between community residents and other health care providers or with public officials. They may also serve a liaison function with individual clients and their families.

Some public health nurses may be involved in client-oriented community health nursing roles. Although the provision of direct care to individuals and families is receiving less emphasis in public health nursing than at some times in the past, many public health nurses still achieve population-level health outcomes in part through direct care to members of the population (Abrams, 2004). Almost all public health nurses are engaged in some manner in the educator function, and they often serve as referral resources for clients or communities in need of specific services. Many public health nurses also engage in case management for clients with long-term conditions (e.g., pregnancy, chronic illness). Table 4◆ compares

TABLE 4	Client-oriented, Delivery-oriented, and Population-oriented Community Health Nursing Roles as Performed by Public Health Nurses and Faith Community Nurses	
Role	Public Health Nurse	Faith Community Nurse
Caregiver	• Plan, implement, and evaluate care delivery systems based on assessed population needs • Sometimes provide direct care to individuals and families	• Provide direct care to individuals and families in the congregation based on needs • Sometimes plan, implement, and evaluate population-based programs to address identified needs
Educator	• Plan population-based health education programs • Occasionally provide health education to individuals and families	• Provide health education to individuals and families or groups within the congregation
Counselor	• Serve as a consultant to communities in addressing health care needs	• Assist members of the congregation with health-related decision making
Referral resource	• Refer individuals, families, and population groups to needed resources	• Refer individuals and families in the congregation to needed health and other services
Role model	• Role-model population-based practice for other health professionals and health profession students, including nursing students	• Role-model health-related behaviors for members of the congregation
Case manager	• Develop case management systems for specific groups within the population	• Provide case management services for members of the congregation
Coordinator	• Coordinate the provision of care by multiple agencies, health and social services providers, and other segments of the community	• Coordinate the activities of the faith community health ministry • Coordinate the health-related activities of volunteer members of the congregation
Collaborator	• Collaborate with broad segments of the community in developing, implementing, and evaluating health care programs based on identified population health needs	• Collaborate with other members of the ministerial team • Collaborate with health and social service providers in the community to meet the needs of specific clients
Liaison	• Assist population groups to connect with needed resources • Present the health-related needs of community members to policy makers	• Assist members of the congregation to obtain needed health care services
Case finder	• Identify trends in diseases and health problems occurring within the population	• Identify members of the congregation with specific health problems
Leader	• Assist communities in taking action to meet identified health needs	• Assist members of the congregation in taking action to meet identified health needs
Change agent	• Motivate and engineer change in health-related policies and health care delivery systems	• Assist members of the congregation to change health-related behaviors
Community mobilizer	• Organize community members to take action to address health-related concerns	• Organize members of the congregation to undertake health-related action
Coalition builder	• Develop associations with other community agencies and individuals to address identified population health needs	• Develop associations between the faith community and other community agencies and individuals to address the identified health needs of the congregation
Policy advocate	• Assist in the development of health-related policy to improve population health	• Assist in the development of health-related policies within the congregation (e.g., a ban on smoking in faith community facilities)
Social marketer	• Participate in the development of social marketing campaigns to change population health-related behaviors or attitudes or health-related policy	• Develop social marketing campaigns to change health-related behaviors or attitudes among members of the congregation
Researcher	• Possibly conduct research related to factors that influence population health or interventions that improve population health • Apply research findings to population-focused practice	• Possibly conduct research related to faith community nursing and its effectiveness • Apply research findings to faith community nursing practice

client-oriented, delivery-oriented, and population-oriented community health nursing roles as they might be executed by a public health nurse and a community health nurse employed in a faith community setting. As can be seen in the table, both public health nurses and faith community nurses are involved in similar roles and functions, but the level at which the roles are executed are quite different, with public health nurses performing roles at a broader population-based level.

The roles of public health nurses may also be examined in terms of the interventions wheel model. The 17 interventions included in the wheel can be implemented at individual-focused, community-focused, and systems-focused levels. At the individual level, the focus is on care provided to individuals and families within the population. At the community level, interventions center on changes in community norms, awareness, attitudes, and behaviors. Systems-level interventions focus on changes in organizations and health care delivery systems and structures (Keller, Strohschein, Schaffer, & Lia-Hoagberg, 2004). The utility of the interventions wheel has been tested in a health-department-based Medicaid Managed Care system. Specific interventions found to be useful in the program were outreach, individual health assessment, screening and surveillance, health education, case management, referral and follow-up, consultation, collaboration, and advocacy (Kaiser, Barry, & Kaiser, 2002). The interventions have also been successfully implemented to direct systems-level, community-level, and individual-level care in other state and local health departments (Keller et al., 2004).

Another role that is relatively unique to public health nurses in official health agencies is the development of community bioterrorism response plans. Although community health nurses in other settings are likely to be involved in developing response plans for their agencies, public health nurses are the ones most likely to participate in the development of response plans for local health departments. Bioterrorism preparedness roles for advanced-practice public health nurses could be adapted to respond to most disasters and include assessment to identify suspected bioterrorism, surveillance for bioterrorism effects, identification of desired response outcomes to a bioterrorist event, participation in the development of policies and response plans, dissemination of information to the public, referral for needed assistance in the event of bioterrorist exposures, and participation in evaluation of the effectiveness of response to a specific bioterrorist incident (Mondy, Cardenas, & Avila, 2003).

The overarching role of the public health nurse, of course, is advocating for the health of the public. Nursing advocacy in a public health setting may be somewhat more difficult than in other community health settings because nurses are functioning in a medically dominated and highly political bureaucracy in which activities are frequently mandated in response to changing political interests. In one study of a large public health agency, for example, public health nurses rated themselves as more influential in controlling their own practice than community members, but less influential than any other group of players (Falk-Rafael, 2005a). In other settings, public health nurses have been constrained by organizational structure or roles from engaging in population-based care and advocacy (Falk-Rafael, 2005b). For example, some authors have contended that failure to fund public health nursing positions on the basis of population needs rather than size has hampered the ability of public health nurses to engage in true population-based practice (Hanafin et al., 2002). Others have noted that the development of other nursing roles in public health departments that do not have a population focus has limited investment in public health nursing (Clarke, 2004). In some cases, public health nurses have themselves been reluctant to assume responsibility for population-based practice and advocacy (Carr & Davidson, 2004). Some research has found that work overload and expectations with respect to the primary care of individuals and families and lack of support has limited public health nurses' abilities to engage in population-level practice and advocacy even when these are organizational expectations. Public health nurses in one study engaged in population-based health projects on their own time and often provided for project needs from their own resources (McMurray & Cheater, 2004).

Public health nurses may need to advocate for their own ability to serve as community advocates and to protect and enhance their role in this area. They may also need to resist pressure to move away from a population focus on health promotion and illness prevention to address more categorically focused health needs (e.g., bioterrorism preparedness and disease prevention) (Falk-Rafael, 2005a). As noted by one author, "Nurses who practice at the intersection of public policy and personal lives are, therefore, ideally situated and morally obligated to include political advocacy and efforts to influence health public policy in their practice" (Falk-Rafael, 2005b, p. 212). This may mean advocating for sufficient funds to support public health nursing activity in official health agencies as well as advocacy for policies that directly affect the health of the population.

Advocacy for population health may involve empowering the communities with which public health nurses work. One study of public health nurses in rural and urban health departments found that the nurses conceptualized empowerment as "an active, internal process of growth . . . toward actualizing one's full potential" that "occurred within the context of a nurturing nurse-client relationship" (Falk-Rafael, 2001, p. 4). The nurses also described three levels of awareness that related to empowerment of individual, family, or community clients. The first level was an awareness of one's own strengths and limitations. The second was an awareness of the right to have control over health issues and to participate in health-related decisions. The third level involved an awareness of political factors and their influence on health and health care services (Falk-Rafael, 2001). Public health nurses can work to create these levels of awareness in community members to empower them to take action with respect to community health issues.

Public health nurses may also engage in population health advocacy and community empowerment through the development of connections among three interacting levels of community: local communities, created communities, and communities of resources (Schulte, 2000). The local community is the geographic divisions of a public health jurisdiction. Created communities are groups of individuals and families connected by blood, marriage, or intended affiliations. The community of resources includes organizations developed to provide goods and services to residents in need of them. Public health nurses work to purposefully develop connections between these levels of

EVIDENCE-BASED PRACTICE

Evidence to support the effectiveness of public health nursing interventions is often lacking, but the Effective Public Health Practice Project of the Ontario, Canada, Ministry of Health has developed a process for systematic research reviews by which public health departments and public health nurses can create an evidence base for their practice. Elements of the process include the following:

- Formulating the question for the evidence review: Identification of the topic on which the review will center. Questions include identification of the population of interest (e.g., clients with HIV infection), an intervention (e.g., home visits), and an outcome (e.g., effects on medication compliance or symptom relief).
- Searching and retrieving relevant literature
- Establishing criteria for relevance of literature retrieved (e.g., specific types of study design, subject populations, etc.)
- Assessing the quality of relevant studies as strong, moderate, or weak, in terms of selection bias, design, control of confounding variables, blinding of participants and outcomes assessors, validity and reliability of data collection methods, and subject retention rates
- Retrieving data related to funding source, number of participants/dropouts, a description of the target populations, the intervention employed, outcomes, and the length of follow-up from studies judged to be of strong or moderate quality
- Writing a report that synthesizes the information retrieved for all studies reviewed
- Disseminating results of the review to policy makers and other appropriate personnel (Thomas, Ciliska, Dobbins, & Micucci, 2004)

Similar reviews have been undertaken by public health nursing administrators in Scotland (Elliott, Crombie, Irvine, Cantrell, & Taylor, 2004).

Identify a topic for a review of evidence that would be relevant to public health nursing practice in your own local health department. Who else might be involved in identifying appropriate topics and questions for systematic reviews?

community. For example, they may link individual clients or families to service organizations, or coordinate the activities of several service organizations to meet the needs of the population. They may also connect several created communities to interact with service providers to design services appropriate to the needs of the population.

COMMUNITY HEALTH NURSING IN A VOLUNTARY AGENCY: A FAITH-BASED ORGANIZATION

As noted earlier, community health nursing may occur in official and voluntary agencies. According to the Public Health Nursing Section of the American Public Health Association (1996), nursing in voluntary agencies constitutes community health nursing when the focus is on the health of population groups that include both those persons who present for services and those who do not.

Health-related organizations within faith communities are a special type of voluntary health agency that present a relatively new practice setting for community health nursing. A **faith community** is "an organization of families and individuals who share common values, beliefs, religious doctrine, and faith practices that influence their lives" (Smith, 2003b). Faith communities may engage in **health ministry**, which is purposeful activity designed to help people in the congregation and surrounding community to achieve an optimal level of "whole person health" (Bay Area Health Ministries, 2001). **Whole person health** is a holistic concept that conceives of health as an integration of physical, psychological, social, and spiritual well-being (Story, 2003).

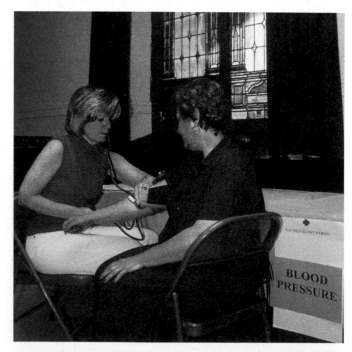

Some faith community nurses provide care to community residents as well as members of the congregation.

Faith communities can provide a significant avenue for influencing the health of populations. In the United States alone, there are 265,000 to 350,000 congregations and 2,000 organized systems of religion. In addition, faith communities influence health and health care through interfaith and ecumenical systems, health institutions owned and operated by religious groups, and institutions that are strongly influenced by religious values and principles, as well as through the everyday activities of members of individual faith communities (Gunderson, 2000). For example, faith communities influence personality development and the development of health-related perspectives, motivate change in unhealthy behaviors, and convey messages of hope in adversity, promoting coping. Faith communities also influence perceptions of pain and disability, encourage caregiving and altruism, and provide a framework that gives meaning to life. Faith communities can influence health by virtue of their stability in the community and in the lives of their members, the respect with which they are viewed, their focus on respect for life and care of others, and their usual receptivity to health promotion interventions (Buijs & Olson, 2001). Faith communities may influence health through their involvement at any of three levels of health-related interventions:

- A recruitment venue for health-related activities provided by secular (nonreligious) sources
- A place for delivering health care services provided by secular agencies (by professionals or lay persons)
- Incorporation of a religious or spiritual focus into health care delivery programs (Holt, Kyles, Wiehagen, & Casey, 2003)

Many faith communities are becoming more actively involved in promoting the health of their members and engaging in activities related to this third level of involvement in health care interventions. These health promotion efforts have been found to be facilitated by the use of "parish" or faith community nurses who can integrate, coordinate, and institutionalize aspects of the faith community's health ministry in a way that is visible both to members of the congregation and to outsiders (Pattillo, Chesley, Castles, & Sutter, 2002). Multiple titles have been advanced for nurses working in this specialty area. The initial terminology, *parish nurse*, has been rejected by many people because many faith-based congregations are not organized as parishes and the term was believed to be too closely tied to certain faith traditions. Other titles used include *congregational nurse, health ministry nurse,* and *faith community nurse* (Pattillo et al., 2002). Because of its global nature and applicability to a broad array of faith traditions, the term *faith community nurse* is used in this text. Faith community nurses practice a newly recognized nursing specialty known as parish or faith community nursing. Faith community or **parish nursing** has been defined as "a health promotion, disease prevention role based on the care of the whole person . . . it is a professional model of health ministry

using a registered nurse" (Solari-Twadell, as cited in O'Brien, 2003, p. 51). Parish or **faith community nurses** are "registered nurses (RNs) with a significant personal religious history who join a church staff, either as volunteers or in paid positions, full- or part-time, and provide services that focus on the intersection of health, faith, and spirituality" (Vandecreek & Mooney, 2002, p. xviii). Faith community nurses focus on the promotion of health in the context of the faith community, building on the strengths of the congregation and providing services that are not otherwise available. They represent the concern of the congregation for members, and sometimes outsiders, who are experiencing health-related problems (Vandecreek & Mooney, 2002).

The number of nurses who function in this capacity is unknown, although the number is increasing. In one study, 57% of U.S. faith-based congregations engaged in some sort of social service programs, including those related to health. Most of these activities centered on primary prevention and health maintenance as well as specific health issues (e.g., smoking cessation, cardiovascular health, nutrition). Nearly one fourth of the programs provided services to members of the surrounding community in addition to members of the congregation (DeHaven, Hunter, Wilder, Walton, & Berry, 2004). Many of the health-related programs provided by U.S. faith communities are supported by the efforts of faith community nurses. Although the criteria for faith community nurses vary somewhat from congregation to congregation, Via Christi Regional Medical Center (n.d.) has identified some criteria that may be useful to congregations seeking to initiate a faith community nursing program. These criteria include the following:

- A registered nurse with a current license
- Willingness to participate in continuing education related to faith community nursing
- Previous clinical experience (preferably in community health, medical-surgical, emergency department, or outpatient department nursing)
- Belief in and willingness to support the healing ministry of the faith community
- Active participation in the faith community
- A holistic philosophy of health
- Expertise in communication and teaching
- Knowledge of health promotion and lifestyle modification strategies
- Familiarity with nursing and health-related issues
- Awareness of and compliance with the state nurse practice act and the nursing code of ethics
- An emphasis on confidentiality
- Ability to collaborate with the pastoral team

Historical Foundations of Nursing in a Faith-based Community

The early history of nursing included healthcare services provided by many religious groups. Faith community nursing traces its roots in the Christian tradition to the deaconesses of the early Christian church. The diaconal role in the early church included not only care for the sick but also the dispensing of alms, teaching, and assistance with liturgical ceremonies and is closely aligned with the modern role of the faith community nurse. The Kaiserswerth Deaconess program, established in 1836 by Theodor Fliedner and his wife Frederika Munster, was a faith-based program that significantly influenced Florence Nightingale in her contributions to modern nursing and community health nursing. The prominence of faith in health work was also seen in the writings of early nurses in the United States (O'Brien, 2003). The roots of care of the sick in parishes in the Roman Catholic tradition lie in the work of the Daughters of Charity, initiated by Vincent de Paul in 1629. The "rules" laid down for the sisters have relevance to modern faith community nursing and include the following:

- The need to be virtuous
- The need to maintain a professional relationship with the spiritual director and to avoid inappropriate relationships in an often intimate situation
- The need to be honest and direct with clients while avoiding incessant preaching
- The need to serve the whole person "so that those who die will leave the world better prepared" and to "assist those you serve to die well and those who recover to lead better lives" (Leonard, quoted in Solari-Twadell & Egenes, 2006, p. 13)
- The need to appropriately manage the nurse's time and to recruit and delegate to volunteers as appropriate
- The need for personal spiritual growth
- The need to care for family members as well as the sick individual, particularly children
- The need to recognize and adhere to the boundaries of practice
- The need to be aware of and set aside personal feelings
- The need to reject monetary gain for one's services

This last rule was not intended to imply that faith community nurses should not be paid for their services if they are employees of the congregation, but that they should direct any gifts in gratitude for services to the congregation (Solari-Twadell & Egenes, 2006).

Throughout history, there have been times of closer relationships between organized religion and public health efforts. For example, the control of tuberculosis at the close of the 19th century relied heavily on the promotion of public health messages of hygiene and sanitation by churches. Women's charitable organizations, many of them church based, supported many of the early health care services for the poor and indigent, and women as well as clergy were actively involved in campaigning for social conditions that would promote health. As public health became more of a scientific discipline dominated by physicians, however, women and the clergy were less involved in public health efforts.

Today, however, the ills that plague society are once again of interest to faith-based groups (e.g., adolescent pregnancy, substance abuse, violence), and faith communities have become more active in promoting healthy behaviors among their members (Gunderson, 2000). Public health agencies have also become more aware of the usefulness of congregations as a source of outreach and access to underserved populations (Holt et al., 2003).

The Reverend Granger W. Westberg saw congregations as playing a key role in illness prevention and in promoting whole-person health and initiated a health focus in the education of those in seminary training. He later implemented training for medical students in the connection of faith and health. In the 1960s, Rev. Granger implemented "holistic health centers," volunteer physician offices housed in church facilities that incorporated the services of a three-member team—pastor, physician, and nurse (Westberg, J., 2006).

The centers proved too costly to maintain, but they had demonstrated that the central feature in their effectiveness was the presence of nurses who spoke both the language of science and the language of faith and could translate between them (Patterson, 2003). Westberg engineered a partnership between Lutheran General Hospital and six Chicago-area churches, each with a faith community nurse, to provide health promotion services to their congregations (Palmer, 2001).

As noted earlier, the concept of faith community nursing has grown since its inception. Although begun in Christian denominations, the concept of faith community nurses has spread to Jewish and Muslim faith communities as well (Fitzgerald, 2000). In 1986, the International Parish Nurse Resource Center was established (O'Brien, 2003), and in 1992, the Interfaith Health Program of the Carter Center was initiated to help encourage best practices in faith community nursing and health ministries. Since then, a number of other organizations have been established to provide resources related to faith community nursing. In 1997, the American Nurses Association recognized faith community nursing as a distinct practice specialty (Fitzgerald, 2000), and began work with the Health Ministries Association to develop a set of standards for practice in the specialty. These standards will be addressed later in this chapter.

Philosophy of Nursing in a Faith-based Community

Faith community nursing focuses on the relationship between mind, body, and spirit in health, illness, and death. In this relationship, spirituality is recognized as a "dynamic force that nurtures and celebrates wholeness" (Swinney, Anson-Wonkka, Maki, & Corneau, 2001, p. 41) and contributes to health and a peaceful death. In the context of faith community nursing, illness is defined as "the experience of 'brokenness,' that is, the disintegration of body, mind, spirit; and disharmony with others, the environment, and God" (American Nurses Association and the Health Ministry Association, as quoted in Pattillo et al., 2002, p. 43). Faith community nursing focuses on total health and healing within the context of spiritual beliefs and values (Dryden, 2004).

The goals of faith community nursing are derived from this philosophical stance and include providing holistic care to members of the congregation and sometimes the larger community, preventing illness, and helping people obtain needed health care services. The faith community health ministry is intended to complement the health care delivery system in the larger community rather than to duplicate services (Swinney et al., 2001).

A health ministry presupposes belief that health is determined by four groups of factors—physical, mental, social, and spiritual—all of which can be modified by intervention. Four areas of interrelationship between faith and health have been identified. The first is the link between personal spirituality and healing. Scientific medicine is just beginning to explore the effect of faith on health and health outcomes. The second relationship is the link between faith structures or communities and public health, a link that is strengthened by the relationship-building efforts of faith community nurses. The third relationship deals with the changing roles and responsibilities for health activities assumed by public, private, nonprofit, and voluntary organizations. The last focus of activity lies in the changing vitality of faith structures, with greater assumption of responsibility for health ministries. This focus is exemplified by the fact that 10% to 15% of religious congregations ground their life in service to and fostering change in communities (Gunderson, 2000). Faith community nurses must themselves have an active spiritual life and must be able to incorporate spiritual interventions into their practice. Helping ability in the spiritual realm is characterized by the ability to access one's own spirituality, respect for spirituality in others, and the ability to offer spiritual as well as material resources to clients in need (Olson & Clark, 2000).

The need for spiritual care is particularly evident in times of transition. Transitions may be developmental or situational in nature (Clark, 2000) and may give rise to a need for spiritual care as well as other interventions. Developmental transitions are expected and arise from normal growth, maturation, and change. They may be

experienced by individual members or families within the congregation or by the congregation as a whole. Marriage, death, or the birth of a child are expected transitions for individuals and families. The replacement of a pastor, priest, imam, or rabbi is an example of a developmental transition for the congregation. Situational transitions, on the other hand, are not expected and usually involve some aspect of loss. Unemployment is an example of a situational transition for an individual member of a congregation, whereas destruction of the church, synagogue, temple, or mosque imposes a situational transition on the congregation as a whole.

The foregoing underpinnings of faith community nursing can be summarized in four philosophical statements derived from the Statement of Philosophy for Parish Nursing endorsed at the First Invitational Educational Colloquium sponsored by the International Parish Nurse Resource Center (Solari-Twadell, 1999). These statements can be summarized as follows.

- Faith community nursing emphasizes the spiritual dimension but also addresses physical, psychological, sociocultural, and environmental dimensions of health.
- Faith community nursing integrates science with theology, and combines service with worship and nursing with pastoral care.
- The faith community nurse facilitates involvement of the faith community in health and healing.
- Spiritual health is central to well-being and may coexist with illness. Similarly, healing may occur in the absence of cure.

Standards and Competencies for Nursing in a Faith-based Community

As in other specialty areas of nursing practice, faith community nursing should be based on specific standards that promote effective, caring practice. The standards of practice for parish nursing summarized below were first published by the Health Ministries Association in conjunction with the American Nurses Association (ANA) in 1998. The standards of care reflect the nursing process and address assessment, diagnosis, outcome identification, planning, implementation, and evaluation. The standards of professional performance address quality of practice, education for competent practice, practice evaluation, collegiality, collaboration, ethics, research, resource utilization, and leadership similar to those put forth for community/public health nursing in general (ANA & Health Ministries Association, 2005). The standards are presented on the next page.

Competencies required of faith community nurses include the general competencies defined by the Institute of Medicine for health care professionals. These competencies include the ability to provide client-centered care, work effectively in interdisciplinary teams, engage in evidence-based practice, foster quality improvement, and effectively use information

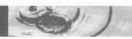

CULTURAL COMPETENCE

*R*eligious rituals are part of the cultural heritage of many faith communities. What are some of the religious rituals of your own faith community or one with which you are familiar? How might these rituals influence health? How do they differ from those of other faith communities? What role might a faith community nurse play in relation to these rituals?

SPECIAL CONSIDERATIONS

FAITH COMMUNITY NURSING: SCOPE AND STANDARDS OF PRACTICE

Standards of Practice for Faith Community Nursing

Standard 1. Assessment: The faith community nurse collects comprehensive data pertinent to the patient's wholistic health or the situation.

Standard 2. Diagnosis: The faith community nurse analyzes the wholistic assessment data to determine the diagnoses or issues.

Standard 3. Outcomes Identification: The faith community nurse identifies expected outcomes for a plan individualized to the patient or the situation.

Standard 4. Planning: The faith community nurse develops a plan that prescribes strategies and alternatives to attain expected outcomes for individuals, groups, or the faith community as a whole.

Standard 5. Implementation: The faith community nurse implements the specified plan.

> *Standard 5A. Coordination of Care:* The faith community nurse coordinates care delivery.
>
> *Standard 5B. Health Teaching and Health Promotion:* The faith community nurse employs strategies to promote wholistic health, wellness, and a safe environment.
>
> *Standard 5C. Consultation:* The faith community nurse provides consultation to facilitate understanding and influence the specified plan of care, enhance the abilities of others, and effect change.
>
> *Standard 5D. Prescriptive Authority and Treatment (Optional for appropriately prepared APRN):* The advanced practice registered nurse, faith community nurse uses prescriptive authority, procedures, referrals, treatments, and therapies in accordance with state and federal laws and regulations.

Standard 6. Evaluation: The faith community nurse evaluates progress toward attainment of outcomes.

Standards of Professional Performance for Faith Community Nursing

Standard 7. Quality of Practice: The faith community nurse systematically enhances the quality and effectiveness of faith community nursing practice.

Standard 8. Education: The faith community nurse attains knowledge and competency that reflects current nursing practice.

Standard 9. Professional Practice Evaluation: The faith community nurse evaluates one's own nursing practice in relation to professional practice standards and guidelines, relevant statutes, rules, and regulations.

Standard 10. Collegiality: The faith community nurse interacts with and contributes to the professional development of peers and colleagues.

Standard 11. Collaboration: The faith community nurse collaborates with the patient, spiritual leaders, members of the faith community, and others in the conduct of this specialized nursing practice.

Standard 12. Ethics: The faith community nurse integrates ethical provisions in all areas of practice.

Standard 13. Research: The faith community nurse integrates research findings into practice.

Standard 14. Resource Utilization: The faith community nurse considers factors related to safety, effectiveness, cost, and impact on practice in the planning and delivery of nursing services.

Standard 15. Leadership: The faith community nurse provides leadership in the professional practice setting and the profession.

technology. Specific competencies required for faith community nursing will vary from one position to another depending on the needs of the faith community, but will generally include core competencies specific to the job description, competencies needed to address specific health issues in the congregation, age-specific competencies, and cultural competency. In addition, faith community nurses require competencies that allow them to intervene effectively in holistic care of body, mind, and spirit (Britt, 2006).

Models for Nursing in a Faith-based Community

Faith community nursing services vary greatly among faith communities, but can generally be grouped into one of several types of models or a blend of several models. The first distinction is between programs in which the faith community nurse is paid and those in which the nurse is an unpaid volunteer. In the paid model, the nurse is paid by either the faith community or by a health care organization that provides services to a faith community. The paid employee model has the advantages of highlighting the professional nature of the health ministry and providing for a specific designated amount of time during which the faith community nurse is available. Paid professionals may also be perceived by members of the congregation as providing more confidential services than volunteer staff. In addition, employing a salaried nurse increases the potential pool of applicants for the position, allowing the congregation some choice in the selection of the nurse. Finally, having a paid position increases the visibility of the health ministry within the congregation (Patterson, 2003).

The use of volunteer faith community nurses, on the other hand, highlights the overall caregiving role of members of the congregation and usually leads to long-term commitment on the part of the nurse who is a member of the congregation. The volunteer faith community nurse is usually already known to and trusted by members of the congregation. Finally, the use of volunteers makes it easier to initiate a health ministry and results in lower costs to the faith community (Patterson, 2003). Despite these advantages, some authors have noted that the best outcomes are usually achieved with paid personnel (Dryden, 2004).

A second approach to differentiating among faith community nursing programs lies in the focus of services. This approach categorizes programs in three models: the mission-ministry model, the marketplace model, and the access model. In the mission-ministry model, the focus is on a ministry of reconciliation, health, healing, wholeness, and discipleship. The faith community nurse in this model is usually a member of the congregation. The role and scope of the nurse's practice is determined by the congregation and may encompass care to members alone or include services to the surrounding community (Smith, 2002, 2003a).

In a marketplace model, services are provided to members of a faith community by professional employees of a health care agency or organization who may or may not be members of the congregation (Smith, 2002). The role and scope of the faith community nurse are defined by the employing agency and often focus on interventions related to specific problems or issues (e.g., cardiovascular disease, smoking cessation). In this model, care is driven by economic values rather than by a value of stewardship as in the mission-ministry model (Smith, 2003a).

Access models are political in nature and focus on advocacy for underserved populations. In this model, the faith community nurse serves as a catalyst and social change agent to promote access to needed health care services either within the congregation or in the larger community (Smith, 2003a). Access models are primarily advocacy models in which the nurse functions as an advocate for the oppressed (Smith, 2002).

Faith community nurses functioning in programs based on the mission-ministry or access models may be either paid staff or volunteers. Those involved in a marketplace model are paid employees of the health system providing services.

Challenges of Nursing in a Faith-based Community

Nursing within a faith community has both advantages and disadvantages. The primary advantage lies in the congruence in belief systems of nurse and clients based on a shared faith. Faith communities also provide easy access to clients with whom the nurse may engage in health-promoting and illness-preventive behaviors. Because the nurse comes into contact with members of the faith community in realms other than those related to health, he or she has the opportunity for case finding and health promotion among people who might otherwise not encounter a health care provider. In addition, this forum for multiple interaction allows members of the congregation to get to know the nurse and develop trust in him or her.

Knowledge of members of the congregation outside the usual defined parameters of health care activities also poses some challenges in faith community nursing. For example, the nurse may have intimate knowledge of clients beyond what he or she might have in a more traditional setting. The intimacy of interaction in multiple spheres of clients' lives may make maintaining confidentiality more difficult. Members of the congregation may fear violation of confidentiality or the loss of the respect of the nurse if they disclose conditions or activities that would be frowned on by other members of the group. For example, an adolescent who believes himself to be gay may hesitate to consult the nurse if he fears her reaction based on the religious beliefs of the group.

An additional challenge in faith community nursing may involve setting parameters, particularly when the needs of the congregation exceed the time available or the role and abilities of the nurse (Carson & Koenig, 2002). Much like community health nurses in rural settings, nurses in faith communities may have difficulty maintaining boundaries and may find themselves "on call" at all times of the day or night. This may be resolved by having several nurses in the congregation who can assume responsibility for addressing members' needs, preventing overload of any one nurse.

Although most faith community nurses share the beliefs and values of the groups they serve, there may be some potential for conflict. The nurse's vision of his or her role may be different from that of the congregation or the pastoral team (Carson & Koenig, 2002). In addition, faith community nurses may find themselves in conflict with doctrinal issues that they believe are interfering with what is best for a given client. Conversely, nurses may find themselves in a position in which a particular client's actions or desires may conflict with the beliefs of the nurse and the religious group. Nurses working in faith community settings must have a highly developed personal code of ethics that will allow them to successfully resolve such conflicts. Faith community nurses may also encounter expectations from the external health care system that do not acknowledge the body-mind-spirit interface and expect the nurse to function as any other community health nurse (Carson & Koenig, 2002). Development of role clarity and clear communication of the role to others within and outside of the faith community can help the nurse to address these challenges (Solari-Twadell & McDermott, 2006a).

Faith community nurses may also encounter initial resistance to the concept of a health ministry on the part of the congregation if this is not part of their previous tradition. There may also be some feelings of jealousy on the part of other congregational staff members that requires the ability to partner without assuming responsibility for the work of others (Solari-Twadell & McDermott, 2006b). Respect for others' areas of responsibility and candid discussion of role overlap and boundaries can assist faith community nurses to deal with these responses (Hahn, Radde, & Fellers, 2002).

ETHICAL AWARENESS

You are covering the practice of a faith community nurse while she is on vacation. You are of a different religious faith than the congregation you are covering. An adolescent girl and her mother seek you out because the girl has been raped by her mother's boyfriend and is pregnant. The mother assures you she has initiated legal proceedings against the boyfriend and seems very supportive of her daughter. They are requesting a referral for abortion services. Your faith holds that abortion is never allowable, even in cases of rape. When you seek guidance from the pastor of this congregation, she suggests that abortion is probably the best option for this girl and would be supported by the tenets of their faith. What will you do?

Other challenges encountered by faith community nurses include allocating limited resources, developing and sustaining relationships with the congregation as well as with other members of the pastoral team, and accepting theological and personal differences while working collaboratively to address health problems. Developing indicators for effective practice is another challenge in faith community nursing. As with much of community health nursing focused on health promotion and illness prevention, it is difficult to document the effects of interventions. Assessing the outcomes of faith community nursing will be addressed in more detail later in this chapter. Finally, because they usually function alone within a congregation, faith community nurses may feel a sense of professional isolation (Carson & Koenig, 2002), which can be addressed by developing and sustaining a network of faith community nurses as well as by participating in organizations devoted to health ministries.

Preparation for Nursing in a Faith-based Community

As a new specialty in nursing practice, educational preparation for faith community nursing is less standardized than for other specialty areas. For example, most faith community nurses take continuing education programs of 30 or more hours related to the specialty (Dryden, 2004). As this specialty grows, education programs are likely to become more standardized. The International Parish Nurse Resource Center has developed a standardized curriculum that is used by many faith community nurse preparation programs. In 1994, the Center initiated a self-regulatory process for educational programs, developed a philosophy of parish or faith community nursing, and differentiated between basic orientation for the role and site-specific orientation to a particular faith community nurse position (McDermott & Solari-Twadell, 2006). The basic faith community nursing education program is intended to provide nurses with an understanding of the integration of faith and health, provide the knowledge and skills required for

beginning practice in this area, provide a peer support network, identify a support network for growth in the practice of faith community nursing, and foster commitment among the nurses to their own continued spiritual growth (Patterson, 2003).

In 2006, Health Ministries USA listed 20 educational programs that prepare faith community nurses. There have been some proposed curriculum changes for multiphase educational programs in this area, with phase one addressing basic role preparation, the context of faith community nursing, organization and administration of programs, and processes involved in faith community nursing. Phase two will address instruction on specific topical areas such as end-of-life care, screening, family and caregiver support, and the consultation process. Phase two will be followed by advanced workshops in areas such as teaching/learning, nutrition counseling, forgiveness facilitation, values clarification, and so on (McDermott & Solari-Twadell, 2006).

There is also movement to educate faith community nurses at the master's level in higher education institutions in nursing. The 2001 *Peterson's Guide to Nursing Programs* (Thomson Learning & American Association of Colleges of Nursing, 2001) did not list parish or faith community nursing or health ministry as an area of specialty practice within any existing graduate nursing programs. By 2006, however, a search for programs with these titles revealed eight programs in seven states and one Web-based program (All Nursing Schools, 2006).

Roles and Functions of Community Health Nurses in a Faith-based Community

The role of the faith community nurse has been described more as one of "being with" clients than of providing direct hands-on care (Carson & Koenig, 2002). The specific roles and functions of particular faith community nurses are dictated by the needs of the faith communities they serve. Because faith community nursing is an innovative field and the faith community nurse is often the only health professional present in the setting, he or she may have more latitude in defining the role than is permitted in more fully developed practice settings. In the first few years of his pilot faith community nursing project, Westberg identified five initial roles for faith community nurses: health educator, personal health counselor, referral agent, coordinator of volunteers, and developer of support groups (Westberg, G., 2006). Most authors consistently add two additional roles: integrator of faith and health and health advocate (Patterson, 2003). Solari-Twadell (2006) conducted a study of interventions from the Nursing Interventions Classification (NIC) system most commonly used by faith community nurses and found that they generally fell into six categories: basic physiologic care (e.g., exercise promotion), behavioral care (e.g., smoking cessation), safety (e.g., risk management and screening for health risks), family care (e.g., family and caregiver support), health system-related care (e.g., referral, consultation), and community care (e.g., health program development). She found that faith community nursing practice did not include hands-on care, medication management, laboratory testing, and similar interventions.

Most of the identified roles for faith community nurses are very similar to those of other community health nurses, so we will focus on a few specific elements of the role. The role of integrating faith and health is unique to faith community nursing and involves recognizing and making others aware of the connection between physical and emotional health and spiritual health (Patterson, 2003). The faith community nurse improves both physical and emotional health by intervening in the spiritual realm as well as with more mundane health care interventions. For example, the nurse might engage in prayer or other rituals as part of the healing function. In addition, faith community nurses model the integration of faith with health beliefs and behaviors.

Although the health educator role of the faith community nurse is very similar to that of all community health nurses, it may have the added feature of writing health messages for church bulletins and other publications (Dryden, 2004). Collaboration is another familiar community health nursing role that has special applications in faith community nursing. Components of the collaborative role for the faith community nurse are similar to those for all nurses: communicating effectively, developing and sustaining connections with clients and other providers, and cooperatively setting goals. The difference arises out of the number and variety of collaborative relationships in which faith community nurses engage. First and foremost, the nurse enters into a collaborative relationship with God. In addition, the nurse collaborates with a variety of individuals within and outside of the congregation. Within the congregation, the nurse must learn to collaborate effectively with pastoral staff, members of the congregation, and existing ministries, as well as with individuals and families to whom care is provided. Collaboration may also be required either within or outside the congregation with coordinators or directors of faith community nursing and with other faith community nurses. Similarly, collaboration with physicians may occur within or outside of the faith community. In addition, the faith community nurse will most likely collaborate with community agencies and possibly with schools of nursing. Finally, faith community health nurses must collaborate in larger world movements that affect the health of members of the congregation and the community at large (Blanchfield & McLaughlin, 2006). Faith community nurses may also be involved in coordination of care for individuals and families with complex needs (Dyess, 2002).

Another role function that deserves special emphasis in faith community nursing is that of working with volunteers. Health needs in all population groups, including faith communities, are usually beyond the capacity of a single person to address. Effective faith community nurses will make appropriate use of volunteer members of the congregation, but this requires skill and planning. The nurse may need to organize volunteer efforts or coordinate, and possibly redirect, existing volunteer programs to achieve desired health outcomes. Working with volunteers may require orienting them to the concept of a health ministry and training them to perform needed functions. Other components of successful volunteer programs include providing volunteers with meaningful work, sharing and confirming them in their faith, and respecting and valuing them for their contribution to the health ministry and as members of the faith community. On a more practical note, the nurse may need to ensure the availability of space for volunteer work and ceremonies that recognize their contributions (O'Brien, 2003).

Faith community nurses have a particularly important role in end-of-life care. Required competencies in this role include the ability to provide physical, emotional, and spiritual comfort; the ability to deal with one's own feelings and attitudes toward death; and the ability to assist the client, family members, colleagues, and oneself to cope with suffering, grief, loss, and bereavement. Faith community nurses working with dying clients assume the role of palliative caregivers, defined by the World Health Organization as persons who:

- Affirm life and accept death as a normal part of life
- Neither hasten nor postpone death
- Provide relief of pain and other symptoms
- Integrate psychological and spiritual care with physical care
- Support clients in their efforts to live as normally as possible for as long as possible
- Support families and others during illness and bereavement (Timms, 2003)

Because of the congruence of beliefs about death between the faith community nurse and clients and their families, faith community nurses can help to promote faith and reduce fears related to death. Because of their connections to the larger community, they can also refer clients and their families to sources of needed services in this critical time.

A final role that may be played by some faith community nurses is that of grant writing. As noted earlier, one of the challenges of faith community nursing is dealing with usually limited resources. Grant writing is one way to increase the resources available for elements of health ministries. Faith community nurses who are writing grant proposals, particularly to government agencies, should be careful, however, to assure that the requested funds are to be used for health-related purposes that do not have religious connotations. Only when the proposed use of funds does not violate the First Amendment provisions for separation of church and state can grant proposals be funded by official government agencies (Zimmerman, 2006).

Developing Faith Community Nursing Programs

Developing a faith community nursing program in a congregation would employ the principles of health program planning. Program development begins with an assessment of the health needs and resources available to the congregation. A congregational health needs assessment is also a way to introduce members of the congregation to the concept of faith community nursing and health ministry. An assessment of a faith community would employ the principles of community assessment and might make use of the community assessment tool included in Appendix G on the Companion Website and in the *Community Assessment Reference Guide* designed to accompany this text. Some of the specific steps in initiating a program include identifying the theological foundation for a health ministry and developing an organizational structure and supervision mechanisms. The nurse and others involved in program development should delineate the long- and short-term goals of the health ministry and describe the role of the faith community nurse. Activities and qualifications of volunteer health ministers should also be identified. Practical issues in program development include finding space and funds for the program, defining lines of accountability, and dealing with possible liability issues. Finally, the planning group should develop a plan for evaluating the effectiveness of the health ministry. The focused assessment provided at right addresses some of the questions that might be asked in planning to develop a faith community nursing program.

Assessing the Outcomes of Nursing in a Faith-based Community

As with every other area of nursing practice, it is essential to evaluate the effectiveness of faith community nursing interventions. Specific outcomes to be assessed will depend on the health needs of the faith community. Possible outcomes might reflect primary, secondary, and tertiary prevention. For example, outcomes at the primary prevention level might address health risk modification (e.g., the extent of smoking cessation, improvements in home safety) or health promotion objectives (e.g., exercise participation among congregation members). Secondary prevention activities might be evaluated based on the level of control achieved in chronic diseases (e.g., hypertension control, reduced hospitalizations among diabetic members of the congregation,

FOCUSED ASSESSMENT

Considerations in Developing a Faith Community Nursing Program

- What are the health needs of the congregation?
- What is the level of health knowledge among members of the congregation? Are there areas where health education is particularly needed?
- What are the attitudes of members of the congregation regarding health and health care services?
- Who will be the focus of care for the faith community nursing program? Members of the congregation? Others in the community? Both?
- What is the theological foundation for the faith community nursing program?
- Should the faith community nursing program employ paid staff or rely on volunteers? What qualifications should staff/volunteers have?
- What organizational structure should the program have? What should the lines of accountability and authority be?
- What are the long-term and short-term goals of the program? What kinds of services will be provided?
- Where will the program be housed? How will it be financed?
- What health-related resources are available to the faith community (e.g., expertise of members of the congregation, collaborative associations with other agencies)?
- How will the faith community deal with issues of professional liability?
- What criteria will be used to evaluate program effectiveness and how will effectiveness evaluation be conducted?

increased breast cancer screening participation), care coordination (e.g., transportation or childcare services provided), crisis intervention outcomes, and reconciliation outcomes. At the level of tertiary prevention, the effectiveness of care might be assessed in terms of improved functional status, spiritual well-being and acceptance of illness, caregiver well-being, or preparation for death. One meta analysis of studies of the effectiveness of faith-based health activities found that programs achieved a variety of significant health effects, including decreased cholesterol levels, decreased blood pressure, decreased weight, improved disease and symptom control, and increased participation in breast cancer screening activities (DeHaven et al., 2004).

BUILDING OUR KNOWLEDGE BASE

*I*n its modern form, faith community nursing is a relatively new phenomenon, and little research has been done regarding its effectiveness. How would you go about designing a study of the effectiveness of a specific faith community nursing program? Would your study be developed differently if you were looking at faith community nursing in general rather than a specific program? If so, how would it be different? What variables might you examine that would cut across faith community programs, and how would you measure them?

PUBLIC AGENCY/FAITH COMMUNITY COLLABORATION

As noted earlier, faith communities are beginning to be seen as important partners with official public health agencies in achieving core functions and essential public health services. Specific collaborative programs between faith communities and local health departments and other agencies are being developed to better meet the health care needs of the diverse populations served by each. Such collaborations can include state and local health departments, local health organizations, and colleges and universities, as well as faith communities (Pattillo et al., 2002). In 2005, U.S. President Bush established the White House Faith-based and Community Initiatives (2005) to support the work of faith-based and community organizations (FBCOs). Goals of the initiative include:

- Identifying and eliminating barriers to FBCO participation in federal grants
- Encouraging corporate and philanthropic support for social programs initiated by FBCOs
- Modifying legislation to permit charitable choice provisions that protect freedom of religion and preserve hiring rights by faith-based charities

Collaborative efforts between faith-based and official health organizations have a number of advantages, including the development of culturally specific interventions and capitalization on the strength of spiritual orientations. Such collaborations are often called faith-based initiatives and differ from faith community nursing in that they bring together faith-based communities and government agencies and funding sources and may include people of several different faiths (Kotecki, 2002).

Authors with experience in public/faith-based collaboration suggest several general considerations. The first of these is the need for a formalized structure for the initiative that includes a mission statement, goals, a statement of values, objectives, and specific activities to be undertaken to achieve the objectives (Pattillo et al., 2002). The formalized structure is best developed in written form when there are employment arrangements or liability considerations involved, when money will change hands, and when the responsibilities of collaborating partners need to be delineated. A written agreement is also beneficial when trust between collaborating partners is in the early stages of development (Zimmerman, 2006).

Other considerations in developing collaborative initiatives between faith communities and official health agencies include identifying groups and organizations that could be a part of the collaborative effort and "going where one is invited," honoring the priorities of the entities involved, finding a common language, promoting buy-in by officials and members of the faith community, addressing the concerns of the larger community in planning, supporting faith communities as co-owners of the program, and employing culturally sensitive staff (DiLeo, Graham, & Solari-Twadell, 2006). Additional recommendations include viewing the collaboration as an element of ministry in and of itself (Pattillo et al., 2002) and incorporating plans for the evaluation of the ministry with its development (DiLeo et al., 2006). One example of a collaborative effort resulted in the recruitment of more faith community nurses and increased competency among existing nurses, increased effectiveness of community resources, increased participation of academic institutions in both research and the education of faith community nurses, and increased visibility of faith community nursing programs (Pattillo et al., 2002).

In the two diverse settings presented here, the local health department and a faith community, community health nurses engage in a variety of similar tasks and functions. In the health department setting, these activities are directed toward accomplishing the three core public health functions—assessment, policy development, and assurance—as well as providing essential public health services. In the faith community setting, activities are determined by the needs of the congregation, but still encompass the aggregate focus on health and health promotion, assessing the needs of the congregation, developing policies and programs to address those needs, and assuring the provision of services through incorporation of the assets of the faith community and existing community services.

GLOBAL PERSPECTIVES

Faith community nursing in this century originated primarily as a North American innovation in nursing practice. How might this area of practice differ if carried out in another country? What effects might the presence of a national health care system have on the role of faith community nurses? How might faith community nursing differ in developed and developing nations?

Case Study

A Public Health/Faith Community Collaboration

You are a faith community nurse who has been approached by the nursing director of the local health department to solicit the participation of the faith community in an initiative to increase physical activity among youth in the larger community.

1. Is this an initiative that is likely to be congruent with the faith community's health ministry? Why or why not?
2. How might the faith community promote achievement of the objectives of the initiative?
3. What role might you, as the faith community nurse, play in this collaborative effort?
4. What criteria might be used to evaluate the effectiveness of the collaboration?

Test Your Understanding

1. How do the legal and regulatory parameters of public health nursing differ from those of community health nursing in other settings?

2. What are the core functions and related essential public health services of official health agencies? How might public health nurses be involved in providing these essential services?

3. What are the core competencies of the public health workforce? How do these core competencies relate to public health nursing practice?

4. What are the roles and functions of public health nurses in carrying out the core functions and essential services in a local health department?

5. What similarities and differences exist between community health nursing roles as performed in public health nursing and faith community nursing?

6. What are the basic philosophical tenets of faith community nursing?

7. What is faith community nursing? How does it differ from other community health nursing practice settings?

8. Describe the standards and competencies for faith community nursing practice.

9. What features differentiate among the models of faith community nursing?

10. What are the key functions of faith community nurses? Give an example of each.

EXPLORE MediaLink

http://www.prenhall.com/clark
Resources for this chapter can be found on the Companion Website.

Audio Glossary
Appendix G: Community Health Assessment
  and Intervention Guide
Exam Review Questions

Case Study: A Nursing Experience
  in a Faith-Based Community
MediaLink Application: Nurse-Managed
  Services (video)

Media Links
Challenge Your Knowledge
Update Healthy People 2010
Advocacy Interviews

References

Abrams, S. E. (2004). From function to competency in public health nursing, 1931 to 2003. *Public Health Nursing, 21*, 507–510.

All Nursing Schools. (2006). *Search results for parish nursing.* Retrieved January 22, 2006, from http://allnursingschools.com

American Nurses Association. (2007). *Public health nursing: Scope and standards of practice.* Silver Spring, MD: nursesbooks.org.

American Nurses Association & Health Ministries Association. (2005). *Faith community nursing: Scope and standards of practice.* Silver Spring, MD: nursesbooks.org

American Public Health Association. (n.d.). *The essential services of public health.* Retrieved June 29, 2006, from http://www.apha.org/ppp/science/10ES.htm

Avila, M., & Smith, K. (2003). The reinvigoration of public health nursing: Methods and innovations. *Journal of Public Health Management, 9*(1), 16–24.

Bay Area Health Ministries. (2001). Promoting health and wellness in congregation and community. Retrieved May 19, 2001, from http://www.bahm.org

Beaulieu, J., & Schutchfield, D. (2002). Assessment of the validity of the National Public Health Performance Standards: The Local Public Health Performance Assessment Instrument. *Public Health Reports, 117*, 28–36.

Blanchfield, K. C., & McLaughlin, E. (2006). Parish nursing: A collaborative ministry. In P. A. Solari-Twadell & M. A. McDermott (Eds.), *Parish nursing: Development, education, and administration* (pp. 65–81). St. Louis: Mosby.

Board of Registered Nursing, State of California. (2004). *Instructions for applying for certification as a public health nurse in California.* Retrieved June 29, 2006, from http://www.rn.ca.gov/pdf/phn-app.pdf

Britt, J. (2006). Competencies for parish nursing practice. In P. A. Solari-Twadell & M. A. McDermott (Eds.), *Parish nursing: Development, education, and administration* (pp. 145–154). St. Louis: Mosby.

Buhler-Wilkerson, K. (2001). *No place like home: A history of nursing and home care in the United States.* Baltimore: Johns Hopkins University.

Buijs, R., & Olson, J. (2001). Parish nurses influencing determinants of health. *Journal of Community Health Nursing, 18*(1), 13–23.

Carr, S., & Davidson, A. (2004). Public health nursing: Developing practice. *Practice Development in Health Care, 3*, 101–112.

Carson, V. B., & Koenig, H. G. (2002). *Parish nursing: Stories of service and care.* Philadelphia: Templeton Foundation Press.

Centers for Disease Control and Prevention. (2005). *Healthy people data.* Retrieved September 6, 2005, from http://wonder/cdc.gov/data2010

Clark, M. B. (2000). Types of transitions in the lives of faith community members. In M. B. Clark & J. K. Olson (Eds.), *Nursing within a faith community: Promoting health in times of transition* (pp. 203–221). Thousand Oaks, CA: Sage.

Clarke, J. (2004). Public health in Ireland: A critical overview. *Public Health Nursing, 21*, 191–198.

Community Health Nurses Association of Canada. (2003). *Canadian community health nursing standards of practice.* Retrieved July 1, 2006, from http://www.communityhealthnursescanada.org/Standards/Standards%20Practice%20jun04.pdf

DeHaven, M. J., Hunter, I. B., Wilder, L., Walton, J. W., & Berry, J. (2004). Health programs in faith-based organizations: Are they effective? *American Journal of Public Health, 94,* 1030–1036.

Derose, S. F., Asch, S. M., Fielding, J. E., & Schuster, M. A. (2003). Developing quality indicators for local health departments. *American Journal of Preventive Medicine, 25,* 347–357.

DiLeo, J. W., Graham, C. S., & Solari-Twadell, P. A. (2006). Working with underserved congregations: A case study. In P. A. Solari-Twadell & M. A. McDermott (Eds.), *Parish nursing: Development, education, and administration* (pp. 297–304). St. Louis: Mosby.

Dryden, P. (2004). Heaven sent—Parish nurses are making a difference. Retrieved May 11, 2004, from http://www.medscape.com/viewarticle/474866

Dyess, S. M. (2002). Parish nursing. In C. C. Clark (Ed.), *Health promotion in communities: Holistic and wellness approaches* (pp. 409–417). New York: Springer.

Elliott, L., Crombie, I. K., Irvine, L., Cantrell, J., & Taylor, J. (2004). The effectiveness of public health nursing: The problems and solutions in carrying out a review of systematic reviews. *Journal of Advanced Nursing, 45,* 117–125.

Falk-Rafael, A. (2001). Empowerment as a process of evolving consciousness: A model of empowered caring. *Advances in Nursing Science, 24,* 1–16.

Falk-Rafael, A. (2005a). Advancing nursing theory through theory-guided practice: The emergency of a critical caring perspective. *Advances in Nursing Science, 28,* 38–49.

Falk-Rafael, A. (2005b). Speaking truth to power: Nursing's legacy and moral imperative. *Advances in Nursing Science, 28,* 212–223.

Fielding, J. E., Luck, J., & Tye, G. (2003). Reinvigorating public health core functions: Restructuring Los Angeles County's Public Health System. *Journal of Public Health Management, 9*(1), 7–15.

Fitzgerald, T. (2000). Body, mind, and soul: RNs reach out to the congregation through parish nursing programs. *NurseWeek, 13*(26), 16.

Fliesser, Y. L., Schofield, R., & Yandreski, C. (2003). Public health nursing: Nursing practice in a diverse environment. *RNAO Practice Page, 3*(2), 1–3.

Gunderson, G. R. (2000). Backing onto sacred ground. *Public Health Reports, 115,* 257–261.

Hahn, K., Radde, J. M., & Fellers, J. E. (2002). Spiritual care: Bridging the disciplines in congregational health ministries. In L. Vandecreek & S. Mooney (Eds.), *Parish nurses, health care chaplains, and community clergy: Navigating the maze of professional relationships* (pp. 130–141). New York: Haworth Press.

Hanafin, S., Houston, A. M., & Cowley, S. (2002). Vertical equity in service provision: A model for the Irish public health nursing service. *Journal of Advanced Nursing, 39,* 68–76.

Head, B., Aquilino, M. L., Johnson, M., Reed, D., Maas, M., & Moorhead, S. (2004). Content validity and nursing sensitivity of community-level outcomes from the nursing outcomes classification (NOC). *Journal of Nursing Scholarship, 36,* 251–259.

Health Ministries USA. (2006). *Training program resource list for parish nurses.* Retrieved January 22, 2006, from http://www.pcusa.org/health/usa/parishnursing/training.htm

Holt, C. L., Kyles, A., Wiehagen, T., & Casey, C. (2003). Development of a spiritually based breast cancer education booklet for African American Women. *Cancer Control, 10*(5), 37–44.

Institute of Medicine. (1988). *The Future of Public Health.* Washington, DC: National Academy Press.

Jakonen, S., Tossavainen, K., Tupala, M., & Turunen, H. (2002). Health and society in Finland: Public health nurses' daily practice. *British Journal of Community Nursing, 7,* 265–272.

Kaiser, M. M., Barry, T. L., & Kaiser, L. L. (2002). Using focus groups to evaluate and strengthen public health nursing population-focused interventions. *Journal of Transcultural Nursing, 13,* 303–310.

Keller, L. O., Strohschein, S., Schaffer, M. A., & Lia-Hoagberg, B. (2004). Population-based public health interventions: Innovations in practice, teaching, and management. Part II. *Public Health Nursing, 21,* 469–487.

Kotecki, C. N. (2002). Developing a health promotion program in faith-based communities. *Holistic Nursing Practice, 16*(3), 61–69.

Manitoba Health. (1998). *The role of the public health nurse within the Regional Health Authority.* Retrieved July 1, 2006, from http://www/gov/mb.ca/health/rha/rolerha.pdf

McDermott, M. A., & Solari-Twadell, P. A. (2006). Parish nursing curricula. In P. A. Solari-Twadell & M. A. McDermott (Eds.), *Parish nursing: Development, education, and administration* (pp. 121–131). St. Louis: Mosby.

McDonald, L. (2000). Florence Nightingale and the foundations of public health care, as seen through her collected works. Retrieved July 18, 2002, from http://www.sociology.uoguelph.ca/fnightingale/online_papers/dalpaper.htm

McMurray, R., & Cheater, R. (2004). Vision, permission and action: A bottom up perspective on the management of public health nursing. *Journal of Nursing Management, 12,* 43–50.

Mondy, C., Cardenas, D., & Avila, M. (2003). The role of an advanced practice public health nurse in bioterrorism preparedness. *Public Health Nursing, 20,* 422–431.

National Public Health Performance Standards Program. (n.d.). *The essential public health services.* Retrieved January 16, 2006, from http://www.cdc.gov/od/nphpsp/EssentialPHServices.htm

National Public Health Performance Standards Program. (2001). *Local public health performance standards.* Retrieved January 16, 2006, from http://www.cdc.gov/od/nphpsp/Documents/LocalModelStandardsOnly.pdf

Nursing & Midwifery Council. (2004). *Standards of proficiency for specialist community public health nurses.* Retrieved July 1, 2006, from http://www.nmc-uk.org/aFrameDisplay.aspx?DocumentID=234

O'Brien, M. E. (2003). *Parish nursing: Healthcare ministry within the church.* Sudbury, MA: Jones and Bartlett.

Olson, J. K., & Clark, M. B. (2000). Characteristics of faith community nurses. In M. B. Clark & J. K. Olson (Eds.), *Nursing within a faith community: Promoting health in times of transition* (pp. 122–140). Thousand Oaks, CA: Sage.

Palmer, J. (2001). Nursing's faith community: Parish nursing, connecting faith and health. *Reflections on Nursing LEADERSHIP, 27*(1), 17–19.

Patterson, D. L. (2003). *The essential parish nurse: ABCs for congregational health ministry.* Cleveland: Pilgrim Press.

Pattillo, M. M., Chesley, D., Castles, P., & Sutter, R. (2002). Faith community nursing: Parish nursing/health ministry collaboration model in Central Texas. *Family and Community Health, 25*(3), 41–51.

Public Health Functions Project. (2000). *The public health workforce: An agenda for the 21st century.* Retrieved May 19, 2001, from http://web.health.gov/phfunctions

Public Health Nursing Section, American Public Health Association. (1996). *The definition and role of public health nursing.* Washington, DC: Author.

Quad Council of Public Health Nursing Organizations. (2004). Public health nursing competencies. *Public Health Nursing, 21,* 443–452.

Rivera, J. C., & Parris, K. M. (2002). Use of nursing diagnoses and interventions in public health nursing practice. *Nursing Diagnosis, 13*(1), 15–22.

Schulte, J. (2000). Finding ways to create connections among communities: Partial results of an ethnography of urban public health nurses. *Public Health Nursing, 17,* 3–10.

Smith, S. D. (2002). Theoretical models of interdisciplinary relationships. In L. Vandecreek & S. Mooney (Eds.), *Parish nurses, health care chaplains, and community clergy: Navigating the maze of professional relationships* (pp. 217–226). New York: Haworth.

Smith, S. D. (2003a). Models for congregational and parish nursing programs. In S. D. Smith (Ed.), *Parish nursing: A handbook for the new millennium* (pp. 79–91). New York: Haworth Pastoral Press.

Smith, S. D. (2003b). Overview of parish nursing. In S. D. Smith (Ed.), *Parish nursing: A handbook for the new millennium* (pp. 25–35). New York: Haworth Pastoral Press.

Solari-Twadell, P. A. (1999). The emerging practice of parish nursing. In P. A. Solari-Twadell & M. A. McDermott (Eds.), *Parish nursing: Promoting whole person health within faith communities* (pp. 3–24). Thousand Oaks, CA: Sage.

Solari-Twadell, P. A. (2006). Uncovering the intricacies of the ministry of parish nursing practice through research. In P. A. Solari-Twadell & M. A. McDermott (Eds.), *Parish nursing: Development, education, and administration* (pp. 17–35). St. Louis: Mosby.

Solari-Twadell, P. A., & Egenes, K. (2006). A historical perspective of parish nursing: Rules for the sisters of the parishes. In P. A. Solari-Twadell & M. A. McDermott (Eds.), *Parish nursing: Development, education, and administration* (pp. 11–16). St. Louis: Mosby.

Solari-Twadell, P. A., & McDermott, M. A. (2006a). Challenges to the administration of the ministry of parish nursing practice. In

P. A. Solari-Twadell & M. A. McDermott (Eds.), *Parish nursing: Development, education, and administration* (pp. 227–331). St. Louis: Mosby.

Solari-Twadell, P. A., & McDermott, M. A. (2006b). Challenges to the ministry of parish nursing practice. In P. A. Solari-Twadell & M. A. McDermott (Eds.), *Parish nursing: Development, education, and administration* (pp. 103–107). St. Louis: Mosby.

State of California. (n.d.). *Title 16. California code of regulations, Division 14. Board of Registered Nursing, Article 9. Public health nurse.* Retrieved June 29, 2006, from http://www.rn.ca.gov/leg/pdf/approvedregs.pdf

Story, C. (2003). Barriers, difficulties, and challenges. In S. D. Smith (Ed.), *Parish nursing: A handbook for the new millennium* (pp. 113–128). New York: Haworth Pastoral Press.

Swinney, J., Anson-Wonkka, C., Maki, E., & Corneau, J. (2001). Community assessment: A church community and the parish nurse. *Public Health Nursing, 18,* 40–44.

Thomas, B. H., Ciliska, D., Dobbins, M., & Micucci, S. (2004). A process for systematically reviewing the literature: Providing research evidence for public health nursing interventions. *Worldviews on Evidence-based Nursing, 1,* 176–184.

Thomson Learning & American Association of Colleges of Nursing. (2001). *Peterson's guide to nursing programs* (7th ed.). Lawrenceville, NJ: Thomson Learning.

Timms, J. (2003). A role for parish nursing in end-of-life care. In S. D. Smith (Ed.), *Parish nursing: A handbook for the new millennium* (pp. 205–216). New York: Haworth Pastoral Press.

Vandecreek, L., & Mooney, S. (Eds.). (2002). *Parish nurses, health care chaplains, and community clergy: Navigating the maze of professional relationships.* New York: Haworth Press.

Via Christi Regional Medical Center, Center for Congregational Health Ministry. (n.d.). *The parish nurse.* Retrieved January 3, 2002, from http://www.via-christi.org/cchmweb...e1cd28625663900615e93!OpenDocument

Westberg, G. (2006). A personal historical perspective of whole person health and the congregation. In P. A. Solari-Twadell & M. A. McDermott (Eds.), *Parish nursing: Development, education, and administration* (pp. 5–10). St. Louis: Mosby.

Westberg, J. (2006). Introduction to: A personal historical perspective of whole person health and the congregation. In P. A. Solari-Twadell & M. A. McDermott (Eds.), *Parish nursing: Development, education, and administration* (pp. 3–5). St. Louis: Mosby.

White House Faith-based and Community Initiatives. (2005). *President Bush's faith-based and community initiative.* Retrieved January 22, 2006, from http://www.whitehouse.gov/government/fbci/overview2005.pdf

Yamashita, M., Miyaki, F., & Akimoto, R. (2005). The public health nursing role in rural Japan. *Public Health Nursing, 22,* 156–165.

Zimmerman, W. (2006). The public-private partnership: Expansion of the ministry. In P. A. Solari-Twadell & M. A. McDermott (Eds.), *Parish nursing: Development, education, and administration* (pp. 83–92). St. Louis: Mosby.

Care of Clients in Urban and Rural Settings

CHAPTER OBJECTIVES

After reading this chapter, you should be able to:

1. Describe various approaches to defining *rural* and *urban*.
2. Analyze barriers to effective health care in urban and rural areas.
3. Identify differences in biophysical, psychological, physical environmental, sociocultural, behavioral, and health system factors as they affect health in urban and rural areas.
4. Analyze differential effects of government policy on urban and rural community health.
5. Discuss assessment of health needs in urban and rural settings.
6. Describe goals for intervention in urban and rural settings.
7. Analyze approaches to evaluating the effectiveness of health care in rural and urban settings.

KEY TERMS

economies of proximity
frontier areas
health disparity population
health professional shortage area (HPSA)
medically underserved area (MUA)
medically underserved populations (MUPs)
metropolitan statistical area (MSA)
organized indigenous caregiving (OIC)
urbanization

MediaLink
http://www.prenhall.com/clark

Additional interactive resources for this chapter can be found on the Companion Website. Click on Chapter 25 and "Begin" to select the activities for this chapter.

From Chapter 25 of *Community Health Nursing: Advocacy for Population Health*, 5/e. Mary Jo Clark. Copyright © 2011 by Pearson Education. Published by Prentice Hall. All rights reserved.

Advocacy in Action

Advocacy in a Rural Nurse-managed Clinic

A rural nurse-managed clinic that received initial funding from the state department of health was required to show proof of local financial support during the second year of the renewal funding application process. The community health nurse appeared before the county commissioners to make a request for funding and was denied because the commissioners understood neither the client population nor the need for the clinic in the community. The commissioners expressed the perception that the clients were unwilling to work and verbalized a negative "welfare stigma" regarding the clients. Their perceptions persisted even after the nurse informed them that the county was designated a medically underserved area 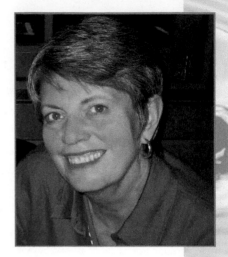 (MUA) and a health professional shortage area (HPSA), and explained that only county residents who lacked access to health care by virtue of being uninsured and who met the 200% level of the federal poverty guidelines could be seen at the clinic.

The community health nurse presented the problem to the clinic's Community Advisory Board, which included client and community representation. After strategizing with the board, the nurse arranged a meeting between the commissioners and some clients. She worked with the clients beforehand to help them advocate for themselves and tell their own stories. The clinic is situated in a community whose primary income base is tourism. The majority of clinic clients work in small shops and restaurants that do not provide health insurance to their employees. The commissioners were surprised to hear the real-life stories of the clients and to learn that they were in fact hardworking, productive community citizens who often held two or more jobs but still lacked access to health care. The advocacy of the clinic community health nurse was instrumental in securing funding from the commissioners, which has been sustained over the past 5 years. The financial support of the local community led in turn to increased funding from the state department of health.

Joyce Splann Krothe, DNS, RN

Associate Professor and Assistant Dean

Indiana University School of Nursing

*T*entalthroughout the world people live in different kinds of environments, from crowded and deteriorating inner cities to planned suburban communities to isolated rural areas. Factors in each of these settings influence health in different ways, some positively and others negatively. Prior to the 20th century, people living in rural areas had generally better health and longer life expectancies than those in cities due to the crowding and poor sanitation that were characteristic of urban life. In large part, advances in public health have been spurred by a focus on the adverse health conditions present in urban areas (Knowlton, 2001), and early community health nursing in the United States was aimed at improving the health of impoverished immigrant populations in urban areas. More recently, however, people in urban areas in developed countries have had access to better health care services and better knowledge of health promotion and illness prevention than those in rural settings (Population Information Program, 2002). Changes in rural and urban environments have resulted in changes in factors that influence health in those settings. In this chapter, we compare and contrast factors that influence health in rural and urban settings and their implications for community health nursing as practiced in those settings.

WHAT IS URBAN? WHAT IS RURAL?

Although an estimated half of the world's population lives in cities, there is no clear definition of what *urban* means. **Urbanization** has been loosely defined by the

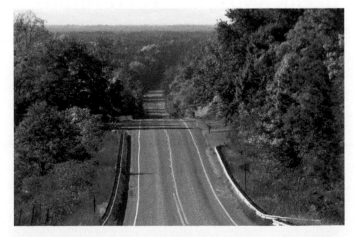

Great distances on poor roads may prevent rural residents from obtaining optimal health care. (©Jeff Greenberg/The Image Works)

National Center for Health Statistics (NCHS) (2005) as "the degree of urban (city-like) character of a particular geographic area" (p. 505). At the international level, the term *urban* can be applied to settlements of all sizes, but is generally reserved for settlements with populations of 20,000 or more people. *City* is a term often used in the international community to indicate "urban centers with large populations" (Population Information Program, 2002, p. 3). *Rural* is frequently defined as "not urban," but the National Rural Health Association maintains that the designation used for rural or urban residence should depend on the purpose for the designation and may legitimately vary from one program to another even in the same area, depending on the purpose of the program (National Rural Health Association, n.d.a).

The U.S. federal government has changed the definitions of urban and rural frequently, and different definitions are used by different agencies within the federal government, making comparisons between rural and urban areas over time and with respect to different aspects difficult. Commonly used definitions of rural and urban have been developed by the U.S. Census Bureau, the Office of Management and Budget (OMB), and the U.S. Department of Agriculture. Several of the approaches to defining urban and rural are summarized in Table 1◆.

The U.S. Census Bureau categorizes geographic areas as urbanized, urban clusters, or rural. Urbanized areas have central cores with populations of 50,000 or more. Urban clusters have core populations of 2,500 to 49,999 people. All other areas are considered rural. In 2000, 21% of the U.S. population lived in areas considered rural by the Census Bureau definition (Hart, Larson, & Lishner, 2005).

The OMB system classifies counties in terms of their metropolitan or nonmetropolitan character and their inclusion of a metropolitan statistical area. A **metropolitan statistical area (MSA)** is "a county or group of contiguous counties that contain at least one urbanized area of 50,000 or more population" (NCHS, 2005, p. 505). In the OMB system, metropolitan counties are classified as large, medium, or small. Large counties are those in an MSA with a million or more people; medium counties are included in MSAs with populations of 250,000 to 1 million people; and small counties are those in MSAs with less then 250,000 population. Nonmetropolitan counties are classified as micropolitan, nonmetropolitan counties or groups of counties that contain an urban cluster of 10,000 to 49,999 people, or nonmicropolitan, counties that do not contain an urban cluster of at least 10,000 people (NCHS, 2005).

A set of 10 rural–urban continuum codes used by the U.S. Department of Agriculture differentiates between metropolitan and nonmetropolitan counties based on the degree of urbanization and nearness to central metropolitan areas (Singh & Siahpush, 2002).

TABLE 1	Approaches to Defining Urban and Rural	
Approach	**Urban**	**Rural**
National Rural Health Association		Designation should depend on the purposes of the programs in which it is used.
U.S. Census Bureau	• Urbanized: Having a central core population of 50,000 or more • Urban clusters: Having a core population of 2,500 to 49,999 people	Areas with fewer than 2,500 people
Office of Management and Budget	• Metropolitan counties: Large: Include an MSA with 1 million or more people • Medium: Counties with MSAs of 250,000 to 1 million people • Small: Counties with MSAs of 50,000 to 250,000 people	• Nonmetropolitan counties: Micropolitan: Counties with an urban cluster of 10,000 to 49,999 people Nonmicropolitan: Counties with no urban cluster of at least 10,000 people
U.S. Department of Agriculture	• Metropolitan counties: Central counties with populations of 1 million or more people Counties on the fringe of central counties with populations of 1 million or more people Counties with populations of 250,000 to 1 million people Counties in metropolitan areas with populations less than 250,000 people	• Nonmetropolitan counties: Urban populations of 20,000 or more people adjacent to a metropolitan area Urban populations of 20,000 or more people not adjacent to a metropolitan area Urban populations of 2,500 to 19,999 people adjacent to a metropolitan area Urban populations of 2,500 to 19,999 people not adjacent to a metropolitan area Completely rural areas or areas with populations of fewer than 2,500 people adjacent to a metropolitan area Completely rural areas or areas with populations of fewer than 2,500 people not adjacent to a metropolitan area
Montana State Rurality Index	An index for an individual resident based on the population density of the county and the distance to the nearest emergency services	An index for an individual resident based on the population density of the county and the distance to the nearest emergency services

Data from: Hart, Larson, & Lishner, 2005; NCHS, 2005; Singh & Siahpush, 2002; Weinert & Boik, 1998. See references for full citations.

These codes are based on the OMB categories and are summarized in Table 1◆.

The Montana State University (MSU) rurality index is another approach to defining rurality. Rather than being county based, this index is person based and categorizes individual residents on the basis of their degree of rurality. The advantage of a resident-based index is that it allows comparisons of people within a county who differ from other people in the same county in terms of their rurality. This index allows comparisons between rural and urban populations within the same county. The index for a given individual is derived by creating a weighted score based on the population density of the county and the distance to the nearest emergency services. In the case of persons within a single county, the index is based on distance to emergency services alone (Weinert & Boik, 1998). Table 1◆ summarizes the features of various approaches to defining rural and urban communities.

For the most part, in this chapter, we will be using the term *rural* to describe groups with very low population densities (fewer than 2,500 people), which includes people in small rural communities, and the term *urban*, or metropolitan, to indicate central metropolitan areas.

URBAN AND RURAL POPULATIONS

Half of the world's present population lives in urban areas, and this is expected to increase to 60% by 2030, with more than 5 billion urban residents throughout the world. In 2000, 388 cities throughout the world had populations greater than 1 million, and the number of cities with populations over a million is expected to increase to 554 by 2015 (Population Information Program, 2002).

In the United States, 30% of the population lived in cities with populations of 5 million people or more at the time of the 2000 census (Knowlton, 2001). In 2004, 83% of the U.S. population lived in urban areas, an increase of roughly 1% since 2000 (Economic Research Service, 2005). The degree of urbanization of the population varies from one area to another. For example, 100% of the Washington, DC, area is considered urban, whereas only 38% of Vermont's population lives in urban areas. States such as California and New Jersey are more than

GLOBAL PERSPECTIVES

*T*he world's population is becoming increasing urbanized. In 1975, only 27% of the population in developing countries lived in urban areas. By 2000, the percentage had grown to 40%, and by 2030 an estimated 56% of the population in developing countries will be urbanized. In developed countries, 75% of the population were already living in urban areas by 2000. The United Nations anticipates that by 2015, there will be 21 "megacities," each with a population in excess of 10 million people, and 17 of these metropolises will be located in developing countries (Population Information Program, 2002).

Many urban areas throughout the world already lack the infrastructure to support existing population levels, with inadequate housing resources and services to meet human needs. An estimated 30% of the world's poor are concentrated in urban areas, and this figure is expected to climb to 50% by 2030. Many of the urban poor live in inadequate housing without access to potable (drinkable) water or sanitation. They also lack access to health care.

Some of the suggested strategies for dealing with the problems of increasing urbanization include the following:

- Improving local governance and shifting decision authority to municipal governments
- Engaging in urban planning to address land use, water, sanitation, waste management, and transportation issues
- Promoting planned industrial and economic development that considers environmental impact
- Upgrading housing stock in slum areas
- Developing and implementing plans for water conservation and managing the demand for water through economic constraints on use
- Developing efficient transportation systems with minimal reliance on private vehicles and cleaner technology to minimize environmental impacts
- Developing and implementing waste recycling programs (Population Information Program, 2002)

Many of these strategies are also appropriate to rural areas. To what extent are these strategies being implemented in your area? What would be required to implement these strategies? How might these requirements be met in developing areas of the world?

increase in urban populations, and reclassification of formerly rural areas as they have been built up (Population Information Program, 2002). Migration may occur because of declining agricultural employment or perceptions of better jobs, service access, or higher standards of living in urban areas. Natural population increases occur when births in the population outnumber deaths.

THE EPIDEMIOLOGY OF HEALTH AND ILLNESS IN URBAN AND RURAL POPULATIONS

Factors influencing the health status of rural and urban populations can be categorized into two types, compositional factors and contextual factors (Phillips & McLeroy, 2004). Compositional factors arise from the characteristics of the people who compose the population in a given area (e.g., proportion of the elderly in the population, presence of ethnic minority group members). Contextual factors are derived from characteristics unique to the setting itself, unique features of rural or urban environments. Both categories of factors may give rise to *health disparity populations*. A **health disparity population** has been defined by the National Institutes of Health as "a population where there is a significant disparity in the overall rate of disease incidence, prevalence, morbidity, mortality, or survival rates in the population as compared to the health status of the general population" (as quoted in Hartley, 2004, p. 1676).

Factors that arise in the biophysical, psychological, physical environmental, sociocultural, behavioral, and health system dimensions of health contribute to compositional and contextual factors influencing the health of both rural and urban populations. The types of factors present in each dimension, however, may differ considerably.

Biophysical Considerations

Biophysical considerations influencing the health of urban and rural populations include age and aging and the extent of physical illness in the population.

Age and Aging

Rural and urban populations differ considerably in their composition, with rural populations including more elderly individuals (Phillips & McLeroy, 2004). In fact, approximately 15% of the 61 million rural residents in the United States are over age 65 (Carty, Al-Zayyer, Arietti, & Lester, 2004). In 2000, 7.4% of the population in isolated rural areas were over 75 years of age, compared to 5.6% of urban populations (Phillips, Holan, Sherman, Williams, & Hawes, 2004). The percentage of elderly people in some rural areas is increasing faster than that in many urban centers as a result of three factors. The

94% urban (U.S. Census Bureau, 2005b). Similar variation is noted worldwide. In the World Health Organization (WHO) European region, for example, 70% of the population lived in urban settings in 2005 compared with only 31% of the population in the Southeast African region (WHO, 2005).

Despite the imbalance between rural and urban populations in various parts of the world, and even in the United States, urban populations are growing, whereas rural ones are shrinking. In 1990, 78% of the U.S. population was considered urban, a figure that had increased to 79% by the next census (U.S. Census Bureau, 2005b). Similar rural-to-urban population shifts are occurring elsewhere in the world. Rapid growth in urban populations throughout the world is the result of three primary factors: migration from rural to urban areas, natural population

MediaLink — Choosing a Career in Rural Health (video)

first and most obvious factor is aging in place—people already living in rural areas are growing older. The second is a decades-long pattern of movement of younger people out of rural areas. The third factor is the more recent phenomenon of older urban dwellers retiring to rural areas (Institute of Medicine, 2005; Rogers, 2002). Persons over age 60 living in nonmetropolitan areas are more likely than their urban counterparts to live alone, to have a high school education or less, and to report worse health. Rural elderly are also more likely than urban elderly to have incomes below poverty level (13.1% vs. 9.3%) and to own their own homes (Rogers, 2002). Community health nurses may need to advocate for income assistance or other services for the unmet needs of both rural and urban elderly poor.

More than 80% of U.S. children live in urban areas. Urban children in the 50 largest U.S. cities are more likely than their rural counterparts to have family incomes below poverty level (26% vs. 20%), to live with a single parent (37% vs. 25%), and to live in families in which no parent has full-time year-round employment (45% vs. 33%). In addition, urban children are more likely to live in a household headed by a high school dropout or to include an adolescent who has dropped out of school. Finally, children in large cities are more than four times as likely to live in a family without a vehicle (21% vs. 5%) (Annie E. Casey Foundation, 2004). This latter figure may be offset by the availability of public transportation in large cities.

Of the 20% of U.S. children who live in rural areas, approximately 1.3 million work and play in farm settings. Another half million nonfarm children work on farms, contributing to a high incidence of injuries to child farmworkers each year (Reed, 2004a). Community health nursing advocacy may be particularly warranted to promote farm safety for both children and adults in rural areas. Nurses may also need to advocate for safe environments in urban areas that are affected by high crime rates or pollution.

Urban and rural populations also display different patterns of disease prevalence with respect to age composition. When five major chronic disease categories are compared (heart disease, hypertension, diabetes, emphysema, and cancer), rural populations have higher percentages of younger people (under age 65) reporting these conditions. Surprisingly, after 65 years of age, self-reported prevalence of many of these conditions is higher in urban populations. This is particularly true of persons over 80 years of age, with the urban elderly having higher reported prevalence of all except diabetes (Wallace, Grindeanu, & Cirillo, 2004). Community health nurses may be active in advocating for preventive services for the physical health conditions that affect rural and urban populations as well as for curative and restorative services for those with existing disease. The types of services needed will be dictated by the kinds of conditions prevalent in any given area.

BUILDING OUR KNOWLEDGE BASE

*R*ural health care providers have identified a set of research priorities to be addressed with respect to the health of rural elderly populations and health care delivery in rural settings (Averill, 2003). Most of these priorities can be applied to the general population in rural areas and include:

- Identification of demographic patterns and trends, health service needs, and existing methods of service delivery
- Examination of systems of care delivery for effectiveness and efficiency
- Tracking of health care delivery outcomes for specific client populations and delivery systems
- Identification of needs of families and caregivers for elderly family members
- Perceptions of elders regarding access to care and the effectiveness of care received

Describe a study that might be designed to address one of these priorities. Would the study need to be modified if it was to be conducted in an urban, rather than rural, setting? Why or why not?

Physical Health Status

Differences between mortality rates in urban and rural areas are difficult to determine given the differing definitions of rural and urban that are used in many studies. For some conditions, rates for the most urban and rural areas are similar, but vary greatly from those encountered in suburban and "near rural" areas (Eberhardt & Pamuk, 2004). *Health United States, 2001, Urban and Rural Health Chartbook*, the rural counterpart of *Health, United States*, gave poorer ratings to rural than urban areas for 21 of 23 health indicators that addressed both physical and behavioral health (Hartley, 2004).

Generally speaking, rural areas have higher rates of premature mortality (before 75 years of age) than urban areas. Infant mortality is lowest in suburban communities, followed by urban areas, then rural areas, and mortality among people 1 to 24 years of age is 31% higher in the most rural counties than in the most urban areas and 65% higher than in suburban areas. Similarly, mortality rates among the 25- to 64-year-old group is 32% higher in rural than urban areas, but mortality in people over age 65 is only 7% higher in rural than urban populations (Eberhardt & Pamuk, 2004). Community health nurse advocacy for adequate prenatal care and education may help to offset differences in infant mortality. Advocacy for other health services in both rural and urban areas will depend on specific causes of morbidity and mortality.

COPD mortality is 32% higher for rural U.S. men than for their most urban counterparts (Eberhardt & Pamuk, 2004), and incidence of cancer is higher. Higher rural cancer mortality may be a result of later stage at diagnosis, particularly among rural ethnic minorities (Gamm, Hutchison, Dabney, & Dorsey, 2003). Rural accident mortality rates are twice as high as those for urban areas (Peek-Asa, Zwerling, & Stallones, 2004). One third of U.S. motor vehicle accidents occur in rural areas, yet rural populations account for two thirds of all motor vehicle accident fatalities (Gamm et al., 2003). Nonfatal injuries in rural areas occur at a rate almost 30 times higher than that seen in urban areas, with the exception of fracture and hip fracture rates, which are lower in rural than urban populations (Peek-Asa et al., 2004). Injuries are particularly prevalent among the farm population due to exposure to hazardous working conditions and work with heavy equipment and fractious animals (Spengler, Browning, & Reed, 2004).

Other nonfatal conditions, such as arthritis, have been found to be more prevalent in rural than urban populations, and rural adults are more likely to experience activity limitation due to chronic illness than urban elders (18% vs. 13%). Edentulism (loss of all teeth) is also more common among the rural elderly (38%) than among their urban counterparts (27%) (Eberhardt & Pamuk, 2004). Diabetes, dental caries, and obesity are also more common conditions in rural than urban populations (Gamm et al., 2003).

Rural–urban mortality differences also vary by gender. For example, heart disease mortality for women is highest in the urban north, followed by the rural south. For men, heart disease mortality is highest in the rural south. In general, however, heart disease, cerebrovascular disease, and hypertension are more prevalent in rural than in urban populations (Gamm et al., 2003).

Worldwide, the health of urban dwellers also tends to be better than that of their rural counterparts due to better access to health care and healthier living conditions. This is not true, however, for the urban poor, who may face more health risks due to inadequate housing, poor sanitation, and lack of other basic necessities in overcrowded urban settlements (Population Information Program, 2002). Community health nurses may be actively involved in advocating for provision of basic health care and health education services to improve the health of both urban and rural populations throughout the world. For example, they may advocate increased humanitarian aid from developed countries or they may be involved in the design of international health care systems that address urban and rural health care needs in developing nations.

A process similar to that used to develop the *Healthy People 2010* national health objectives was used among rural health care agencies and providers to identify an initial set of 10 top priorities for improving the health of rural populations. This initial set of priorities included heart disease and stroke, diabetes, mental health and mental disorders, oral health, tobacco use, substance abuse, maternal/child/infant health, nutrition and overweight, and cancer (Gamm et al., 2003). Additional priority issues that have been added since

then include injury and violence prevention, immunization and infectious diseases, public health infrastructure development, health education and community-based programming, and long-term care and rehabilitation (Gamm & Hutchison, 2004). Similar sets of priorities have been developed for specific subpopulations in rural settings. For example, priority diseases for rural American Indian/Alaskan Native populations include cardiovascular disease, cancer, diabetes, HIV/AIDS, sexually transmitted diseases (STDs), respiratory diseases, communicable diseases, malaria, and diarrhea. Other priority health concerns identified for this rural subpopulation included mental health and violence, child and adolescent health, women's health, tobacco use, maternal health and safety, emergency preparedness and response, immunization, nutrition, and safety of food and blood supplies (Baldwin et al., 2002). Community health nurses can be actively involved in advocacy efforts to address these rural health priorities at both state and local levels. For example, they may campaign for equitable allocation of state funds for health care services, particularly preventive services, in rural areas.

Psychological Considerations

In assessing an urban or rural population, the community health nurse will examine factors in the psychological dimension that influence population health. Actual rural and urban prevalences of mental health problems are probably similar, although rural men may have slightly higher prevalence of negative mood (Eberhardt & Pamuk, 2004). Migrant workers also display a higher incidence of depression than other rural residents. They, and members of other ethnic groups, are also less likely to seek treatment (Gamm et al., 2003; Monts, 2002). Community health nurses in areas that employ significant numbers of migrant workers are often those most likely to identify evidence of mental health problems in this population. Their advocacy may be required to assure access to care for mental illness among the migrant population.

Residents in both urban and rural areas are subjected to considerable levels of stress. For example, the rural farm population is faced with financial uncertainty, intense time pressures at certain seasons, uncertain weather, and intergenerational conflict that may lead to problems in interpersonal relationships, substance abuse, family violence, and suicide. Conversely, it is hypothesized that stressful conditions in urban areas, such as increased noise levels, sensory stimulation and overload, interpersonal conflict, and the vigilance needed regarding crime victimization and accidents, may also contribute to mental health problems (House et al., 2000). In fact, research has indicated that higher crime rates in urban areas are associated with increased incidence of asthma symptoms. Individuals

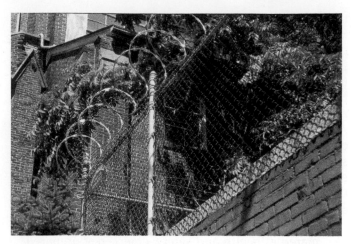

Unsafe neighborhoods with high crime rates create stress and poor health conditions.

with asthma who live in high-crime areas have greater symptom frequency than those who live in low-crime areas (Wright et al., 2004).

Areas in which differences do exist include the adequacy of mental health services and suicide rates. Rural mental health services are far less adequate than those available in urban areas. For example, 95% of metropolitan counties have available mental health services compared to only 80% of nonmetropolitan counties. Similarly, 87% of federally designated mental health professional shortage areas are in rural portions of the country. Three fourths of small rural counties lack the services of a psychiatrist and 95% have no access to child psychiatric services (Gamm et al., 2003).

Finally, rural areas have higher suicide mortality rates than urban settings. Rural counties have firearm-related suicide rates 1.5 times those of urban counties (Branas, Nance, Elliott, Richmond, & Schwab, 2004). For most age groups, rural men have suicide rates twice those among urban men. Rural suicide rates are 85% higher than those in urban areas for young women and 22% higher for working women (Singh & Siahpush, 2002). Reasons given for differences in rural and urban suicide rates include a rural cultural value on self-reliance, travel distance to and availability of mental health services, and greater social stigma attached to mental illness in rural cultures (Eberhardt & Pamuk, 2004; Gessert, 2003). Social stigma and the lack of anonymity in rural areas have even been suggested as reasons for purposeful underdiagnosis of mental health problems by health care providers, as well as for failure to seek assistance (Gamm et al., 2003). Community health nurses can advocate with providers to increase diagnosis and effective treatment of mental illness in rural, as well as urban, areas. They may also need to educate rural populations regarding mental illness in order to decrease the stigma that may prevent residents from seeking care for mental health problems. For both rural and urban dwellers, community health nurses

may need to actively advocate for access to affordable mental health services. For example, they may be active in political campaigns to increase coverage of mental illness and substance abuse under state Medicaid programs or to support the availability of tax-funded treatment services in both rural and urban areas of need. In Tennessee, for example, the Rural Health Association of Tennessee (2005), which includes rural nurses as well as other health professionals, was instrumental in negotiating the use of tobacco settlement funds for health and agricultural priorities.

Physical Environmental Considerations

Both the built and natural environments affect health status. The built environment consists of buildings, spaces, and products created or modified significantly from their natural state by people, and the natural environment involves natural features of the area, including plant and animal life, terrain, and so on. The community health nurse assessing the health status of a particular rural or urban population would consider the effects of both the built and natural environments and interactions between them on the health of the population.

Differences between the built and natural environments are perhaps the most obvious differences between rural and urban settings. Elements of the built environment are probably more significant influences on health than those of the natural environment in urban settings. Health risks in the urban environment include noise exposure, crowding, and increased potential for environmental pollutants such as air pollution and heavy metals (Perdue, Stone, & Gostin, 2003). For example, approximately half of U.S. urban dwellers are exposed to excessive ozone levels, and many U.S. cities have particulate-matter air pollution levels one and a half to two times the national standard (Population Information Program, 2002). Central urban areas, however, have the advantage of being more energy efficient than rural or suburban areas. In fact, "suburban sprawl" has been described as being wasteful of both space needed for agricultural purposes and energy used to commute between widely separated residential, commercial, and industrial centers. Energy use increases threefold with movement from center city to suburban fringe areas as a result of greater motor vehicle use, and traffic congestion in small urban and rural areas is growing by 11% per year, twice the rate of increase in urban areas (Sierra Club, n.d., 2001). Urban areas have also been touted as safer in terms of accidents since the accident fatality rate involved for public transit is one twentieth the rate associated with personal automobile use (Hancock, 2000). Unfortunately, more than 140 million people in the United States live more than a quarter mile from a transit stop, and 41% of populations in small urban and rural areas do not have any access to public transit (Sierra Club, n.d.). Motor vehicle accident fatalities in rural areas are, in part, due to narrow two-lane roads that lack crash reduction features such as controlled entrances and exits, wide divided lanes, and traffic control devices. High speeds typical of travel on rural roads are also a factor (Peek-Asa et al., 2004). In addition, urban centers encourage exercise when destinations are within walking distance and contribute to less social isolation than more sparsely settled areas. Community health nurses can be active advocates for planned urban development that promotes physical activity. They can also advocate for changes in rural environments that increase access to needed transportation services or that promote safety (e.g., divided roads). For example, community health nurses may help to organize transportation cooperatives that improve access to goods and services for isolated rural residents.

In rural settings, the natural environment contributes to a variety of health risks. The presence of plants and wild and domesticated animals in the rural environment contributes to the potential for plant and animal allergens and zoonoses (diseases transmitted from animals to people) (National Center for Infectious Diseases, 2001). Dust and extreme weather conditions are other significant aspects of the natural environment in the rural setting that have health consequences. For example, weather conditions have been shown not only to decrease access to health care facilities, but also to impede home care in rural areas (Gallagher, Alcock, Diem, Angus, & Medves, 2002).

Deteriorated housing and lack of affordable housing may affect the health of urban residents, contributing to high levels of homelessness. In rural areas, this component is more apt to reflect the effects of substandard housing that is in poor repair, particularly among the elderly (National Coalition for the Homeless, 2005). Higher rates of fire-related mortality

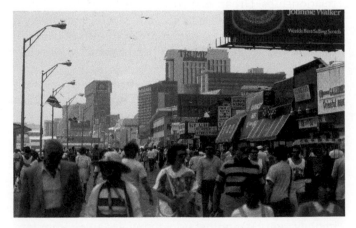

Crowding in urban areas can increase stress, leading to a variety of health effects. (Patrick J. Watson)

Think Advocacy

Millersville is a small town of 3,000 people in rural Arizona. The main street of town is part of a four-lane undivided highway to Phoenix. The part of town traversed by the highway comprises about 20 blocks, four of which are lined by local stores and diagonal parking on either side. Except when it is raining, which is infrequent, most of the town's children ride their bicycles to the local elementary school, which is located on the highway three blocks south of the main shopping area. In the past 2 years, three children have been killed and seven others injured by cars speeding through town on the highway. There is a stop sign in the middle of town, but it does not seem to have reduced speeds or accidents. Research suggests that bicycle lanes divided from motor vehicle traffic by concrete barriers reduce child bicycle injuries. Although you have suggested creation of bicycle lanes on the section of the highway that bisects the town, the idea has been resisted by local merchants who do not want to give up the parking in front of their stores. They are afraid that if people from the outlying ranches have to park elsewhere and walk to the stores, they will take their business to the city 40 miles away. How would you go about advocating for a bicycle lane in town?

in rural areas have been associated with older homes and use of high-risk heating mechanisms. In addition, rural homes are less likely to have functioning smoke detectors (86%) than urban residences (93%) (Peek-Asa et al., 2004). An estimated 30% of rural homes have at least one major problem (National Coalition for the Homeless, 2005). In 2003, for example, 30% or more of households in 300 nonmetropolitan counties lacked adequate kitchen or bathroom facilities (U.S. Department of Agriculture [USDA], 2005). Safety education is one important form of community health nurse advocacy in both rural and urban areas. The types of issues addressed, however, are likely to differ, with rural safety focusing on issues of farm and traffic safety. Elimination of safety hazards in the home and use of smoke detectors will be relevant in both settings.

In the United States, rural housing issues are particularly serious for migrant and seasonal farmworkers who generally live in "camps," which often consist of temporary shelters erected for short periods of time. Although migrant camps are supposed to meet OSHA standards for housing and plumbing facilities, a survey by the Housing Assistance Council found that 52% of farmworker housing was crowded and 53% was deficient in bathtub/shower and laundry facilities. In addition, the lack of adequate sanitary facilities for workers in the fields promotes the spread of disease. Workers are often required to pay for the inadequate housing provided in camps, thus decreasing the funds available for food, health care, and other basic necessities (Culp & Umbarger, 2004). Community health nurses working with migrant workers can advocate for adequate housing.

For example, they may report OSHA violations by farms that employ large numbers of migrant workers and do not provide adequate living facilities.

Worldwide, both urban and rural areas present physical environmental hazards to health. According to the World Health Organization (WHO, 2003), 600 million urban and 1 billion rural residents live in inadequate housing. Approximately one fourth of urban housing in developing countries is temporary in nature, and one third of it does not meet local housing codes. In some areas, such as sub-Saharan Africa, as much as 60% of urban housing is temporary quarters, and half of it does not meet building safety codes. Such temporary housing is often built in areas prone to natural disaster or with other unhealthy attributes. Legal housing is often too expensive for the urban poor to afford or not available at all. It is estimated that low-income households in many countries would need to save 30% to 50% of their income for 15 to 30 years to be able to afford legal housing that meets minimum safety standards (Population Information Program, 2002). Community health nurses can advocate for construction of safe housing units as well as for reasonable safety codes that do not price housing beyond the affordable range for most residents.

Although 100% of both urban and rural residents in the United States and other developed nations have access to improved water sources and sanitation, the same is not true for many developing countries. In many of these countries rural residents have far lower rates of access to these basic necessities than urban dwellers, and the greatest difference is noted in such countries as Papua New Guinea, where 88% of urban dwellers and 32% of rural residents have access to improved water, and Niger, where 79% of the urban population but only 4% of rural residents have adequate sanitation (WHO, 2004). Community health nurses can advocate development of safe water systems in both rural and urban areas. They can also educate rural and urban dwellers regarding inexpensive water purification methods and help to assure that the necessary supplies are available to and affordable for even the most needy. In the United States, many rural residents rely on wells as their primary source of drinking water, and many wells are contaminated with a variety of pollutants, particularly with agricultural runoff that includes pesticides and other hazardous substances.

The built environment also contributes to health risks in rural areas in the use of pesticides and other chemicals used in agriculture. For instance, in 2002, more than 483 million pounds of pesticides were applied to U.S. crops (U.S. Census Bureau, 2005b). Improper use of such chemicals and failure to follow safety instructions have resulted in human exposures to toxic and carcinogenic substances. In addition, 85% of fruits and vegetables are picked by hand, increasing the risk of toxic exposures for farmworkers (Culp & Umbarger, 2004). These exposures are compounded by lack of adequate shower and laundry facilities to wash away pesticide accumulations on skin or clothing. Exposure to high noise levels also occurs as a result of some aspects of the built rural environment (e.g., operation of farm machinery) (Reed, 2004b).

Finally, the built and natural elements combine to create sources of water pollution in rural areas. Agricultural runoff contaminated with chemical pesticides and heavy metals pollutes drinking water sources as well as local lakes and rivers. According to the Environmental Protection Agency, 91% of drinking water violations involve small water systems serving 25 to 3,300 people, many of which are in rural areas (U.S. Department of Health and Human Services [USDHHS], 2001). Urban sprawl also increases water runoff and potential contamination of water sources. Runoff is an increasing problem with the development of impervious surfaces in urban and suburban areas. Runoff is actually one and a half to four times higher in suburban than rural areas (Gaffield, Goo, Richards, & Jackson, 2003).

Sociocultural Considerations

Differences in sociocultural dimension factors between rural and urban settings, although not as immediately obvious as physical environmental factors, are nevertheless quite influential in their effects on population health status. Areas to be considered in assessing rural and urban populations include social values and conditions, economic issues, cultural factors, occupational factors, and factors related to health knowledge and values.

Rural cultures have been described as high-context cultures in which people experience sustained interactions with others (Phillips & McLeroy, 2004). Urban cultures, on the other hand, tend to be low-context cultures in which individuals are more socially isolated and experience greater mobility and frequent changes in relationships. Urban and rural areas also differ in terms of the potential number of social ties, which are likely to be more numerous in urban areas due to population density and greater opportunity to interact with others (Leyden, 2003).

Despite the enduring nature of interpersonal relationships in rural settings, long distances and lack of public transportation may lead to social isolation, particularly among the elderly. Social isolation may be particularly prevalent among migrant farmworkers from outside the United States. Many migrant workers are not able to return home to visit with families due to fears of being unable to return to the United States. In the past, most migrant workers would return home approximately every 9 months; now many are away from families for up to 4 years at a time (Monts, 2002).

Rural residents are more likely than urban dwellers to be married and tend to adhere to traditional gender roles. People in urban and rural settings also differ in terms of the likelihood of exposure to strangers and to unconventional norms, including gender norms. Urban areas are more heterogeneous in their population and residents are more likely to be exposed to attitudes and values different from their own (Fitzpatrick, 2000). Depending on the context of these encounters, they may lead to greater tolerance of differences or exhibitions of prejudice and discrimination. Rural areas are experiencing a growth in the diversity of their populations that may lead to tensions among racial and ethnic groups. Community health nurses may need to be actively involved in promoting cultural competence among residents. For example, they may advocate for cultural sensitivity training for employers of migrant workers or in rural and urban school settings.

Sustained interpersonal relationships in rural settings lead to the development of trust and informal support networks. These relationships may also result in the lack of anonymity and privacy discussed earlier and lead to less help-seeking for problems one does not want known by one's neighbors (Gamm et al., 2003). Urban society, on the other hand, may be characterized by stimulus overload and increasing complexity of interpersonal interactions that may result in a sense of "diffused responsibility" or failure to respond in the face of another's obvious need. Urban residents are twice as likely as rural dwellers to be victims of violence, and firearms-related homicide rates are three times higher in urban than rural areas (Branas et al., 2004). Gun safety education and advocacy are important aspects of health education by community health nurses.

Poverty affects health in both urban and rural settings, but those in rural areas are more likely to be poor than their urban counterparts. Per capita income for rural residents is nearly $10,000 less than among urban dwellers, and rural poverty rates are higher than those

in urban areas (13.9% vs. 12.2%) (Economic Research Service, 2005). Within metropolitan areas, however, central-city populations are more likely to be poor (17.5%) than those living in non-central-city areas (9.1%) (U.S. Census Bureau, 2005a). Rural poverty is particularly prevalent among ethnic minorities and migrant or seasonal workers. Rural Black and Native American residents are three times as likely and rural Hispanics twice as likely to be poor as their rural White counterparts (Probst, Moore, Glover, & Samuels, 2004). Community health nurses may advocate for assistance to individual poor rural or urban families. They may also advocate for economic changes that will benefit the poor in either setting. For example, they may campaign for state legislation or local ordinances increasing the minimum wage to a living wage.

Each year, U.S. produce growers employ 750,000 to 5 million migrant and seasonal workers (Gamm et al., 2003). The 1983 Migrant and Seasonal Agricultural Worker Protection Act (AWPA) defined a seasonal worker as "a person employed in agricultural work of a seasonal or other temporary nature who is not required to be absent overnight from his or her permanent place of residence" (as quoted in Culp & Umbarger, 2004, p. 384). A migrant agricultural worker, on the other hand, was defined as "a person employed in agricultural work who is required to be absent overnight from his or her permanent place of residence, except for immediate family members of an agricultural employer or a farm labor contractor" (as quoted in Culp & Umbarger, 2004, p. 384). Under these definitions, then, adolescents who work on a farm during the summer months but return to their homes in town each night would be considered seasonal workers. People who move to an agricultural area for several months but have a home base elsewhere are considered migrant workers. For example, some migrant workers live in the Southwest, but travel to Midwestern states during peak planting and harvesting periods.

Migrant and seasonal workers are less likely than others in rural areas to be highly educated and more likely to live in poverty. In 2003, for example, 81% of 753,000 hired farmworkers had a twelfth-grade education or less. Nearly 83% of this population worked full-time, but the median weekly earnings were only $373 (U.S. Census Bureau, 2005b).

Poverty is also more prevalent among rural than urban elderly populations. In 2000, for example, more than 13% of people over 60 years of age living in non-metropolitan areas had incomes below poverty level, compared to just over 9% of the urban elderly (Rogers, 2002).

Worldwide, 70% of poor people live in rural areas, but urban poverty may have more severe consequences than rural poverty due to the dependence on cash income for goods and services in urban areas. Many rural families raise at least a portion of their food, and

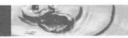

CULTURAL COMPETENCE

Traditionally, refugee and immigrant families enter the United States through major metropolitan areas, and the large majority of them remain in these or similar urban centers throughout the country. More recently, however, some refugee groups have begun to relocate to more rural areas. For example, many Laotian Hmong families have moved from San Diego to areas of North Carolina.

- What do you think might be some of the reasons for this migration?
- What are the social implications of an in-migration of a unique cultural group such as the Hmong into the rural culture of the Southeast?
- What are the implications for community health systems in the North Carolina area?

urban residents throughout the world pay about 30% more for food than rural residents (Population Information Program, 2002). Other goods and services may be less expensive in urban areas due to **economies of proximity**, in which the cost of public services is decreased in areas of greater population density (Awofeso, 2003).

According to World Bank estimates, 330 million urban poor in the developing world earned less than US$1 per day in 1988. By 2000, this number had increased to 495 million. Approximately 20% of urban residents in half of the world's developing nations have incomes below the defined poverty level for their countries, and this figure rises to 50% in some countries (Population Information Program, 2002). Again, community health nurses may advocate for international aid or for economic changes within developing nations to offset poverty.

The economic situation of migrant workers in the United States is further complicated by political inequities. For example, although migrant workers are covered by minimum wage provisions of the 1966 Fair Labor Standards Act, they are specifically excluded from overtime compensation requirements. In addition, agricultural employers with fewer than 7 employees or 500 worker days of labor are exempted even from the minimum wage requirements. The Act also permits children as young as 10 to work in the fields. Because this legislation is often not enforced and migrant families may not have access to childcare, children may be working beside their parents at much earlier ages (Culp & Umbarger, 2004).

Again, community health nurses may advocate for public assistance for low-income families or for measures like the living wage that enable urban and rural families to afford basic necessities of life. Such advocacy may be particularly needed for migrant populations who may not advocate for themselves due to language barriers or fear of deportation or other retaliation. For example, community health nurses may work to see that the provisions of minimum wage legislation are upheld for migrant workers as well as for other employees. They may also work to change legislation so migrant workers are eligible for overtime pay.

Political inequities also occur for other segments of the rural population. For example, rural populations received approximately $261 less per capita in federal funding in 2000 than urban populations. Farming-dependent counties, however, receive slightly higher per capita rates of federal funding, primarily due to higher levels of loan funding (Reeder & Calhoun, 2002).

Rural populations are also less highly educated than urban dwellers. For example, in the 2000 census, nearly 60% of rural residents age 25 and older had a high school education or less, compared to 46% of the urban population. Conversely, more than a quarter of urban residents (26.4%) had completed college versus 15% of the rural population (Economic Research Service, 2005). Lack of education is more prevalent among some segments of the rural population than others.

Significant poverty also exists in urban settings, and urban poor families are more likely to be headed by single parents than those in rural areas. Rates of homelessness due to poverty and other factors are higher in urban than in rural areas, but the number of homeless people in rural settings is increasing. Rural homeless are apt to be less visible because of the lack of social services and shelters where they might congregate. The rural homeless are also more likely than their urban counterparts to double or triple up in housing with family or friends, increasing their virtual invisibility (National Coalition for the Homeless, 2005).

Urban settings are more culturally diverse than rural settings, which can be both an advantage and a disadvantage depending on the character of relationships among population groups. Foreign-born persons are more likely to reside in urban than rural settings, but a significant proportion of this population is now migrating to rural areas (USDA, 2005). Because these immigrants tend to have more health-related needs than their U.S.-born counterparts, they are placing considerable strain on rural health care systems that are already overburdened. Movement of U.S.-born retirees with existing chronic illnesses and health care needs to rural areas has a similar effect on the social and health care infrastructures in rural settings (Phillips & McLeroy, 2004).

Primary occupations in rural areas include agriculture, mining and other extractive industries, and manufacturing. Agricultural occupations are of two types: agricultural production and agricultural services. Agricultural production encompasses general farming and ranching; agricultural services occupations include custom crop and animal care, horticulture, and landscaping.

The primary differences between agricultural occupations and other rural and urban occupations is the absence of regulatory efforts. The Occupational Health and Safety Act of 1970 excluded agricultural workplaces, and this exclusion led to great differences in federal spending for health and safety in rural and urban settings. Exclusion from OSHA also means that occupational health and safety regulations are unenforceable on the 90% of U.S. farms that are family-owned or employ few paid workers (U.S. Census Bureau, 2005b). In addition, children engaged in work on family farms are not covered by the Fair Labor Standards Act, which leaves them at risk for hazardous working conditions and injury. Approximately 12,000 injuries occur to child farmworkers each year as a result of heavy machinery, work with animals, and other hazardous activities performed with little experience or training. Children are also more prone to agricultural injury than adults because of their limited strength and flexibility (Reed, 2004a). Another disparity lies in the fact that workers' compensation programs do not apply to rural workers in many states. Community health nurses can join other advocacy groups to address this inequity by reformulating workers' compensation legislation in their states.

Family violence and abuse are another consideration in examining the epidemiology of health and illness in urban and rural populations. Intimate partner violence may be more prevalent in rural areas due to isolation, lack of available services, and cultural differences in societal attitudes and norms. In one study, nearly 3% of rural women and nearly 5% of men reported at least one incident of severe physical abuse by an intimate partner. In addition, nearly 48% of rural women and 30% of men reported being victims of emotional abuse. Both physical and emotional abuse were found to be more common among young and unmarried couples. Interestingly, men engaged in farmwork reported more physical abuse and controlling abuse directed at them than other rural men, possibly due to the greater stress and economic insecurity of farmwork. Farm women, on the other hand, reported less abuse than nonfarm rural women (Murty et al., 2003).

The last sociocultural dimension factor to be considered in assessing factors influencing health in rural and urban settings lies in differences in the definitions of health and illness accepted by rural and urban residents. Definitions of health and illness differ widely in urban groups due to the greater heterogeneity of the population as well as greater cultural diversity. Rural definitions tend to be more homogeneous, reflecting a perception that health is synonymous with the ability to work (Gessert, 2003). This definition may lead rural residents to give work needs a higher priority than health needs and to put off seeking health care until conditions become severe. The self-reliance characteristic of rural culture, although often a strength, may also lead to rejection of needed health care services. Rural residents also tend to get fewer preventive health services than urban residents. Community health nursing advocacy

may be required to assure provision of adequate health care services for both urban and rural populations. Advocacy may also be required among members of the population, particularly in rural areas, to change attitudes to health and health care.

Behavioral Considerations

Rural and urban populations also differ with respect to elements of the behavioral dimension as they affect health status. Areas for the community health nurse to consider in assessing a specific rural or urban population include diet, use of tobacco, use of alcohol and other drugs, physical activity, sexual activity, and health-related behaviors.

With respect to diet, rural residents are more likely than their urban counterparts to be overweight, and rural diets tend to contain more fat and calories than those of more urban populations. Rural populations also have little access to nutritionists and fewer weight control programs available to them (Gamm et al., 2003). Rural and urban populations may also differ in terms of meal patterns, particularly in the case of rural farm families who may plan meals in the traditional pattern connected with the workday, with the heaviest meal at noon. Urban families and nonfarm rural families are more likely to eat their largest meal in the evening.

Adequate nutrition may be particularly problematic for migrant farmworkers, who may rely on convenience foods while working and who have limited budgets for providing adequate diets. In addition, English language difficulties may force many families to rely on children to read labels and make food choices, with children selecting foods with high sugar content and few vegetables and fruits. The absence of transportation, adequate refrigeration, and cooking facilities may further hamper efforts to provide adequate family nutrition. Community health nurses may need to advocate for access to affordable healthful food sources for this population. For example, a nurse might organize transportation for a weekly shopping trip to a grocery store with reasonable prices for migrant farm families or encourage cooperative buying to achieve some economy of scale.

Tobacco use rates tend to be higher in rural populations than in urban settings. For example, cigarette smoking rates are 19% higher among rural than suburban youth and 32% higher among adults (Eberhardt & Pamuk, 2004). Rural youth are also more likely than their urban counterparts to use smokeless tobacco, and pregnant women in rural areas are less likely to refrain from smoking (Gamm et al., 2003).

Alcohol and tobacco are the most likely substances to be abused in rural areas. For example, more rural residents report five or more drinks on a single occasion than urban dwellers (Gamm et al., 2003), and prevalence of abuse may be as high as 29% among migrant

ETHICAL AWARENESS

*R*esearch has indicated that operation of heavy farm machinery—particularly tractors—by children is a serious risk factor for fatal injury. In your rural community, you are aware of several farm families whose use of children in this capacity places them at very high risk. This occurs primarily on small family farms where much of the machinery in use is aging and is not equipped with more modern safety devices, such as rollover protection on tractors. Would you become involved in political activity to ban operation of farm machinery by children less than 16 years of age? Why or why not? If not, what other action might you take to protect these children?

farmworkers, possibly as a result of social isolation and depression (Monts, 2002). Illicit drug use among adults, on the other hand, tends to be higher in large metropolitan areas. Among youth, however, rural adolescents have a higher prevalence of illicit drug use (14%) than youth in small and large metropolitan areas (10% each). Drug and alcohol abuse may have more severe consequences in rural areas due to lack of access to adequate treatment and the greater stigma attached to substance abuse (Gamm et al., 2003). Community health nursing advocacy can help to assure that treatment facilities are available and that substance abuse treatment is covered by health insurance. Nurses may also need to advocate among members of rural populations to change the perceptions of stigma attached to substance abuse diagnoses.

Lack of exercise is another common feature of rural residence. For example, lack of leisure-time physical activity has been found to be 50% higher in rural than suburban areas (Eberhardt & Pamuk, 2004), and rural schools are less likely than their urban counterparts to include physical education in the curriculum or to have exercise facilities (Gamm et al., 2003). Community health nurses can advocate inclusion of physical education in school curricula as well as the availability of low-cost avenues for physical activity. For example, a nurse might help to create an exercise club in a rural church or school or promote "mall walking" in an urban area.

Health-related behaviors are the final behavioral consideration in assessing the health of rural or urban populations. As noted earlier, rural residents tend not to receive preventive health care. In part, this is the result of lack of access to convenient services, but also reflects the definition of health as the ability to work. Rural residents have also been shown to be less likely than their urban counterparts to engage in health-promotive behaviors. Older persons in rural settings are less likely to receive influenza and pneumonia immunizations than those in urban areas, and older rural women are less likely than their urban counterparts to receive mammograms or Papanicolaou smears (Slifkin, Goldsmith, & Ricketts, 2000). Younger rural women, particularly those in ethnic minority groups, may also be less likely to obtain prenatal care or more likely to obtain care late in their pregnancies than those in urban areas (Baldwin et al., 2002; Gamm et al., 2003).

Rural residents may also be somewhat less likely than their urban counterparts to engage in the use of complementary or alternative medicines (CAM). For example, in one study, only 58% of rural residents reported use of CAM for pain relief compared to 77% of urban and 82% of suburban residents (Vallerand, Fouladbakhsh, & Templin, 2003). In another study, 17.5% of rural elders sought care from complementary providers, primarily for chronic health problems. Another 36% reported using self-directed CAM therapies

for health promotion purposes (Shreffler-Grant, Weinert, Nichols, & Ide, 2005).

Health System Considerations

Significant differences in health care systems in rural and urban areas influence the health of populations in these settings. Areas for consideration in assessing this dimension of health include the availability of and access to health care services, barriers to service use, and the influence of health policies and delivery systems on population health.

Health care services for many rural residents are less accessible, more costly to deliver, narrower in range and scope, and fewer in number than those available to their urban counterparts. This is true for most professional services, including those of physicians, dentists, nurses, and social workers, and is particularly true of services for the elderly in rural areas.

Nearly three fourths (70%) of federally designated health professional shortage areas in the United States are rural (National Rural Health Association, n.d.b). A **health professional shortage area (HPSA)** is defined as "a geographic area, population group, or medical facility that has been designated by the Secretary of the Department of Health and Human Services as having a shortage of health professionals" (National Health Service Corps, 2005, p. 1). HPSA designations may be made for shortages related to primary care, dental care, and mental health. Designation as a HPSA is based on one of two criteria: a ratio of population to full-time-equivalent primary care providers greater than 3,500:1 or a ratio between 3,500:1 and 3,000:1 and "an unusually high need for primary care services or insufficient capacity of existing primary care providers" (Center for Rural Health, n.d., p. 2).

Another designation for populations lacking access to health care services is that of a medically underserved area or population. A **medically underserved area (MUA)** is "a county or group of contiguous counties, a group of county or civil divisions or a group of urban census tracts in which residents have a shortage of personal health services." **Medically underserved populations (MUPs)** are "groups of people who face economic, cultural, or linguistic barriers to health care" (Bureau of Health Professions, n.d., p. 1). A given population may have a sufficient number of providers, therefore not qualifying for designation as a HPSA, and still contain MUPs. For example, if a significant group of Hispanics in the population cannot get adequate health care due to language barriers, the community may be designated a MUP even though it may have large numbers of health care providers overall. HPSAs, MUAs, and MUPs all exist in both rural and urban settings, but tend to be more common in rural communities.

There is a severe shortage of health care providers in many rural areas that does not occur in many urban populations. For example, the physician-to-population ratio is 139% higher for urban than rural counties. The ratio is 150% higher for dentists in urban counties and 130% higher for hospital-based registered nurses. From 1990 to 2000, nearly one fourth of nonmetropolitan counties lost primary care physicians, compared to only 7% of metropolitan counties. Although the number of physicians per population decreased in both rural and urban counties, the decrease in rural areas (37%) was more than twice that for urban populations (15%) (Ricketts, 2005). Approximately 65% of all rural counties are part of HPSAs, and this figure increases in counties with large ethnic minority populations (e.g., 81% of rural counties with large Hispanic populations, 83% of counties with primarily African American residents, and 92% of counties with populations consisting primarily of American Indians/Native Alaskans) (Probst et al., 2004).

Although 17% of the U.S. population lives in rural areas, fewer than 9% of all physicians and 14% of primary care physicians practice there. Rural and urban populations seem to fare equally well with respect to having a regular source of health care, but rural residents are less likely than their urban counterparts to have access to a regular source of care at night or on weekends. Approximately 30% to 40% of rural residents rely on care from a physician outside of their own local area. Factors contributing to the difficulty of attracting providers to rural areas include lack of sufficient population density to support specialty practices, differences between general practice and specialty reimbursement rates, professional isolation, and heavy workloads for the few providers in the area (Gamm et al., 2003).

The lack of specialty providers and rural cultural values of loyalty to local providers may influence primary care practice patterns, forcing providers to take on roles for which they are not prepared. This increases the risk for litigation for rural health care providers, particularly rural mental health nurses (Gibb, Livesey, & Zyla, 2003). These factors, as well as low population density, make it difficult for managed care organizations (MCOs) to maintain fiscal viability in rural areas (Waitzkin et al., 2002; Weeks et al., 2004). In addition, rural providers may find it difficult to participate in MCOs due to their lack of familiarity with managed care, lack of expertise in negotiating contracts, absence of alternative revenue sources, and increased use of mid-level providers (e.g., nurse practitioners) that may not be recognized for reimbursement by some MCOs. Many rural providers also lack the information systems capabilities needed for participation in an MCO (Waitzkin et al., 2002). Lack of providers is particularly noticeable with respect to specialty care.

As we saw earlier, similar disparities between urban and rural settings are noted with respect to the availability of mental health services. For example, the percentage of rural hospitals that have substance abuse treatment facilities in rural areas (10.7%) is less than half that of urban areas (26.5%). Likewise, the ratio of dentists to population is twice as high in large urban areas (60 per 100,000 people) as rural ones (30 per 100,000). In part, the lack of providers in rural areas is offset by the use of nonphysician primary care providers such as nurse practitioners, nurse midwives, and physician's assistants, and rural areas have slightly higher provider-to-population ratios for these categories of providers than urban areas (Gamm et al., 2003). The U.S. federal government also allows foreign physicians who do not meet licensure requirements to practice in HPSAs and provides Medicare bonus payments for physicians in these areas (Ricketts, 2005).

In addition to the shortage of physician providers faced by rural residents in general, members of minority populations in rural settings frequently do not have access to providers who understand their cultures and backgrounds. The problems of recruiting Caucasian providers to rural areas are compounded for ethnic minority providers, who may be faced with lack of acceptance and an even greater perception of being "outsiders."

Rural areas may fare slightly better than urban areas with respect to the public health workforce. For example, in one study of three states with large rural populations, rural health departments reported professional full-time-equivalent employees at a rate of 32.2 per 100,000 population, compared to only 29.2 per 100,000 in urban areas in those states. Rural health departments in these states reported almost twice as many nurses per 100,000 population as their urban counterparts (20.8 vs. 11.2). Unfortunately, nurses in rural health departments were more likely than those in urban areas to lack public health training or related clinical learning experiences, and many were employed only part-time. Rural health departments employed nearly twice as many nurse practitioners per 100,000 population as those in urban areas (1.7 vs. 1.1) (Rosenblatt, Casey, & Richardson, 2002).

Rural health departments may engage in a broader array of services than their urban counterparts, meeting needs that are not addressed by the private sector. For example, rural health departments provide 81% of all immunizations for children and adults in their jurisdictions. Urban health departments, on the other hand, provide only 64% of child and 65% of adult immunization services. Rural health departments also provide more personal care services with less privatization of services, do more community assessments, and provide more community outreach and education than urban departments. Only 7% of rural health departments, however, provide comprehensive primary care services versus 15% of urban health departments. Despite their generally broader array of services, rural health departments had lower funding levels, fewer medical specialists, less access to grant funding, and more difficulty recruiting personnel than urban health departments. Rural health departments also tended to be handicapped by lack of information technology, inadequate laboratory facilities, larger service areas with limited transportation availability, smaller hospitals for acute care needs, and greater fragmentation of resources (Berkowitz, 2004).

The bulk of services provided in rural U.S. health departments were provided by public health nurses (Berkowitz, 2004). This pattern is similar throughout the world, where the most frequent providers of health services in rural areas are nurses. In one study, for example, 84% of the systems responding employed nurses, 56% used physicians, 44% employed nurse practitioners, and 46% used nurse midwives. An additional 11% of systems employed lay health care workers and 10% employed traditional healers (Carty et al., 2004).

Generally speaking, rural areas worldwide have fewer health care providers than urban areas. According to WHO (2002) data, for example, the provider-to-population ratio in Cameroon is 1:400 in urban areas, but 10 times that in rural areas (1:4,000). Similarly, 85% of the population of Cambodia lives in rural settings, yet only 13% of health care workers are employed there. In Angola, 65% of the population is rural, but only 15% of health care workers are stationed in rural areas. The use of **organized indigenous caregiving (OIC)** strategies, which involves the training of local lay people for specific provider extender roles, has been advocated as a means of meeting rural service needs in the United States as well as overseas (May, Phillips, Ferketich, & Verran, 2003).

Emergency medical services (EMS) are another area in which rural populations may experience a deficit. Longer waits for emergency response, longer transport distances to hospitals, and lack of sophisticated emergency departments in rural hospitals increase the risk of trauma-related deaths. In fact, a 30-minute wait for EMS response has been found to increase the risk of death sevenfold. The average EMS response time in the rural United States is 18 minutes, more than eight times the response time in urban areas (Gamm et al., 2003). In addition, EMS personnel in rural areas are more likely than their urban counterparts to be volunteers and to lack adequate protocols for triage and transfer decisions (Peek-Asa et al., 2004). For example, 90% of EMS teams in rural **frontier areas** (those with a population density of fewer than seven people per square mile) are volunteers with only basic training (Gamm et al., 2003).

Health care in rural areas is also influenced by the relatively great distances to facilities and the lack of specialized facilities to meet particular needs (e.g., facilities for cancer therapy). Furthermore, small rural hospitals are at risk for low patient census and closure, further reducing availability of services. From 1990 to 2000, for example, 208 rural hospitals closed, and 29% of the rural

elderly must travel 21 to 30 miles to obtain acute care services. An additional 5% of this population travel more than 30 miles for acute care (Sanford & Townsend-Rocchiccioli, 2004).

Even when health facilities and providers are available, people in rural areas may have more difficulty making use of them than those in urban settings. Distance has already been mentioned as a barrier to health care. Other barriers that are relevant to both urban and rural residents, but are often more prevalent in rural areas, include cost and inconvenience. Rural residents are less likely than their urban counterparts to be insured. In 2003, nearly 19% of the rural population was uninsured, compared to 16% of people living in metropolitan statistical areas (NCHS, 2005). Poor and near-poor residents of rural areas are less likely to have Medicaid coverage (21%) than their urban counterparts (30%), and fewer rural residents receive health insurance benefits from employers (62% vs. 75%) (Eberhardt & Pamuk, 2004). Rural elderly are also less likely than older urban residents to have supplemental insurance in addition to Medicare coverage (Probst et al., 2004).

Many rural workers, especially those involved in agriculture, do not have "sick days" and may be unable to take time from work to obtain health care during the hours when facilities are typically open.

Community health nurses can advocate for the establishment of health care services that meet the needs of the population, particularly in rural areas. For example, a community health nurse may assist a rural community designated as a MUA to apply for federal funding for a rural health clinic (RHC) under the Rural Health Services Clinic Act. Both rural and urban populations may be assisted by community health nurses to obtain funds for community health centers (CHCs) or federally qualified health centers (FQHCs). Community health nurses might also assist local residents living in HPSAs and interested in health professional careers to apply for National Health Service Corps Scholarship and Loan Repayment programs with the understanding that they would practice in their own or another underserved area (Indiana State Department of Health, n.d.).

URBAN AND RURAL COMMUNITY HEALTH NURSING

Rural nursing has been defined as "the provision of health care by professional nurses to persons living in sparsely populated areas" (Long & Weinert, 1998, p. 4). Rural community health nursing originated in 1896, when Ellen M. Wood established an initial rural nursing service in Westchester County, New York. In 1911, Lydia Holman established an independent nursing service in Appalachia (Griffin, 1999), and in 1912, the American Red Cross founded the Rural Nursing Service, which later became the Town and Country Nursing Service. This organization was credited with decreasing infant and overall mortality and improving sanitation, hygiene, and nutrition in rural populations. The Town and Country Nursing Service continued until 1947, when it was disbanded due to the rise of official nursing agencies in state and local health departments. Other rural nursing services were provided by organizations such as the Frontier Nursing Service established by Mary Breckenridge in 1928 (Kalisch & Kalisch, 2004). More recent developments in rural nursing include the Migrant Health Act of 1962, which established the Migrant Health Program (Goldberg & Napolitano, 2001), and the passage of the Rural Health Clinic Service Act in 1977 (Oregon Health & Science University, 2006). Both of these pieces of legislation provided funding for health care services in rural areas that have addressed some of the health needs of the rural population and increased the use of nurse practitioners as providers of care. The Rural Health Clinic Service Act, in particular, mandated the use of mid-level practitioners such as nurse practitioners in underserved rural areas (Aday, Quill, & Reyes-Gibby, 2001).

Urban community health nursing in the United States began primarily with the efforts of Lillian Wald and others in the late 19th century. Occupational health nursing, which was primarily focused on urban manufacturing, also began about this time. Although occupational health risks related to agriculture were recognized as early as 1555, when the effects of breathing grain dust on the lungs of threshers were noted, little attention has been given to occupational health in rural areas until relatively recently. One other exception was the identification of anthrax among sheep handlers in the 1800s (Bell, 2002). Thackrah's 1832 report on The Effects of Arts, Trades, and Professions addressed the effects of occupational postures on the health of the working poor, but there was no mention of agricultural occupations—in which bending, twisting, and heavy lifting are common occurrences—as contributing factors (Schenker, 1995).

Recent concerns about health influences in rural areas have led to the development of beginning theory related to rural nursing. Key concepts of rural nursing theory include work beliefs and health beliefs, isolation and distance, self-reliance, lack of anonymity, insider/outsider, and old-timer/newcomer (Long & Weinert, 1998). These key concepts and their relationships are summarized at right and discussed where relevant throughout the remainder of this chapter. No comparable theory of urban nursing has been noted in the literature.

Rural nurses tend to be generalists who may be required to deal with any type of health problem that arises. They are expected to be competent in multiple areas and expert in a few. Rural community health nurses should have generalized expertise related to childbearing, child health, injury prevention, health education, and so on. Urban nurses, on the other hand,

SPECIAL CONSIDERATIONS

KEY CONCEPTS AND RELATIONSHIPS IN A THEORY OF RURAL NURSING

- **Work beliefs and health beliefs:** Work and health are related. Work is of primary importance, and health is assessed in relation to the ability to work. Health needs are often secondary to work needs.
- **Isolation and distance:** Rural residents often live great distances from health care and other services. Despite these differences, however, they do not generally see themselves as isolated.
- **Self-reliance:** Rural residents are characterized by a strong desire to do and care for themselves. This may result in reluctance to seek help from others, reliance on informal support networks when care is sought, and resistance to seeking care from "outsiders."
- **Lack of anonymity:** Rural communities are close-knit and rural residents may feel a lack of privacy. For rural nurses, this means multiple different relationships with clients that are interrelated. For example, the nurse's credibility as a professional may be linked to perceptions of her performance as a wife and mother as well as to evidence of professional competence. The role diffusion caused by multiple roles within the community may lead to a broader diversity of tasks expected of rural nurses, including expansion into the practice realm of other disciplines.
- **Insider/outsider:** Rural residents prefer to receive services from people well known to them. Rural nurses must become actively involved within their communities in other than professional roles. This may be uncomfortable for nurses who try to maintain a clear separation between their personal and professional lives.
- **Old-timer/newcomer:** Rural residents may continue to perceive people who have lived in the area for several years as "newcomers," and rural nurses new to the area should expect a long period of being considered a newcomer before they are completely accepted by the population.

Data from: Long, K. A., & Weinert, C. (1998). Rural nursing: Developing the theory base. In H. J. Lee (Ed.), Conceptual basis for rural nursing (pp. 3–18). New York: Springer.

may have more opportunity for specialization because of the array of other providers available to fulfill other needs in urban areas.

Rural and urban nursing may also differ in the scope of practice. Because of the dearth of health professionals in many rural areas, rural community health nurses may be the only source of health care for many clients. Again, this demands a generalist perspective, but may also mean that the boundaries between nursing and medicine are less distinct than in urban settings. Rural nurses may often be required to engage in what would elsewhere be considered medical practice until a physician arrives, particularly in emergency situations (Gamm et al., 2003).

Care of population groups in both urban and rural settings relies on the nursing process as an organizational framework. However, the factors assessed as influencing health, the health problems identified, and intervention approaches may often differ.

Assessing Factors Influencing Health in Urban and Rural Populations

The first step in meeting the health care needs of urban and rural populations is to identify those needs through population health assessment. In addition, a community assessment tool that would be appropriate in the assessment of either rural or urban populations is provided in Appendix G on the Companion Website and in the Community Assessment Reference Guide 📋 designed to accompany this text.

Information about population composition, morbidity, and mortality for both rural and urban populations may be obtained from state agencies (e.g., departments of vital statistics or state health departments). Rural statistics may also be available from local, state, national, and international agencies dealing with rural concerns and issues. At the federal level, for example, the Office of Rural Health Policy of the Health Resources and Services Administration (HRSA) and the USDA provide a wide array of information about rural populations. Many states also have rural policy agencies (e.g., the California Rural Health Policy Council). Local governments in largely rural areas also collect population data. Generally these local agencies would be county health departments or other agencies. Finally, several voluntary organizations, such as the National Rural Health Association, collect information on rural populations. Similar organizations, such as the International Council of Nurses' (2005) Rural and Remote Nursing Network, the Rural Health Association of Tennessee (2005), the Australian Rural Nurses, Inc. (2003), and the Rural Nurse Organization (n.d.) may be found at U.S. state or national levels, in other countries, or internationally.

With respect to urban populations, city or county governments or other local agencies (e.g., Chambers of Commerce) collect a variety of data, and state and national data can be found by urban census tract or other designation (e.g., MSA). In addition, national and international voluntary agencies, such as the Urban Health Institute and the International Society for Urban Health, may provide a wealth of data on national or worldwide urban populations. The World Health Organization also collects data related to both urban and rural populations.

Other types of information included in an assessment of an urban or rural population may be derived from service agencies operating in the area. For example, crime statistics might be available from an urban police department, county sheriff's department, or state police agency. Similarly, information regarding morbidity and mortality

as well as the extent of health insurance coverage might be obtained from local health care organizations.

Community health nurses might obtain still other forms of data from surveys of area residents. For example, the extent of depression in a rural or urban community can only be partially determined from treatment records because many people do not seek help for depression. Surveys of urban or rural dwellers would be apt to give a clearer picture of the extent of depression in the population. Finally, some information is best obtained through actual observation (e.g., housing conditions in the area, traffic hazards, and so on).

Diagnostic Reasoning and Care of Urban and Rural Populations

In rural areas, the etiology of nursing diagnoses is frequently related to a lack of resources and limited access to health care in the community. A nursing diagnosis of "potential for poor infant outcome due to extended travel time to nearest maternity delivery service" is common in today's rural health system and requires that the rural nurse providing prenatal care be most astute in assessing this client during her pregnancy. A second nursing diagnosis might be "increased suicide risk due to lack of access to and use of mental health services." This diagnosis may be attributable to limited access to health care as well as to perceptions of stigma frequently attached to mental illness among rural populations.

Nursing diagnoses developed for urban populations might also reflect unique factors affecting health in that setting. As an example, the nurse might make a diagnosis of "lack of physical activity due to fear of walking in high-crime neighborhoods." Another diagnosis related to urban populations might be "potential for hearing loss among children in schools adjacent to airport."

EVIDENCE-BASED PRACTICE

*H*uttlinger, Schaller-Ayers, and Lawson (2004) have advocated a population-based approach to health care delivery in rural areas. Population health is defined as "an approach [that] focuses on interrelated conditions and factors that influence the health of populations over the life course, identifies systematic variations in the patterns of occurrence, and applies the resulting knowledge to develop and implement policies and actions to improve the health and well-being of those populations" (Kindig & Stoddart, as quoted in Hartley, 2004, p. 1675). A population-based approach would work equally well to address health needs in urban settings. Population-based health care planning, however, must be based on an understanding of the health care needs of the particular population. Select an urban or rural population with which you are familiar. Then examine the literature for any information regarding the health problems and care needs of that population. Is there sufficient evidence on which to base health system planning? If not, how might that evidence base be developed?

Planning and Implementing Care for Urban and Rural Populations

Nursing interventions in rural and urban settings can be directed toward meeting the needs of individual clients, families, or population groups. Community health nurses play pivotal roles in planning intervention strategies for urban and rural populations. A key feature of planning interventions to address the health needs of either urban or rural populations would be the development of partnerships with community members and other groups and organizations in the setting. The development of such partnerships would employ principles of coalition building and strategies for empowering communities.

Overall goals for care in urban and rural settings are similar and include:

- Increasing access to health care services and decreasing barriers to their use
- Eliminating or modifying environmental risk factors
- Modifying social conditions that adversely affect health
- Increasing clients' abilities to make informed health decisions
- Developing systems of care that are population appropriate
- Developing equitable health care policies that address the diverse needs of urban and rural populations

Although the goals of care are similar for rural and urban populations, the means by which they are accomplished may be quite different. For example, increasing access to health care in rural settings may revolve primarily around increasing the number and variety of available providers or changing reimbursement rates and other characteristics of practice to attract providers to rural areas. In both urban and rural settings, increasing access may involve dealing with problems of cost, increasing insurance coverage, and developing systems that provide low-cost quality health care to these populations.

Interventions designed to decrease barriers to use of health care services may also differ significantly between urban and rural settings. For example, in urban settings, actions may be needed to increase the ability of providers to communicate with clients from multiple ethnic groups and cultures. With the movement of immigrants to rural areas, some actions along this line will be needed in rural settings as well, but providers are unlikely to be called on to communicate in multiple different languages and with multiple ethnic groups as occurs in urban areas. Decreasing barriers to care in rural settings may involve providing access to transportation services, changing times when services are provided, or finding creative ways to deliver services at great distances in cost-effective ways.

Activities to eliminate or modify environmental risks will also differ greatly between rural and urban settings. For example, skin cancer prevention education should be a high-priority focus among agricultural workers, whereas interventions to address high urban noise levels or reduce violent crime and gang activity may be more appropriate to urban settings.

In urban settings, action to modify social factors that adversely affect health may involve assisting clients to develop support systems or linking them to available health and social services. Community health nurses may also be involved in activities to promote the availability of affordable housing or to decrease unemployment levels. In rural settings, more focus is needed on providing support and respite for members of informal care networks and changing attitudes to the need for and use of health care services, particularly preventive services.

Increasing clients' abilities to make informed health decisions usually focuses on the type of decisions to be made and the health problems prevalent in the setting. For example, a rural community health nurse may focus on assisting clients with farm safety issues or use of preventive services. In the urban setting, on the other hand, community assessment data may suggest a need to focus on personal safety and crime prevention.

As noted earlier, the urban model of managed care may not be appropriate to meeting the needs of rural populations, and modified delivery systems may be required. Nurses may be involved in the development and implementation of creative modes of health care delivery in either urban or rural settings. For example, school-based clinics may be an effective mode of providing care in the urban environment. When children travel long distances to consolidated schools, however, the concept of the school as a central community structure that can support health services becomes less meaningful. It may be that faith community nursing or some other form of locally based nursing services may be a more appropriate vehicle for delivering nursing services in rural areas.

Finally, community health nurses should be actively involved in developing and promoting national and state health care policies that are equitable and address the diverse needs of both urban and rural populations. For example, nurses may advocate for higher reimbursement rates for providers in rural settings or for other incentives that attract and retain providers in rural communities, or community health nurses might become involved in revisions to policies that prevent both rural and urban immigrants from having access to certain health and social services.

Evaluating Health Care for Urban and Rural Populations

Nurses providing services in rural and urban settings must evaluate the outcomes of care as well as its cost-effectiveness. Outcomes of care in rural and urban settings may also be evaluated in terms of the accomplishment of the national health objectives. Several of the *Healthy People 2010* objectives deal with disparities in health care and

HEALTHY PEOPLE 2010
Goals for Population Health

OBJECTIVE	BASELINE	MOST RECENT DATA	TARGET
■ 1-1. Increase the proportion of people with health insurance:			
Metropolitan statistical areas (MSAs)	83%	84%	100%
Non-MSAs	80%	81%	100%
■ 1-5. Increase the proportion of people with a usual primary care provider:			
MSAs	77%	78%	85%
Non-MSAs	78%	80%	85%
■ 1-6. Reduce the proportion of families with difficulty in getting care:			
MSAs	12%	10%	7%
Non-MSAs	12%	12%	7%
■ 7-6. Increase the proportion of employees who participate in employer-sponsored health promotion:			
MSAs	66%	59%	75%#
Non-MSAs	73%	62%	75%#
■ 11-1. Increase the proportion of people with Internet at home:			
MSAs	26%	51%	80%
Non-MSAs	22%	49%	80%
■ 20-2d. Reduce injuries in agriculture, forestry, and fishing (per 100 full-time workers over age 16)	7.6	6	5.3
■ 22-1. Reduce the proportion of people with no leisure-time physical activity:			
MSAs	39%	37%	20%
Non-MSAs	43%	41%	20%

 # Objective moving away from target

Data from: Centers for Disease Control and Prevention. (2005). Healthy people data. Retrieved September 5, 2005, from http://wonder.cdc.gov/data2010

health care outcomes between rural and urban populations. These objectives and their current status may be viewed on the *Healthy People 2010* Web site, which may be accessed at http://wonder.cdc.gov/ data2010. Data regarding the status of some of these objectives are presented above. Similarly, the priority areas for rural health identified in *Rural Healthy People 2010* can be used as the basis for evaluating the effectiveness of rural health care.

Community health nursing in urban and rural settings displays some similarities but many differences. Effective community health nurses will be aware of these similarities and differences and will develop health care interventions accordingly. They will recognize that, although a particular intervention has demonstrated effectiveness in one setting, that effectiveness may not translate to other settings.

Case Study

Nursing in a Rural Setting

You are a rural community health nurse assigned to the county health department mobile van visiting a large migrant community at a local farm. Mr. Robert Kelbert is a 64-year-old African American migrant worker who comes into the mobile unit to have his blood pressure medication refilled. He will be in the county for the next 3 to 4 weeks to harvest the soybean crop. He usually attends a rural health clinic in the northern part of the state where he has been receiving his care and medications free.

Today, his blood pressure is 154/98, pulse 88, height 69 inches, and weight 198 pounds. He states he is "worn out" from the heat. He chews tobacco and drinks alcohol "some." He travels and stays with his son and family. His daughter-in-law does the cooking. During your interview, Mr. Kelbert tells you he is worried because two of the migrant workers have been given medicine for lung congestion and one of them has been coughing up blood.

1. In what ways is Mr. Kelbert's situation typical of that of rural clients in general? Of migrant farmworkers? In what ways is it different?

2. What are some of the biophysical, psychological, physical environmental, sociocultural, behavioral, and health system factors operating in this situation?

3. List three nursing diagnoses that you would identify for Mr. Kelbert.

4. What are your objectives for today's client visit?

5. How might your care for Mr. Kelbert differ from that provided to a client you see regularly at the rural health department?

6. What primary, secondary, and tertiary prevention measures are appropriate for Mr. Kelbert?

7. How will you follow up on this visit?

Test Your Understanding

1. Discuss differences in the definitions of *rural* and *urban*. What implications do these definitions have for health care policy? For research?

2. What are some of the differences in factors that affect health in rural and urban settings?

3. In what ways do policy inequities influence health in urban and rural settings?

4. How might you go about assessing factors influencing health in urban and rural settings?

5. What are the primary goals for nursing intervention in urban and rural settings? How might accomplishment of these goals differ between settings?

6. How would you go about evaluating the effectiveness of nursing interventions in a rural setting? Would your approach to evaluation differ in an urban setting?

EXPLORE MediaLink

http://www.prenhall.com/clark
Resources for this chapter can be found on the Companion Website.

Audio Glossary
Appendix G: Community Health Assessment and Intervention Guide
Exam Review Questions
Case Study: Community Health Care in a Rural Area

MediaLink Application: Choosing a Career in Rural Health (video)
MediaLink Application: The Urban Health Initiative (video)
Media Links

Challenge Your Knowledge
Update *Healthy People 2010*
Advocacy Interviews

References

Aday, L. A., Quill, B. E., & Reyes-Gibby, C. C. (2001). Equity in rural health and health care. In S. Loue & B. E. Quill (Eds.), *Handbook of rural health* (pp. 45–72). New York: Kluwer Academic/Plenum.

Annie E. Casey Foundation. (2004). *City & rural kids count data book.* Retrieved March 25, 2006, from http://www.aecf.org/publications/data/city_rural_databook.pdf

Australian Rural Nurses, Inc. (2003). *Mission and objectives.* Retrieved July 8, 2006, from http://www.aarn.au/about/mission.htm

Averill, J. (2003). Keys to the puzzle: Recognizing strengths in a rural community. *Public Health Nursing, 20,* 449–455.

Awofeso, N. (2003). The healthy cities approach—reflections on a framework for improving global health. *Bulletin of the World Health Organization, 81,* 222–223.

Baldwin, L.-M., Grossman, D. C., Casey, S., Hollow, W., Sugarman, J. R., Freeman, W. L., et al. (2002). Perinatal and infant health among rural and urban American Indians/Alaska Natives. *American Journal of Public Health, 92,* 1491–1497.

Bell, J. H. (2002). Anthrax and the wool trade. *American Journal of Public Health, 92,* 754–757.

(Reprinted from J. H. Bell, Anthrax: Its relation to the wool industry. In *Dangerous trades: The historical, social, and legal aspects of industrial occupations as affecting health, by a number of experts,* pp. 634–643, by T. Oliver, Ed., 1902, London: John Murray.)

Berkowitz, B. (2004). Rural public health service delivery: Promising new directions. *American Journal of Public Health, 94,* 1678–1681.

Branas, C. C., Nance, M. L., Elliott, M. R., Richmond, T. S., & Schwab, C. W. (2004). Urban–rural shifts in intentional firearm death: Different causes, same results. *American Journal of Public Health, 94,* 1750–1755.

Bureau of Health Professions. (n.d.). *Shortage designation.* Retrieved March 26, 2006, from http://bhpr.hrsa.gov/shortage

Carty, R. M., Al-Zayyer, W., Arietti, L. L., & Lester, A. S. (2004). International rural health needs and services research: A nursing and midwifery response. *Journal of Professional Nursing, 20,* 251–259.

Center for Rural Health, University of North Dakota. (n.d.). *Health professional shortage areas (HPSAs) and Medically underserved areas (MUAs).* Retrieved March 26, 2006, from

http://www.med.und.nodak.edu/depts/rural/pdf/hpsa.pdf

Centers for Disease Control and Prevention. (2005). *Healthy people data.* Retrieved September 5, 2005, from http://wonder.cdc.gov/data2010

Culp, K., & Umbarger, M. (2004). Seasonal and migrant agricultural workers. *AAOHN Journal, 52,* 383–390.

Eberhardt, M. S., & Pamuk, E. R. (2004). The importance of place of residence: Examining health in rural and nonrural areas. *American Journal of Public Health, 94,* 1682–1686.

Economic Research Service. (2005). *Data fact sheets: United States.* Retrieved March 25, 2006, from http://www.res.usda.gov/StateFacts/US.htm

Fitzpatrick, K. M. (2000). *Unhealthy places.* New York: Routledge.

Gaffield, S. J., Goo, R. L., Richards, L. A., & Jackson, R. J. (2003). Public health effects of inadequately managed stormwater runoff. *American Journal of Public Health, 93,* 1527–1533.

Gallagher, E., Alcock, D., Diem, E., Angus, D., & Medves, J. (2002). Ethical dilemmas in home care case management. *Journal of Healthcare Management, 47(2),* 85–97.

Gamm, L., & Hutchison, L. (2004). *Rural Healthy People 2010—Evolving Interactive Practice. American Journal of Public Health, 94,* 1711–1712.

Gamm, L., Hutchison, L., Dabney, B., & Dorsey, A. (Eds.). (2003). *Rural healthy people 2010: A companion document to healthy people 2010* (vol. 1). College Station, TX: Texas A&M University System Health Science Center, School of Rural Public Health, Southwest Rural Health Research Center.

Gessert, C. E. (2003). Rurality and suicide. *American Journal of Public Health, 93,* 698.

Gibb, H., Livesey, L., & Zyla, W. (2003). At 3 am who the hell do you call? Case management issues in sole practice as a rural community mental health nurse. *Australasian Psychiatry, 11*(Suppl.), S127–S129.

Goldberg, B. W., & Napolitano, M. (2001). The health of migrant and seasonal farmworkers. In S. Loue & B. E. Quill (Eds.), *Handbook of rural health* (pp. 103–117). New York: Kluwer Academic/Plenum.

Griffin, J. (1999). Parish nursing in rural communities. In P. A. Solari–Twadell & M. A. McDermott (Eds.), *Parish nursing: Promoting whole person health within faith communities* (pp. 75–82). Thousand Oaks, CA: Sage.

Hancock, T. (2000). Healthy communities must also be sustainable communities. *Public Health Reports, 115,* 151–156.

Hart, L. G., Larson, E. H., & Lishner, D. M. (2005). Rural definitions for health policy and research. *American Journal of Public Health, 95,* 1149–1155.

Hartley, D. (2004). Rural health disparities, population health, and rural culture. *American Journal of Public Health, 94,* 1675–1678.

House, J. S., Lepkowski, J. M., Williams, D. R., Mero, R. P., Lanz, P. M., Robert, S. A., et al. (2000). Excess mortality among urban residents: How much, for whom, and why? *American Journal of Public Health, 90,* 1898–1904.

Huttlinger, K., Schaller-Ayers, J., & Lawson, T. (2004). Health care in Appalachia: A population-based approach. *Public Health Nursing, 21,* 103–110.

Indiana State Department of Health, Local Liaison Office. (n.d.). *Health professional shortage area and medically underserved area designations.* Retrieved March 26, 2006, from http://www.in.gov/isdh/publications/llo/shortages/shortage.htm

Institute of Medicine. (2005). *Quality through collaboration: The future of rural health.* Washington, DC: National Academies Press.

International Council of Nurses. (2005). *Rural and Remote Nursing Network (ICN-RRNN).* Retrieved December 15, 2005, from http://www.icn.ch/rrn_network.htm

Kalisch, P. A., & Kalisch, B. J. (2004). *American nursing: A history.* Philadelphia: Lippincott Williams & Wilkins.

Knowlton, K. (2001). Urban history, urban health. *American Journal of Public Health, 91,* 1494–1496.

Leyden, K. M. (2003). Social capital and the built environment: The importance of walkable neighborhoods. *American Journal of Public Health, 93,* 1546–1551.

Long, K. A., & Weinert, C. (1998). Rural nursing: Developing the theory base. In H. J. Lee (Ed.), *Conceptual basis for rural nursing* (pp. 3–18). New York: Springer.

May, K. M., Phillips, L. R., Ferketich, S. L., & Verran, J. A. (2003). Public health nursing: The generalist in a specialized environment. *Public Health Nursing, 20,* 252–259.

Monts, R. (2002). Depression among migrant farm workers. *Community Health Forum, 3*(5), 52–54.

Murty, S. A., Peek-Asa, C., Zwerling, C., Stromquist, A. M., Burmeister, L. F., & Merchant, J. A. (2003). Physical and emotional abuse reported by men and women in a rural community. *American Journal of Public Health, 93,* 1073–1075.

National Center for Health Statistics. (2005). *Health, United States, 2005 with chartbook on trends in the health of Americans.* Retrieved December 23, 2005, from http://www.cdc.gov/nchs/data/hus/hus05.pdf

National Center for Infectious Diseases. (2001). Outbreaks of *Escherichia coli* O157:H7 infections among children associated with farm visits—Pennsylvania and Washington, 2000. *Morbidity and Mortality Weekly Report, 50,* 293–297.

National Coalition for the Homeless. (2005). *Rural homelessness.* Retrieved November 29, 2005, from http://www.nationalhomeless.org/publications/facts

National Health Service Corps. (2005). *Health professional shortage areas.* Retrieved March 26, 2006, from http://nchs.bhpr.hrsa.gov

National Rural Health Association. (n.d.a). *How is rural defined?* Retrieved July 8, 2006, from http://www.nrharural.org/about/sub/ruraldef.html

National Rural Health Association. (n.d.b). *What's different about rural health?* Retrieved March 26, 2006, from http://www.nrharural.org/about/sub/different.html

Oregon Health & Science University. (2006). *Oregon Office of Rural Health: Rural health clinics.* Retrieved October 6, 2006, from http://www.ohsu.edu/oregonruralhealth/rclinpg.html

Peek-Asa, C., Zwerling, C., & Stallones, L. (2004). Acute traumatic injuries in rural populations. *American Journal of Public Health, 94,* 1686–1693.

Perdue, W. C., Stone, L. A., & Gostin, L. O. (2003). The built environment and its relationship to the public's health: The legal framework. *American Journal of Public Health, 93,* 1390–1394.

Phillips, C. D., Holan, S., Sherman, M., Williams, M. L., & Hawes, C. (2004). Rurality and nursing home quality: Results from a national sample of nursing home admissions. *American Journal of Public Health, 94,* 1717–1722.

Phillips, C. D., & McLeroy, K. R. (2004). Health in rural America: Remembering the importance of place. *American Journal of Public Health, 94,* 1661–1663.

Population Information Program, Center for Communication Programs. (2002). Retrieved July 25, 2003, from http://www.jhucpp.org

Probst, J. S., Moore, C. G., Glover, S. H., & Samuels, M. E. (2004). Person and place: The compounding effects of race/ethnicity and rurality on health. *American Journal of Public Health, 94,* 1695–1703.

Reed, D. B. (2004a). Collaboration between nurses and agricultural teachers to prevent adolescent agricultural injuries: The Agricultural Disability Awareness and Risk Education Model. *Public Health Nursing, 21,* 323–330.

Reed, D. B. (2004b). The risky business of production agriculture: Health and safety for farm workers. *AAOHN Journal, 52,* 401–409.

Reeder, R. J., & Calhoun, S. D. (2002). Federal funds in rural America: Payments vary by region and type of county. *Rural America, 17*(3), 74–76.

Ricketts, T. C. (2005). Workforce issues in rural areas: A focus on policy equity. *American Journal of Public Health, 95,* 42–48.

Rogers, C. C. (2002). The older population in 21st century rural America. *Rural America, 17*(3), 2–10.

Rosenblatt, R. A., Casey, S., & Richardson, M. (2002). Rural–urban differences in the public health workforce: Local health departments in 3 rural western states. *American Journal of Public Health, 92,* 1102–1105.

Rural Health Association of Tennessee. (2005). *About us.* Retrieved July 8, 2006, from http://www.rhat.org/About-Us.php

Rural Nurse Organization. (n.d.). *The history of RNO.* Retrieved July 8, 2006, from http://www.rno.org/about.htm

Sanford, J. T., & Townsend-Rocchiccioli, J. (2004). The perceived health of rural caregivers. *Geriatric Nursing, 25,* 145–148.

Schenker, M. B. (1995). Preventive medicine and health promotion are overdue in the agricultural workplace. *Wellness Lecture Series.* Davis, CA: University of California.

Shreffler-Grant, J., Weinert, C., Nichols, E., & Ide, B. (2005). Complementary therapy use among older rural adults. *Public Health Nursing, 22,* 323–331.

Sierra Club. (n.d.). *America needs more transit.* Retrieved March 1, 2006, from http://www.sierraclub.org/sprawl/reports/transit_fact sheet.pdf

Sierra Club. (2001). *Clearing the air with transit spending.* Retrieved March 4, 2002, from http://www.sierraclub.org

Singh, G. K., & Siahpush, M. (2002). Increasing rural–urban gradients in US suicide mortality, 1990–1997. *American Journal of Public Health, 92,* 1161–1167.

Slifkin, R. T., Goldsmith, L. J., & Ricketts, T. C. III. (2000). *Race and place: Urban–rural differences in health for racial and ethnic minorities.* Chapel Hill, NC: North Carolina Rural Health Research Program.

Spengler, S. E., Browning, S. R., & Reed, D. B. (2004). Sleep deprivation and injuries in part-time Kentucky farmers. *AAOHN Journal, 52,* 373–383.

U.S. Census Bureau. (2005a). *Poverty: Historical poverty tables.* Retrieved March 22, 2006, from http://www.census.gov/hhes/www/poverty/histpov/histpov8/html

U.S. Census Bureau. (2005b). *Statistical Abstract of the United States: 2004–2005.* Retrieved May 12, 2005, from http://www.census.gov/prod/2004pubs/04statab

U.S. Department of Agriculture. (2005). *Rural America at a glance.* Retrieved March 25,

2006, from http://www.ers.usda.gov/publications/EIB4

U.S. Department of Health and Human Services. (2001). Health equity benefits everyone. *Prevention Report, 15*(2), 1–2.

Vallerand, A. H., Fouladbakhsh, J. M., & Templin, T. (2003). The use of complementary/alternative medicine therapies for the self-treatment of pain among residents of urban, suburban, and rural communities. *American Journal of Public Health, 93,* 923–925.

Waitzkin, H., Williams, R. L., Bock, J. A., McCloskey, J., Willging, C., & Wagner, W. (2002). Safety-net institutions buffer the impact of Medicaid managed care: A multi-method assessment in a rural state. *American Journal of Public Health, 92,* 598–610.

Wallace, B. R., Grindeanu, L. A., & Cirillo, D. J. (2004). Rural/urban contrasts in population morbidity status. In N. Glasgow, L. W. Morton, & N. E. Johnson (Eds.), *Critical issues in rural health* (pp. 15–26). Ames, IA: Blackwell.

Weeks, W. B., Kasiz, L. E., Shen, Y., Cong. Z., Ren, X., Miller, D., et al. (2004). Differences in health-related quality of life in rural and urban veterans. *American Journal of Public Health, 94,* 1762–1767.

Weinert, C., & Boik, R. J. (1998). MSU rurality index: Development and evaluation. In H. J. Lee (Ed.), *Conceptual basis for rural nursing* (pp. 449–471). New York: Springer.

World Health Organization. (2002). *Scaling up the response to infectious diseases.* Retrieved April 2, 2002, from http://www.who.int/infectious-disease-report/2002/investigating health.html

World Health Organization. (2003). *Right to water.* Geneva, Switzerland: Author.

World Health Organization. (2004). *World health report, 2004: Changing history.* Retrieved November 23, 2004, from http://www.who.int/whr/2004/annex/en

World Health Organization. (2005). *World Health Statistics, 2005.* Retrieved September 21, 2005, from http://www.who/int/healthinfo/statistics/whostat2005en1.pdf

Wright, R. J., Mitchell, H., Visness, C. M., Cohen, S., Stout, J., Evans, R., et al. (2004). Community violence and asthma mortality: An inner-city asthma study. *American Journal of Public Health, 94,* 625–632.

Care of Clients in Correctional Settings

From Chapter 26 of *Community Health Nursing: Advocacy for Population Health,* 5/e. Mary Jo Clark. Copyright © 2011 by Pearson Education. Published by Prentice Hall. All rights reserved.

Advocacy in Action

Facilitating Reentry

Women who have been incarcerated are often at a loss when they are released from a correctional facility. They have often exhausted their social support networks and don't know where to turn for assistance with issues of housing, employment, and ongoing physical and mental health care. Welcome Home Ministries (WHM) is an organization started by a nurse/minister that attempts to assist women with the reentry process. Working one-to-one with women was effective in helping them to address their needs, but there was a need for basic information on services available to these women that could be provided to a wider audience, not just those who sought services at WHM.

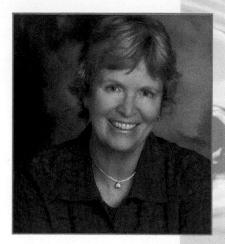

Community health nursing students of a local university undertook a project to identify services for which women were eligible and to produce a directory that could be distributed to women being released from the local jail and state prison. The students began by identifying categories of resources that women in reentry would need. They obtained this information in consultation with several recently released women who described their needs. The students explored services available in the community in each of the categories identified. They then interviewed staff at each of the agencies to get information on services provided, eligibility requirements, and how to obtain services. They were particularly careful to identify services for which previously incarcerated women would be eligible and that were in geographic areas that were easily accessible to the women.

Based on the information collected, the students created a services directory. WHM had a small grant that paid to print the directory. The directory was disseminated through WHM, as well as by the local sheriff's department and county jail personnel to women being released back into the community. With the students' assistance these women had a better chance of successfully reintegrating themselves into the community.

Diane Hatton, DNSc, RN

Professor, Hahn School of Nursing and Health Science

University of San Diego

Care of Clients in Correctional Settings

CHAPTER OBJECTIVES

After reading this chapter, you should be able to:

1. Discuss the impetus for providing health care in correctional settings.
2. Differentiate between basic and advanced nursing practice in correctional settings.
3. Describe biophysical, psychological, physical environmental, sociocultural, behavioral, and health system factors that influence health in correctional settings.
4. Identify major aspects of primary prevention in correctional settings and analyze the role of the community health nurse in each.
5. Describe approaches to secondary prevention in correctional settings and analyze community health nursing roles with respect to each.
6. Discuss considerations in tertiary prevention in correctional settings and analyze related community health nursing roles.

KEY TERMS

detainees
diversion
forensic nurses
jails
juvenile detention facilities
lockdown
lockup
medical parole
parolee
prisons
probationer
recidivism
reentry
search and seizure
TB prophylaxis

 MediaLink

Additional interactive resources for this chapter can be found on the Companion Website. Click on Chapter 26 and "Begin" to select the activities for this chapter.

*T*he concept of prisons as a place to contain wrongdoers began as early as the 1600s with workhouses that were used to punish people who violated the law. Unfortunately, workhouses were also used to confine family members who were likely to impugn the family's honor through their activities, whether or not those activities were actually criminal in nature (Fagan, 2003). Criminalization still occurs within populations that society would prefer to ignore, such as the homeless.

Correctional populations may be particularly vulnerable to a variety of health problems. In many instances, members of this population have not had access to effective health care services. In other cases, they have not seen health as a priority and frequently do not engage in practices that are conducive to good health. In addition, drug and alcohol use, which may result in incarceration, have both physical and psychological consequences for health. Incarceration, in and of itself, may have adverse health consequences.

Because of the great potential for coercion, correctional populations are also considered highly vulnerable to exploitation as research subjects. In addition to active coercion for participation, other more subtle forms of coercion may be employed. For example, inmates may agree to participate in research studies in order to obtain special privileges or gain additional time outside of cellblocks. For all these reasons, community health nurses working in correctional settings may be called on to engage in even greater advocacy efforts than might be required in other settings.

Correctional facilities provide a relatively new practice setting for community health nursing compared to the settings discussed in previous chapters. Correctional nursing, however, is congruent with the primary focus of community health nursing—the health of groups of people and the general public (Norman & Parrish, 2000). Corrections nursing frequently involves challenges not encountered in other community health nursing settings. Practice in a correctional setting requires autonomy and excellent assessment skills. Nurses are often responsible for triaging inmates during sick call and identifying those who need to be seen by physicians, nurse practitioners, or other providers. Nurses may also provide routine treatments, including medication, under agency protocols. Nursing in correctional settings operates within the constraints of the security system, which may contribute to increased job stress and frustration. Another source of stress is the fear of litigation by a population that is prone to threats of lawsuits (Morgan, 2003). Although there is some risk to the nurse's physical safety, many correctional nurses feel safer than they would in other settings such as emergency departments.

Another source of stress in the correctional setting is the potential for conflict between nursing values and

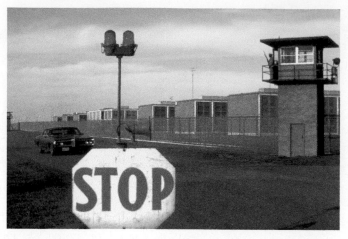

Providing health care to inmates of correctional settings presents multiple challenges. (John Bryson/Getty)

those of corrections personnel. Differences in values frequently give rise to the need for community health nursing advocacy in correctional settings to ensure that health care needs are balanced with custodial and security needs. For example, the primary concerns of the nurse are health care and meeting the health needs of inmates. For custodial personnel, however, the primary concern must be security. The priority placed on security may often make it difficult for the nurse to meet inmates' needs. For instance, giving medications such as insulin in a timely fashion may be impeded by security measures like lockdowns, when nurses are not ordinarily allowed into the areas where inmates are housed. Similarly, nurses may be expected to share information obtained while taking a health history (e.g., past drug use) with custodial or law enforcement personnel, when confidentiality and privacy are primary values of the nursing profession.

Correctional nursing takes place in three general types of facilities: prisons, jails, and juvenile detention facilities. **Prisons** are state and federal facilities that house persons convicted of crimes, usually those sentenced for longer than one year (Wolfe et al., 2001). Municipal or county facilities are usually called **jails** and house both convicted inmates and detainees. Convicted inmates in jails are usually serving sentences under a year in length. **Detainees** are people who have not yet been convicted of a crime. They are being detained pending a trial either because they cannot pay the set bail or because no bail has been set. They may also have violated the terms of probation or parole (National Center for HIV, STD, and TB Prevention, 2005). **Juvenile detention facilities** house children and adolescents convicted of crimes and those who are awaiting trial but who cannot be released in the custody of a responsible adult. Jails and juvenile detention facilities tend to be smaller and house fewer inmates than prisons.

Whatever the size of the facility or the terminology used, nurses working in correctional facilities must be committed to the belief that inmates retain their individual rights as human beings despite incarceration and that they have the same rights to health care as any other individual. Society does not categorically deprive any other group of individuals of access to adequate health care. In fact, there are carefully monitored standards of health care in such institutions as nursing homes, mental health facilities, and orphanages. It has only been as recently as 1979, however, that a program for accrediting health services in prisons was developed by the American Medical Association. Development of accreditation standards occurred at the request of the U.S. Department of Justice following a landmark court decision that depriving inmates of access to health care violated their civil rights (Stringer, 2001). Only since 1985 have published standards for nursing practice in such settings been available (American Nurses Association, 1985).

THE CORRECTIONAL POPULATION

On any given day, more than 2 million people are housed in U.S. correctional institutions, but as many as 10 million people may pass through the local, state, and federal correctional systems each year (Paris, 2005). At midyear 2004, there were 2.1 million inmates in U.S. prisons and jails, with approximately two thirds of this number housed in state and federal prisons and one third in local jails (Bureau of Justice Statistics [BJS], 2005d).

Incarceration rates have increased dramatically in the United States. From 1925 to 1973, rates remained relatively stable at 110 per 100,000 population (Travis, Solomon, & Waul, 2001). By the end of 2004, this figure had risen to 486 per 100,000 population or one of every 138 Americans (BJS, 2005e, 2005f; Golembeski & Fullilove, 2005), and if current rates of incarceration continue, 6.6% of all people born in the United States in 2001 will spend some time in prison during their lives (BJS, 2003a). Despite increases in bed capacity, local jails are operating at 94% of their capacity (BJS, 2005c). Federal and state facilities are over capacity with many facilities engaging in "double celling," a practice of placing more inmates in cells than are allowed based on national standards (Restum, 2005).

There are several reasons for this marked increase in correctional populations. First, there have been significant changes in sentencing guidelines, with mandatory sentences for specific crimes. In addition, criminal justice agencies have taken a more punitive approach to crime reduction, incarcerating more first-time offenders than in the past (Golembeski & Fullilove, 2005). Other reasons for the increase include longer sentences and less opportunity for discretionary release by parole boards, resulting in more inmates serving their entire sentences than in the past (BJS, 2003b). As a result, the United States now has the dubious distinction of having the highest rate of incarceration in the developed world (Restum, 2005).

From 1994 to 2004, the rate of incarceration for violent crime decreased significantly, with more convictions for drug and property offenses than for violent crimes (BJS, 2005a). Based on 2004 figures, incidence rates for rape were 1 per 1,000 population, and for assault with injury and robbery 2 per 1,000. Murder rates were 6 per 100,000 population in 2003 (BJS, 2005b).

THE NEED FOR HEALTH CARE IN CORRECTIONAL SETTINGS

Health care in correctional facilities is an appropriate endeavor for several reasons. First, the right to adequate health care is a constitutionally recognized right arising from the Eighth Amendment, which prohibits "cruel and unusual punishment" of those convicted of crimes. Detainees also have a constitutional right to health care under the Fifth and Fourteenth Amendments, which prohibit punishment of any kind without "due process" (e.g., conviction through the normal legal processes of the nation). In 1976, the U.S. Supreme Court handed down a decision that failure to provide adequate health care to correctional populations constituted unusual punishment and violated their constitutional rights (Weiskopf, 2005).

In addition to the constitutional right to health care, correctional care is good common sense for a variety of other reasons. Because of poverty, lower education levels, and unhealthy lifestyles that frequently involve substance abuse, inmates may enter a correctional facility with significant health problems. Because many of these individuals cannot afford to pay for care on the outside, the cost of care will be borne by society. Societal costs for this care will be lower if interventions occur in a timely fashion, before health problems become severe. Provision of care within the correctional facility also saves taxpayers the cost of personnel and vehicles to transport inmates to other health care facilities. Primary prevention in correctional settings is also cost-effective.

Another possible societal cost of failure to provide adequate health care to inmates lies in the potential for the spread of communicable disease from correctional facilities to the community (Inmate Infections Spread, 2005). Environmental conditions and behaviors within correctional facilities lend themselves to the transmission of communicable diseases such as tuberculosis. When inmates are released back into society, they may constitute a source of infection for the rest of the population.

Finally, correctional settings have been described as "inherently unhealthy environments" (Brodie, 2000, p. 15) and may themselves give rise to a variety of health problems. Correctional environments limit inmate autonomy;

MediaLink Interview with Author of *Acres of Skin* (video)

promote social isolation and communicable diseases; limit exercise; and foster boredom, stress, hostility, and depression. Services are needed to deal with these effects of incarceration as well as the myriad health problems inmates bring with them to correctional settings.

THE EPIDEMIOLOGY OF HEALTH AND ILLNESS IN CORRECTIONAL SETTINGS

Factors in each of the six dimensions of health influence the health status of clients and staff in correctional settings. The nurse assesses factors related to the biophysical, psychological, physical environmental, sociocultural, behavioral, and health system dimensions to identify health problems and to direct interventions to resolve those problems.

Biophysical Considerations

In the biophysical dimension, the nurse in the correctional setting needs to assess individual clients for existing physical health problems. He or she also needs to identify problems that have a high incidence and prevalence in the overall institutional population. Particular areas to be considered include the age, gender, and ethnic composition of the population and evidence of existing physical health problems as well as the population's immune status.

Age and Aging

Correctional populations vary greatly in their composition. The age group most likely to have ever been incarcerated is people aged 35 to 39 years (BJS, 2003a). Despite this majority, however, there are growing numbers of youth and the elderly in U.S. correctional facilities. In 2003, 2.2 million juveniles were arrested and 1.1 million cases were referred to juvenile courts. At any given time, more than 104,000 youth are incarcerated in juvenile correctional facilities (Teplin, Abram, McClelland, Washburn, & Pikus, 2005). Children and adolescents account for 17% of all arrests and 15% of arrests for violent crimes in the United States. Although these figures may seem high, the number of juvenile arrests for violent crimes actually decreased 47% from 1994 to 2002. In contrast, arrests for driving while under the influence of alcohol or drugs (DUI) increased 46% from 1993 to 2002, and drug abuse violations increased by 59% (Snyder, 2004). At midyear 2004, more than 7,000 youth were being held in local jails, and 2,477 state prisoners were under 18 years of age (BJS, 2005d). Juveniles are more apt to commit crimes in groups rather than alone and are more likely than adults to be arrested for violations (Snyder, 2004).

Juvenile inmates tend to have higher prevalence rates of a variety of physical and mental health conditions than their counterparts in the general population and usually have less access to care prior to incarceration. In one study, for example, 43% of juveniles

in detention centers had no previous health care provider and reported high rates of sexual abuse and sexual activity. Asthma was noted in 27% of the population, dental caries in 19%, sexually transmitted diseases in 12%, and scrotal masses were found in 11% of the youth (National Commission on Correctional Health Care [NCCHC], 2001b). Other studies have noted high incidence and prevalence rates for fractures, injuries, and chlamydial infection (Head, Kelly, Bair, Baillargeon, & German, 2000), as well as menstrual disorders, pregnancy, somatic complaints, and skin problems (American Academy of Pediatrics [AAP], 2001).

Incarcerated youth also display significant levels of mental illness and substance abuse. An estimated 15% of juvenile inmates display major mental disorders with functional impairment, but only about 15% of these receive treatment while incarcerated (Teplin et al., 2005). Identifying and treating mental health problems in juveniles in correctional settings may be complicated by their tendencies to minimize or exaggerate or fabricate symptoms. Many juvenile offenders may minimize mental health problems out of fear of being victimized if they are seen as weak or "crazy" or a desire to avoid administrative measures such as increased surveillance. Conversely, some youth may fabricate mental illness to receive psychotropic drugs or to induce peers to avoid them (Boesky, 2003).

Because of the move to try more juveniles as adults, particularly for violent crimes, the number of youth incarcerated in adult correctional facilities is growing. Because of the potential for victimization by older and stronger inmates, younger inmates should be in areas segregated both visually and auditorily (Shimkus, 2004b).

Incarcerated youth have different needs than adult inmates. For example, they have greater nutritional needs than adults (Shimkus, 2004b). In addition, correctional protocols are often based on the needs of adult inmates. For example, juvenile suicide prevention plans and staff training are often modeled on information from adult prisoners or from youth in the community and may not be effective with incarcerated youth (Hayes, 2004). Because of these differences, the National Commission on Correctional Health Care (NCCHC) (1999) has developed standards for juvenile detention facilities separate from those for adult facilities. Elements of these standards are presented as special considerations on the next page. In addition, the standards for adult correctional facilities include an appendix addressing the special needs of youth incarcerated in adult facilities (Shimkus, 2004b). The American Academy of Pediatrics (2001) has adopted a statement on care of juvenile offenders that includes the following recommendations:

• Incarcerated youth should receive care in keeping with AAP general guidelines for health supervision of children and adolescents, including immunization, care for psychosocial issues, and development of a "medical home."

- All youth should receive regular preventive services during incarceration.
- Incarcerated youth should receive prenatal services, parenting classes, and tobacco, alcohol, and other drug cessation services as needed.
- Pediatricians should be involved in policy development for incarcerated youth.
- Correctional personnel dealing with juvenile offenders should be specifically trained to address their needs.
- Youth incarcerated in adult settings should be segregated from the adult population by both sight and sound and should receive developmentally appropriate services.

Community health nurses may need to advocate for the application of these sets of standards and recommendations in the care of the juvenile correctional population.

The fastest-growing segment of corrections populations is the elderly, primarily because of extended sentences, with a large proportion of the population growing old in the correctional setting (Hills, Siegfried, &

SPECIAL CONSIDERATIONS

AREAS ADDRESSED BY NCCHC STANDARDS FOR JUVENILE CORRECTIONAL FACILITIES

- Access to care
- Communication and confidentiality
- Continuity of care
- Credentialing and orientation of staff
- Diet
- Emergency plans and procedures
- Employment of juvenile workers
- Environmental health and safety
- Exercise
- Grievances
- Hygiene
- Infection control
- Informed consent
- Kitchen sanitation
- Pharmaceuticals and medication administration
- Policies and procedures
- Research
- Reporting and notification
- Services (assessment, screening, diagnosis, treatment, oral health, mental health, health education and promotion, family planning, emergency, special needs)
- Staffing levels
- Sexual assault
- Substance abuse
- Suicide prevention
- Therapeutic restraint

Data from: National Commission on Correctional Health Care. (1999). A summary guide to revisions in the 1999 Standards for Health Services in Juvenile Detention and Confinement Facilities. Correct Care, 13(2), 18–19.

Ickowitz, 2004). The number of elderly inmates in state prisons increased more than 200% over a 10-year period (Richardson, 2003). People over 50 years of age are considered "old" in correctional systems due to the accelerated aging that occurs in correctional populations. In fact, the biological age of inmates over age 50 is, on average, 11.5 years more than their chronological age. This accelerated aging process is due to life histories that often include substance abuse and withdrawal, poor health care, and high-risk behaviors as well as the stress of incarceration (Shimkus, 2004a).

In 2004, people over 55 years of age constituted 5% of the state and federal prison population (BJS, 2005f) and nearly 4% of persons held in local jails (BJS, 2005d). Both medical and mental health problems increase in older clients. For example, approximately 40% of inmates over age 45 have been found to have medical problems, compared to 12% of those under age 24 years. Similarly, the incidence of mental health problems in inmates over 45 years of age was 48%, compared to 24% in the younger group (Maruschak & Beck, 2001). Common problems include incontinence, sensory impairments, limited mobility, respiratory disease, cardiovascular disease, and cancer. Other conditions experienced by this group are similar to those found in older populations in the community and include arthritis, hypertension, ulcers, and prostate disease (Shimkus, 2004a). Correctional facilities are often unprepared to address the health care needs of older inmates, nor are budgets designed to accommodate these needs. For example, it is estimated that health care costs for elderly inmates are approximately three times those for younger age groups (Hills et al., 2004) and may rise to as much as $60,000 to $70,000 per person per year (Shimkus, 2004a). Community health nurses may need to be actively involved in assuring that facilities and services are available to meet the needs of elderly inmates as well as to protect them from victimization by younger inmates.

Gender and Ethnicity

In 2004, women constituted 10% of the state and federal correctional population and 12% of the local jail population, but the rate of incarceration for women is growing faster than that for men. For example, the rate of incarceration among women has increased by 5% per year since 1995, compared to a 3.3% increase among men. The rate of incarceration among U.S. women in 2004 was 123 per 100,000 women; the rate for men was 1,348 per 100,000 (BJS, 2005d). Overall, there was a 313% increase in incarceration among women from 1981, compared to a 182% increase for men.

Similar differences are noted among incarcerated youth, with boys accounting for 71% and girls for 29% of juvenile arrests, but arrest rates are increasing faster for female juveniles than males. For example, DUI arrests from 1993 to 2002 rose 94% for girls versus 37% for boys. Similarly, drug abuse violations increased 120% for girls and only 51% for boys, and aggravated assault arrests increased 7% among adolescent girls, but decreased by 29% among boys in the same time period (Snyder, 2004). Women tend to be arrested more often for minor property crimes and drug offenses than violent crimes (Braithwaite, Treadwell, & Arriola, 2005).

Women inmates often have high rates of physical and mental health problems such as histories of physical and sexual abuse and early initiation of sexual intercourse and drug and alcohol use. Incarcerated women also have more unplanned and frequent pregnancies than women in the community and higher rates of STD, depression, suicide attempts, and dental problems (Newkirk, 2003). Female prisoners have twice the rates of mental illness as males, and in approximately one fourth of women, alcohol or drug use was associated with the offense for which they were arrested (Wagaman, 2003).

Incarcerated women are more likely to be unmarried, divorced, or separated than their community-dwelling counterparts, and have lower educational and economic levels than male inmates. Approximately 65% of women inmates are parents of minor children (Wagaman, 2003), and an estimated 1.3 million U.S. children have a mother who has been incarcerated. As many as 5% to 10% of women enter correctional systems pregnant, but few of them have received prenatal care prior to incarceration (Braithwaite et al., 2005). Prenatal services while incarcerated may be inadequate, with little prenatal education or availability of abortion or contraceptive services if desired. Conversely, some pregnant inmates report pressure to have an abortion when it is not desired. Women inmates have higher rates of low-birth-weight (LBW) babies than the general population, but the incidence of LBW among this population is similar to that of other high-risk populations (Mertens, 2001).

Women inmates have special needs not experienced by men. For example, they require both routine and nonroutine gynecologic care and have more difficulty with sleep disturbances due to anxiety and apprehension than men. In addition, their nutritional needs differ, and women tend to gain weight in correctional settings because the typical correctional diet is designed for more active men. Similarly, pain management needs may be influenced by higher levels of depression. Women's substance abuse treatment needs also differ from men's, and treatment often must address their histories of trauma and abuse (Wagaman, 2003). Women are more likely to request health care and mental health services than men, so staff levels in these areas may need to be higher than in facilities for men (Newkirk, 2003). Unfortunately, because they are fewer in number, incarcerated women are less visible than men (Braithwaite et al., 2005) and services may be less available. Because of gender socialization, women inmates may also be less able to articulate and advocate for themselves (Hills et al.,

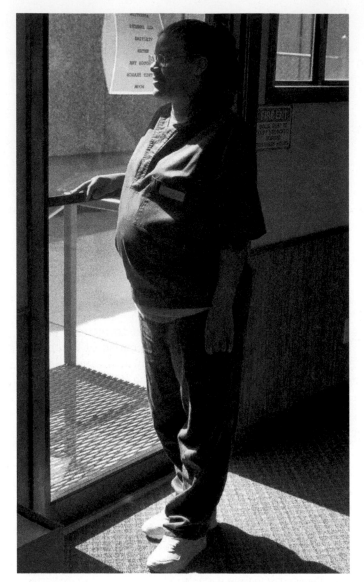

Women in correctional settings may have special needs, including care during pregnancy. (© Sean Cayton/The Image Works)

2004), leading to a need for community health nursing advocacy to assure that their health and social service needs are met.

Men and women also respond differently to the experience of being incarcerated. Men have been found to be most distressed by the loss of freedom, social rejection and loss of social status, autonomy, and self-control. Women, on the other hand, have similar concerns, but consider separation from family to be the most difficult aspect of incarceration. Other areas of concern for women include the constant stress of living in close proximity to others and lack of privacy with respect to personal property, modesty, and invasion of personal space. Men tend to view incarceration as an interruption in their lives, which will proceed normally on their release. Women are more likely to view incarceration as a significant change in their lives (Wagaman, 2003). Women, in particular, need support in dealing with family separation and in maintaining family relationships. Unfortunately, because of fewer numbers, women's correctional facilities are less likely to be located close to their place of residence than men's facilities (Braithwaite et al., 2005).

Another issue related to gender in correctional settings is the presence of transgendered individuals in the population. Concerns around transgendered individuals include housing decisions, safety, mental health issues, and maintenance of hormone therapy (American Public Health Association [APHA], 2003). Decisions need to be made whether to place these inmates in male or female housing. It is recommended that they be housed in the general correctional population if possible, with attention given to privacy for hygiene, appropriate clothing, and protection from assault by other inmates (Fry, 2003). These decisions will best be made in light of where the inmate is in the process of transition. Mental health services may also be needed to address issues of gender dysphoria or stigma (APHA, 2003).

Members of ethnic minority groups are disproportionately represented in correctional settings. Approximately 70% of the U.S. correctional population is comprised of minority group members (Paris, 2005), and one fourth of those housed in correctional facilities are African American. Black men are incarcerated at a rate seven times that of White men, and an estimated one in three African American men is under correctional supervision at any point in time (Cooke, 2004). In 2004, for example, 8.4% of all Black males age 24 to 29 were in prison (BJS, 2005f). The 2004 incarceration rate for Black men was 3,218 per 100,000 population compared to 1,220 per 100,000 and 463 per 100,000 for Hispanic and White men, respectively (BJS, 2005e). Similarly, two thirds of incarcerated women are members of ethnic minorities (Braithwaite et al., 2005). These and other similar figures have prompted concerns for inequities and prejudice within the justice system. Whether this is indeed the case, the fact remains that correctional populations are ethnically diverse, which may result in racial tensions within facilities as well as the need for culturally sensitive health care. Community health nurses may need to actively advocate for correctional health care services that meet the needs of a culturally and linguistically diverse population as well as advocate for fair treatment for all inmates regardless of ethnicity.

Physiologic Function

Environmental conditions and behavioral patterns in correctional settings foster the spread of communicable diseases. Although many communicable diseases are found in this population, four of particular concern are tuberculosis (TB), HIV infection and AIDS, hepatitis, and other sexually transmitted diseases (STDs). Nearly

4% of all TB diagnosed in the United States occurs among correctional inmates. Overall TB incidence is 5 times higher in state and federal prisons than in the general public (MacNeil, Lobato, & Moore, 2005), and may be as much as 6 to 15 times higher in some states (Francis J. Curry National Tuberculosis Center, 2003). Overcrowding and generally poor health status are two of the factors that promote the spread of tuberculosis (TB) in inmate populations. Moreover, co-infection with both TB and HIV is occurring in large segments of some correctional populations (Francis J. Curry National Tuberculosis Center, 2003). Additional complicating factors in the problem of tuberculosis in correctional facilities are the prevalence of multi-drug-resistant (MDR) tuberculosis and the tendency of inmates not to complete a full course of treatment. In some studies, for example, the rate of treatment completion among inmates is 59%, compared to 73% in the general population (MacNeil et al., 2005).

A large portion of all persons with tuberculosis will enter a correctional facility at some point. For example, in one year 40% of all persons with TB were admitted to a correctional facility during that year (Hammett, Harmon, & Rhodes, 2002). This makes correctional facilities ideal settings for minimizing the spread of TB in the general population. Community health nurses working in correctional settings should assess inmates for signs of tuberculosis as well as provide routine screenings for TB according to agency policy. Tuberculin skin test screening in jails may be inappropriate for many inmates who stay only one or two days, so the nurse should ask about TB symptomatology and history of exposure during the intake assessment to isolate potentially infectious inmates.

HIV infection and confirmed cases of AIDS are another growing problem in correctional facilities. Many inmates are at increased risk of infection because of injection drug use, and the potential for exposure during incarceration via continued drug use and homosexual activity is high. HIV prevalence peaked at rates 13 times those of the general population (Golembeski & Fullilove, 2005), but current rates are approximately five times those of the general population (Heines, 2005). Overall, rates for confirmed cases of AIDS are four times higher in correctional populations than on the outside (Braithwaite & Arriola, 2003). HIV infection rates are higher among incarcerated women than among men (Bauserman et al., 2003). For example, 3.4% of female prisoners in state correctional facilities in 2001 were HIV positive, compared to 2.2% of men (Bauserman, Ward, Eldred, & Swetz, 2001). Like TB, approximately 40% of people with HIV infection pass through correctional systems each year (Paris, 2005), making this setting a good place to identify them and initiate treatment.

Rates of HIV infection and AIDS diagnoses vary from one area of the country to another, and nurses should be aware of the overall prevalence of infection in their jurisdictions. Corrections nurses should assess all inmates for a history of HIV infection, high-risk behaviors, and a history or symptoms of possible opportunistic infections. In addition, community health nurses should advocate for effective treatment for HIV-infected inmates during incarceration and following their release into the community.

Drug use behaviors contribute to the increased incidence of tuberculosis and HIV infection in inmates. Such behaviors also place inmates at risk for other STDs and hepatitis B (HBV) and C (HCV). In addition to drug use, sexual activity and tattooing are other risk factors for HBV and HCV common in correctional populations. The prevalence of HBV infection in adult inmates ranges from 13% to 47% in different populations. As many as 1% to 3.7% of inmates may develop chronic HBV infection, a rate two to six times that of the general population. The incidence of new HBV infections in correctional settings may be as high as 3.8% per year, arguing for spread of disease during incarceration (Division of Viral Hepatitis, 2004c). Hepatitis C infection rates are nine to ten times higher in correctional populations than in the general public (Heines, 2005; Travis et al., 2001). In one study, prevalence rates for HIV, HBV, and HCV infection in a correctional population were 1.8%, 20.2%, and 23.1%, respectively (Macalino et al., 2004). In assessing individual inmates for health problems, the nurse should ask about a history of STDs and hepatitis B and C and should be alert to the presence of physical signs and symptoms of these diseases.

Other communicable diseases are also prevalent in correctional populations. For example, methicillin-resistant *Staphylococcus aureus* (MRSA) is a common occurrence in institutional settings, including jails and prisons (Tobin-D'Angelo et al., 2003). Similarly, *Chlamydia trachomatis* infection has been found in 22% of girls and 9% of boys admitted to juvenile detention facilities (Head et al., 2000). Higher syphilis rates are also found in correctional settings than in the general population (Wolfe et al., 2001).

Chronic illnesses of particular concern in correctional settings include diabetes, hypertension, heart disease, and chronic lung conditions such as asthma. Seizure disorders are also common, and inmates may also exhibit seizure activity during withdrawal from drugs and alcohol. Diabetes may be particularly difficult to control given the rigid structure of the correctional routine and the need to time hypoglycemic medications, meals, and exercise periods appropriately. The availability of vending machines and the use of commissary privileges as a reward may also complicate dietary control for inmates with diabetes. Many inmates with chronic conditions, particularly those with substance abuse problems, enter the correctional facility after prolonged periods without medications or may not know what medications they have been taking. In many instances, the nurse has to exert considerable ingenuity

to obtain an accurate health history from clients, family members, and health care providers in the community. Because of poor overall health status, inmates may also be especially susceptible to exacerbations of chronic conditions. The nurse should assess individual inmates for existing chronic conditions and should also identify problems with high incidence and prevalence in the correctional population with whom he or she works.

Injury is another area of physiologic function that should be assessed by the nurse. Injury may result from activities preceding arrest, from actions taken by arresting officers, or from accidents or assaults occurring during incarceration. The nurse should be aware of the potential for internal as well as visible injuries and should assess inmates for signs of trauma. Slightly more than one fourth of state and federal inmates reported injuries that occurred during their incarceration. Approximately two thirds of injuries were due to accidents, and the balance were related to fighting (Maruschak & Beck, 2001).

Dental health problems are also common among inmates. One particular problem that nurses in correction settings may encounter is a condition called "meth mouth." Meth mouth is characterized by severe erosion and decay of teeth and usually requires emergency dental services. Meth mouth results from several factors associated with methamphetamine use including gnashing of the teeth, poor oral hygiene, and dry mouth, which increases the acidic effects of methamphetamine. Methamphetamine use also leads to cravings for high-caffeine, high-sugar soft drinks that further contribute to tooth decay. In some correctional systems, meth mouth has been credited with doubling correctional health care costs over a 4-year period. The high demand for emergency dental services has also resulted in long waits for routine services by other inmates (Brunswick, 2005).

Pregnancy is the final biophysical consideration in assessing the health of correctional populations. As noted earlier, the number of female inmates increases annually. Because of prior drug use and poor health care, pregnant women in correctional settings may be at higher risk for poor pregnancy outcomes than women in the general population. Conversely, incarceration may improve pregnancy outcomes because it interrupts drug use and provides access to prenatal care that the women might not otherwise have. Care of pregnant women in correctional settings, however, is often hampered by lack of special diets to support pregnancy, lack of exercise, and inappropriate work assignments. Fetal health may also be compromised by problems encountered in drug and alcohol withdrawal in the correctional setting. Finally, the timely transfer of women in labor to obstetrical facilities is often hampered by the security constraints of the correctional facility (Fulco, 2001).

In assessing female inmates, the nurse should ask about the last menstrual period and solicit any symptoms of possible pregnancy. Because drug use can interfere with menses, menstrual history is not always reliable for indicating pregnancy or for suggesting length of gestation when pregnancy is confirmed. The nurse should also ask about high-risk behavior that may affect the fetus such as smoking, drug and alcohol use, and so on. The pregnant inmate's nutritional status should also be assessed. Other physical problems common in this population that may affect pregnancy outcomes include urinary tract infections and STDs, and the nurse should assess for symptoms of these conditions. Depression and anxiety are also common phenomena among these women. Advocacy may be required to assure adequate prenatal and perinatal care for pregnant inmates. For example, community health nurses may need to convince correctional personnel of the necessity of keeping outside appointments for high-risk pregnancy care, even when these require pulling security personnel away from the correctional facility.

Psychological Considerations

Psychological dimension factors can have a profound influence on health in correctional settings. The presence of mental illness in the correctional population is one of the major psychological factors influencing the health of this population. An estimated 16% of state prison inmates have serious mental illness or have been previously hospitalized for a psychiatric condition, and another 15% to 20% require some mental health care. Mentally ill inmates are often significantly disabled by their conditions and have a more difficult time adjusting to prison life than other inmates. Inmates are nearly four times more likely than the general population to experience schizophrenia, and approximately 6% of inmates have bipolar disorder. Major depression is present in approximately 9% of inmates and general anxiety disorders (including post-traumatic stress disorder [PTSD]) in 6%. Psychiatric disorders are more common in women inmates than men, with 34% of women experiencing PTSD and 17% experiencing major depression. Overall, as much as 80% of women inmates may have a lifetime history of one or more psychiatric disorders (Hills et al., 2004).

Juvenile inmates also experience high rates of mental illness, including attention deficit hyperactivity disorder (ADHD), conduct disorder, oppositional-defiant disorder, depression, and PTSD. Oppositional-defiant disorder is characterized by a consistent pattern of negative, hostile, and defiant behavior, whereas conduct disorder is the result of a basic disregard for rules and norms of behavior and for the rights of others (Boesky, 2003). Attempted suicide is a particularly prevalent problem among incarcerated youth, and as noted earlier, suicide prevention programs may not be designed to effectively address the needs of young inmates.

The high rates of PTSD in women and youth can be explained, in part, by past history of abuse. Approximately 25% to 31% of incarcerated youth have a history of abuse and neglect (American Academy of Pediatrics, 2001), and 50% to 80% of women inmates have been abused at some point in their lives (Wagaman, 2003).

Another 7% to 15% of young offenders may be mentally retarded, and an additional 17% to 53% may experience learning disabilities and other developmental disorders (American Academy of Pediatrics, 2001). The prevalence of mental retardation in correctional settings is two to three times that of the general population (Hills et al., 2004). Mentally retarded individuals, particularly youth, may be persuaded to participate in group crimes in order to be accepted by their peers without fully realizing the consequences of their actions. Developmentally disabled inmates may display deficits in both cognitive/intellectual function and adaptive capabilities, leading to greater difficulty adjusting to life in a correctional facility (Richardson, 2003). Because of their diminished mental capabilities, this group of inmates may have difficulty understanding instructions and display impulsivity and low frustration tolerance, earning them frequent punishment for infractions in the correctional setting (Hills et al., 2004). Mentally retarded inmates may be a subgroup in the correctional setting that requires particular advocacy on the part of community health nurses to assist them in their adjustment and to help correctional personnel recognize their limitations.

The increasing proportion of mentally ill persons in correctional institutions has several explanations (Broner, Borum, & Gawley, 2002; Fagan, 2003). "Get tough" philosophies and public initiatives that target nuisance crimes lead to more incarcerations, including among those with mental illness. Deinstitutionalization and the resulting closure of many locked psychiatric wards shifted mentally ill persons who could not cope with community living to jails and prisons. It is proposed by some that there may be as many as three times the number of mentally ill individuals in correctional settings as in mental hospitals (Bell, 2005). Some authors have described correctional institutions as a "safety net" for the care of the mentally ill (Cutler, Bigelow, Collins, Jackson, & Field, 2002). In addition, the federal "war on drugs" and the extent of co-occurring mental illness and substance abuse disorder put many mentally ill persons at increased risk of incarceration for drug offenses. Approximately 70% of mentally ill inmates also abuse alcohol and other drugs (Bell, 2005). Homelessness among the mentally ill and inability to compete for existing low-income housing also leads to their arrest and conviction, often for minimal crimes. Some studies have indicated that the mentally ill are more likely to be incarcerated than non-mentally ill offenders (Heines, 2005). Finally, the mentally ill have few legitimate economic opportunities, putting them at risk for criminal behavior to survive. In fact, in one study, 64% of persons

MediaLink Puppetry in Prison (video)

discharged from mental hospitals were involved in some sort of criminal activity shortly after their discharge (Cutler et al., 2002).

By law, inmates are entitled to mental health services as well as medical treatment. Mental health services, however, may be lacking in some correctional systems, or the need for these services may go unrecognized. This is particularly true among women inmates, the elderly, and youth. An estimated 75% to 85% of state prisons provide mental health screening, assessment, and treatment services with medication management (Bell, 2005).

Incarceration itself is stressful and can lead to psychological effects, including depression and suicide. Incarceration also exacerbates existing mental illness. Correctional nurses should be alert to signs of depression and other mental or emotional distress in inmates, and assessment of suicide potential is a critical part of every intake interview. Suicide is the leading cause of death in jails and "lockups," and is the cause of nearly 100% of deaths among incarcerated juveniles. A **lockup** is a temporary holding facility in which inmates are placed prior to transportation to a jail or other facility. Suicide rates in prisons, on the other hand, are more or less comparable to those in the general population.

Finally, state and federal prison systems may house a number of inmates who have been sentenced to death, creating a need for emotional and psychological support. Corrections nurses working in systems with "death-row" inmates should assess them for evidence of psychological problems and refer them for counseling as appropriate.

Because of the increasing age of corrections populations, nurses may also encounter clients with terminal conditions in the correctional setting. These clients have the same end-of-life care needs as people in the general population. End-of-life care for terminally ill inmates is discussed in more detail later in this chapter.

Mental health challenges in dealing with correctional populations are many and varied. Some of these challenges include determining who has mental health problems and how they should be treated, managing behavior and symptoms associated with psychiatric illness, and recognizing and dealing with the negative mental health effects of incarceration. Other challenges include understanding the difficulty adjusting to incarceration that might be experienced by inmates with mental illness and determining the need for and providing specialized services (Hills et al., 2004). For example, few correctional settings deal effectively with the mental health needs of older inmates. Similarly, women and youth exposed to psychological trauma need therapy to deal with issues of abuse as well as co-occurring substance abuse. Community health nurses in correctional settings can engage in advocacy to assure that appropriate services are provided to these vulnerable population groups.

Physical Environmental Considerations

Factors in the physical environmental dimension also influence the health of correctional populations. The physical environment of the correctional setting is constrained by the need for security. Inmates may be relegated to specific spaces at specific times of the day. Because of the tremendous growth in the incarcerated population, jails and prisons are extremely overcrowded and few jurisdictions are not in violation of space standards for inmates. For example, at the end of 2003, local jails were at 94% of their capacity. State prisons were at capacity to 16% over capacity, and federal prisons were 39% over capacity (BJS, 2005d). Other physical environmental problems common in correctional settings include poor ventilation, lack of temperature control, and unsanitary conditions. Lack of funds for maintenance may lead to buildings in poor repair, creating safety hazards for both inmates and staff. Other areas that should be assessed by the nurse include the safety of recreational areas, fire protection, lighting, plumbing, solid waste disposal, and safety of the water supply. Additional considerations include vermin control, noise control, and the presence of high levels of radiation.

Because correctional facilities are often situated in areas away from the general population, they may be located in sites with disaster potential such as flooding, earthquake, and so on. The nurse should assess the potential for such disasters as well as the adequacy of the facility's disaster response plan. Disaster potential may also arise from prison industries. Inmate occupations may also present other physical hazards for individual clients that need to be assessed.

Sociocultural Considerations

A wide variety of sociocultural dimension factors influence the health status of correctional populations. An estimated 80% of law enforcement activity addresses social problems, yet police personnel are often ill-equipped to deal with them because of lack of understanding of the underlying dynamics of social problems. Like health care providers in correctional settings, law enforcement personnel may experience conflict between their law enforcement role and a role in resolving social problems. In addition, social problems that lead to criminal activity are given low priority at the societal level (Patterson, 2002). For example, the estimated cost of adequate treatment for persons with mental illness is one third to one half of the cost of incarceration for mentally ill offenders (Meyer, 2003). Sociocultural factors contribute to incarceration, and correctional systems have sociocultural effects on inmates and on the general society.

Particular elements of the sociocultural dimension that influence health in correctional settings include socioeconomic and cultural factors that lead to incarceration, family relationships, the correctional culture, and the potential for violence in the setting.

Socioeconomic and Cultural Influences

To a large extent, correctional populations tend to be at the low end of economic and educational spectrums. It is estimated that every 10% decrease in income is associated with a 10% to 20% greater likelihood of criminal activity and incarceration (Travis et al., 2001). Women offenders, in particular, often come from poverty-stricken neighborhoods with low levels of social capital (Reisig, Holtfreter, & Morash, 2002). Lower socioeconomic status is also associated with worse health status among inmates. For example, unmarried and homeless inmates and those of lower socioeconomic levels have been found to be at higher risk of TB infection than other inmates (Kim & Crittenden, 2005).

Housing is another socioeconomic issue that may contribute to incarceration. Many activities performed by homeless individuals in ensuring their survival have been criminalized, with the result that they are often arrested for activities that would be tolerated in other members of society. The homeless are overrepresented in correctional populations, and recently released prisoners often become homeless due to poor reentry planning. Incarceration may also lead to homelessness due to the disruption of family and community ties and decreased employment and housing opportunities associated with the stigma of incarceration. In one study, one fourth of homeless individuals had a history of imprisonment, and homeless people who had been incarcerated had higher levels of health risk than other homeless individuals (Kushel, Hahn, Evans, Bangsberg, & Moss, 2005).

As we saw earlier, correctional populations include many minority group members who are frequently culturally and linguistically, as well as economically and educationally, disadvantaged (Paris, 2005). Many more inmates are being incarcerated as a result of immigration offenses than in the past. In fact, from 1995 to 2003 there was a 394% increase in federal incarcerations for immigration offenses, comprising 10% of all federal convictions in 2003 (BJS, 2005f). At midyear 2004, 20% of federal prisoners in the United States were noncitizens (BJS, 2005d).

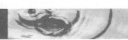

CULTURAL COMPETENCE

You are working in a correctional setting in the southwestern United States. You see a corrections officer grab an inmate by the collar and jerk his head up, saying "Look at me when I talk to you. I want to know when you're lying." You know that in the inmate's culture, it is considered inappropriate to look others in the eye while speaking to them. How would you handle this situation?

BUILDING OUR KNOWLEDGE BASE

Approximately 2% of U.S. children have a parent who has been incarcerated in a state or federal prison, yet there is little knowledge of the effects of parental incarceration on children's health and well-being. How might you go about conducting a study to identify some of the effects of parental incarceration on child health?

Family Relationships

Concerns for children can be a source of stress for many inmates. Approximately 75% of women inmates have children under 18 years of age (Hills et al., 2004), and the percentage of inmates with minor children increased by 55% over an 8-year period (Thigpen, Hunter, & Watson, 2002). As we saw earlier, separation from families was the most difficult aspect of incarceration for women, yet only slightly more than half of correctional systems consider place of residence and distance from families in placement decisions within the system. Approximately one third of institutions provide family visitation assistance, including help with lodging or transportation. Visitation assistance is more apt to be available in facilities that house men than in those that house women, although women's facilities are more likely to provide special family visitation space (Thigpen et al., 2002).

Women's facilities are twice as likely as men's to provide parenting education, but most such programs are provided without children present, prohibiting inmates from modeling learned skills with their own children (Thigpen et al., 2002). In one study, one third of children with mothers in state prison systems lived with their fathers during their mothers' incarceration; the rest lived with other family members or were placed in foster care. To date little research has been done on the effect of parental incarceration on children (Travis et al., 2001).

Problems caused by separation of children from their mothers have led some correctional facilities to allow young children, particularly newborns, to remain with their mothers in custody. According to a Bureau of Justice report (Thigpen et al., 2002), one fifth of state and large metropolitan departments of corrections house infants and small children with their incarcerated mothers, but only 17% are able to provide outside housing for pregnant women. Areas for concern in these types of programs that need to be addressed by correctional nurses and other correctional personnel include the security of children, liability issues, costs and mechanisms for providing health care and other services for children, the effects of incarceration on child development, charges of discrimination if pregnant and recently delivered inmates receive special consideration, and lack of interest in parenting by some incarcerated women (Fulco, 2001).

Family dynamics may also lead to incarceration, either directly or indirectly. For example, 15% of state prison inmates have been convicted of a violent crime against a family member (Durose et al., 2005). Family violence may also contribute to other criminal activity. In one study, for instance, South African men who observed abuse of their mothers during childhood were more likely to be arrested for physical violence against their partners as adults and for illegal firearms possession (Abrahams & Jewkes, 2005).

The Correctional Culture

The primary purpose of correctional institutions is custody and punishment, not health care. This custodial culture may pose considerable challenges to health care providers who must balance their health care and advocacy roles against security concerns and create a therapeutic environment without being perceived as a "soft touch" by either inmates or corrections personnel (Norman & Parrish, 2000).

Security concerns may also hamper provision of health care. In some institutions, nurses do not have immediate access to inmates unless security personnel are present. In other instances, transportation of inmates for outside services may be postponed if there are insufficient security personnel available to accompany them. There is also the potential for violence against health care providers and their use as hostages.

The nurse should be alert to the use of excessive force or punitive conditions to which inmates may be subjected. Correctional nurses will also assess the extent of social support available to inmates. Social support may arise from interactions and programs available within the correctional system or from continued interactions with persons or agencies outside the system (e.g., family). Development of social support systems may be particularly important for clients about to be released from the facility.

Some correctional facilities have assets that promote rehabilitation and permit inmates to earn some money. In some states, there are even provisions for inmates to work to repay the victims of their crimes. Such opportunities are less readily available to women inmates than men and are rarely adequate to meet the rehabilitation needs of all inmates. The presence of occupational opportunities, however, may contribute to a variety of occupational risks to health that should be assessed by nurses in correctional facilities. Occupational hazards for correctional facility staff, as well as those for inmates, should be considered. Corrections personnel, for example, are at higher risk for infectious disease exposure, with an estimated 3,000 bloodborne disease exposures among corrections personnel each year (Gershon, 2002). Physical and psychological safety considerations also present the need for constant vigilance among health care and other personnel in correctional settings (Weiskopf, 2005).

Violence and Abuse

As noted earlier, violence may lead to incarceration. Similarly, exposure to violence and abuse in one's past may increase the risk of incarceration, particularly among women and youth. Violence also occurs within correctional settings. Younger, smaller inmates or those with nonheterosexual orientations may be subjected to abuse by other inmates or by correctional personnel. Rates of sexual abuse of homosexual inmates may be as high as 41%, approximately four times that of the general inmate population (Coolman & Eisenman, 2003). Elderly, mentally ill, and mentally retarded inmates are also vulnerable to abuse within correctional settings. Inmates subjected to violence may need to be segregated from other inmates to ensure their safety, but isolation may result in creation or exacerbation of poor psychological response to incarceration. Community health nurses can be advocates for protection of these inmates in ways that promote rather than impair their mental health.

Inmates may also be abused by correctional staff (Braithwaite et al., 2005), and community health nurses working in correctional settings should be alert to signs of abuse. Women inmates in particular may be coerced to provide sexual favors in return for privileges (Coolman & Eisenman, 2003).

Behavioral Considerations

Behavioral dimension factors that influence the health of inmates and staff in correctional settings include diet, substance abuse, smoking, opportunities for exercise and recreation, and sexual activity. Inmates are more likely than the general public to engage in tobacco use and alcohol and drug use and abuse. With little to occupy their time, inmates may find themselves smoking more after incarceration than before. Smoking coupled with overcrowding, lack of exercise, and inadequate diet may increase inmates' risk of both communicable and chronic diseases. Access to tobacco is also a traditional reward for compliant behavior in correctional settings. Approximately 75% of all inmates smoke, far higher than the 23% of the general population, and only a few correctional facilities have or enforce smoking bans or promote smoke-free environments. Even when such bans do exist, 79% of them involve tobacco use only by inmates and do not include staff. Health care providers tend to see other addictive behaviors as having higher priority than smoking cessation, and 80% of corrections systems surveyed in one study do not provide smoking cessation programs or cessation aids (e.g., nicotine patches) (Porter, 2005). In 2004, California banned smoking, chewing tobacco, and snuff by inmates and staff in all state prisons and youth correctional facilities (NCCHC, 2004b).

Alcohol and other substance abuse is also common among correctional populations. One fourth of state prison inmates have been incarcerated for drug-related offenses (Brunswick, 2005), and 80% of the state correctional population has a history of drug and alcohol use, half of them at the time of commission of the crime for which they were incarcerated (Travis et al., 2001). Similarly, drug offenses accounted for 55% of federal convictions in 2003 (BJS, 2005f). In 2004, in 30% of all victimizations involving violent crimes, the perpetrator was using alcohol, and two thirds of intimate partner violence involves alcohol. In 20% of these crimes other drug use was also implicated (BJS, 2005a). An estimated 12% of all arrestees are alcohol dependent and as many as 4% may be addicted to opiates, yet only 28% of U.S. jail administrators surveyed reported detoxification of arrestees (Fiscella, Pless, Meldrum, & Fiscella, 2004).

The correctional nurse should assess substance use and abuse in individual clients as well as in the inmate population as a whole. The nurse should also assess nutritional status and particular dietary needs for individual inmates (e.g., those with diabetes). Nurses may need to advocate for special diets to accommodate medical or religious needs. Types of diets that may be needed include kosher diets, low-salt diets, diabetic diets, consistency-modified diets, allergy diets, bland diets, and diets to address specific renal problems or gastric reflux. Recently, there has been a trend toward the use of heart-healthy diets for the general inmate population as well (Wakeen & Roper, 2002), and community health nurses can advocate for such general dietary changes in correctional settings.

Sexual behaviors prior to and during incarceration can also influence inmate health status. Early initiation of sexual activity is common among inmate populations (e.g., before age 13) (Head et al., 2000), and 85% of infections such as HIV, HBV, and HCV are associated with preincarceration behaviors including sexual behavior and injection drug use (IDU) (Macalino et al., 2004). Among incarcerated youth, 90% of males in one study were sexually active, and more than 60% reported multiple sexual partners. Boys were more likely than girls to engage in high-risk sexual behaviors, but overall 95% of the study population engaged in three or more high-risk behaviors and 65% engaged in 10 or more such behaviors (Teplin, Mericle, McClelland, & Abram, 2003).

Sexual activity also occurs within the correctional setting. Such behavior may be consensual or nonconsensual, and high-risk behaviors such as anal intercourse are common (Restum, 2005). As many as 33% of inmates may be sexually assaulted while incarcerated (Macalino et al., 2004). Some authors note that "same-sex encounters during incarceration are defined as situational in nature and therefore not an individual or sustained sexual orientation" (Braithwaite & Arriola, 2003), so prevention messages targeted toward the gay and bisexual population may not be perceived as relevant to the general inmate population. Lack of access to condoms and the prevalence of STDs in correctional populations promotes the spread of disease to others in the setting. For example, a 3.6% rate of new cases of HBV in one correctional study provides strong evidence for in-house transmission of disease (Kahn et al., 2005). The nurse should assess the extent of sexual activity among the correctional population and the availability and use of condoms within correctional systems. Nurses may also need to advocate for provision of condoms to sexually active inmates.

Other behavioral dimension factors that should be assessed include opportunities for and participation in exercise and recreational activities. Potential safety hazards posed by exercise and recreation activities should also be assessed.

Health System Considerations

Factors in the health system dimension also influence the health status of correctional populations. Correctional facilities are the only settings in which people have a constitutional right to health care (Treadwell & Ro, 2002). Because many inmates enter the correctional setting with multiple health problems, the adequacy of the correctional health care system has a significant influence on the health status of the population. Depending on several factors, including size and financial capabilities, correctional facilities may take one of two approaches to the provision of health care services for inmates. Services may be provided in-house by staff employed by the facility, or the agency may contract with other provider agencies for needed services. In many institutions, a combination of both approaches is used.

Whatever the approach used, a public health model of correctional health services would address assessment and early detection of health problems, treatment for existing conditions, prevention, health education, and continuity of care (Conklin, Lincoln, Wilson, & Gramarossa, 2003). Table 1◆ presents emphases related to each of these areas.

Specific areas to be addressed in the correctional health care system include health promotion and illness prevention services, medical and dental services, mental health services, and emergency response capabilities. Health promotion services will be discussed in more detail in the section on primary prevention in correctional settings. Minimum medical services should include screening, diagnostic, treatment, and follow-up services. Services begin with an initial health screening on admission to the facility. This initial screening is a brief immediate evaluation of whether it is safe to admit the inmate to the facility given his or her current health status. The initial screening also facilitates correct placement of the inmate within the facility, initiates planning to meet identified health needs, and provides aggregate data for use in overall program planning. Areas to be addressed in this screening include, at a minimum, evidence of infectious disease, existing health problems,

233

TABLE 1 Components and Emphases in the Public Health Model for Correctional Health Care

Component	Emphases	Component	Emphases
Detection and assessment	• Initial booking assessment • Dental health assessment • Mental health assessment • Information on accessing services in correctional system	Prevention (cont.)	• Immunization • Cessation counseling and relapse prevention to prevent long-term consequences of tobacco and other substance use • Dental health education • Prenatal care for pregnant inmates • Occupational health and safety for inmate workers and staff • Facility-wide smoking ban • Suicide prevention training for staff • Exercise and nutrition education for inmates and staff
Treatment	• Individualized treatment plan for identified health needs • Provision of pharmacy medications • Daily "sick call" triage system for new problems • Nursing clinic and treatment teams • Disease-specific education programs (group and individual) • On-site substance abuse and mental health treatment • Emergency services (on-site or contracted with local hospitals) for medical, psychiatric, and dental emergencies • Contracted surgical services at local hospitals	Health education	• Chronic disease management • HIV/AIDS education • Inmate wellness education programs
		Continuity of care	• Discharge planning beginning at admission • Collaboration between case manager and discharge planner • Planning to meet medical and social needs (e.g., housing, job training/placement, family reintegration, financial assistance) • Establishment of "medical home"
Prevention	• Communicable disease prevention education • Chronic disease screening and management to prevent complications		

Data from: Conklin, T., Lincoln, T., Wilson, R., & Gramarossa, G. (2003). Innovative model puts public health services into practice. Correct Care, 17(3), 1, 14–15.

current medications, evidence of disability or activity limitation, suicide risk, and other special needs (e.g., dietary restrictions, pregnancy, need for dialysis).

The correctional health care system should also make adequate provision for diagnostic and treatment services with access to health personnel evaluation in a timely fashion. In some situations, this may mean curtailing the discretion of corrections personnel in determining whether an inmate should be brought to the attention of health care providers. If necessary diagnostic and treatment services are not available within the facility, arrangements should be in place for securing these services elsewhere. The need for diagnostic and treatment services extends to dental health and mental health needs as well as to physical health problems.

Mental health services are also an important component of correctional health. Elements of effective mental health programming include the following:

• A correctional environment that supports program goals and provides a social climate and staff that promote mental health
• A view of mental health programming as congruent with institutional mission and values
• Service providers with appropriate background and training
• Program goals that address attitudes, associations, and behaviors that contribute to criminal activity
• Emphasis on the development of cognitive-behavioral problem-solving skills that relate actions to consequences

• Provision of post-program support within the correctional setting and at release into the community (Fagan, 2003)

Mental health services in correctional settings may occur at three levels: basic mental health services available to all inmates, services targeted to specific groups of inmates with similar problems or mental health treatment needs (e.g., youth, the elderly, inmates with substance abuse), and institutional-level services. Basic mental health services should include an initial intake assessment, crisis intervention, brief counseling, individual therapy, detention or segregation review, and record maintenance (Fagan, 2003). The initial intake assessment should address the risk or presence of mental illness, suicide risk, and potential danger to others. Crisis intervention activities may be required for inmates who are suicidal, the seriously mentally ill, victims of assault, mentally retarded inmates who are having difficulty adjusting to the correctional setting, or inmates experiencing other crisis events (Morgan, 2003).

The primary goal of counseling and therapeutic services in correctional settings is to stabilize the inmate and promote adaptation to the correctional setting, rather than to cure their mental illness. Therapeutic services may be individual or group oriented. Individual therapy tends to be provided for seriously disturbed inmates, whereas group therapies tend to be more problem focused (e.g., anger management, substance abuse) (Morgan, 2003).

Detention and segregation evaluations are part of the administrative support provided by mental health professionals in correctional settings. For example, mental health providers might evaluate an inmate for placement in the general housing population or recommend segregated housing. Another example of care at this level is evaluation of the suitability of parole (Morgan, 2003).

Record maintenance is a critical component of mental (and other) health services in correctional settings for several reasons. First, accurate documentation may help to prevent or at least minimize the consequences of litigation by inmates. Second, effective documentation promotes continuity of care for inmates who may be seen by multiple providers or be transferred among multiple correctional settings. Finally, documentation of treatment effects can help to demonstrate the worth of mental health services to system administrators (Morgan, 2003).

Level-two mental health services include specific treatment programs for particular subsegments of the correctional population. For example, services may be provided to women substance abusers who have a history of physical or sexual abuse. Other examples are treatment programs for inmates convicted of family violence crimes, counseling for "death row" inmates, and integrated treatment programs for inmates with dual diagnoses of mental illness and substance abuse. Mental health services for correctional personnel might also be included in this level of services (Fagan, 2003).

Institutional-level services would include consultations regarding system development or research. For example, mental health providers might assist in the development of initial assessment protocols or suicide prevention plans or the design of conflict management training for personnel.

A 3-year study by the National Commission on Correctional Health Care, entitled *The Health Status of Soon-to-be-released Inmates*, prompted a series of recommendations to the U.S. Congress related to correctional health care systems. These recommendations included the following:

- Surveillance for selected communicable and chronic diseases and mental illnesses in correctional populations
- Use of nationally accepted evidence-based clinical practice guidelines
- Establishment of a national vaccine program for incarcerated inmates
- Development and maintenance of a national literature database on correctional health care
- Initiation of a national ethical advisory panel for correctional health care
- Elimination of barriers to public health practice in correctional settings, including reducing barriers to the implementation of in-house public health programs, maintaining Medicaid enrollment during incarceration, mandating immediate Medicaid eligibility on release, supporting correctional system research, promoting improvement in inmate health care, and encouraging primary and secondary prevention in correctional settings
- Promotion of prerelease planning to address needs for continuing health care services on release from correctional facilities (NCCHC, 2003)

Correctional health services tend to be chronically underfunded, and some authors have suggested Medicaid as a source of payment for services for eligible inmates (Conklin, 2004). At present, federal law prohibits people in correctional and mental institutions from obtaining care under Medicaid or Medicare, and most states terminate Medicaid benefits when someone is incarcerated. In 2004, however, the Center for Medicare and Medicaid Services (CMS) requested states to suspend, rather than terminate, Medicaid enrollment for those in correctional institutions (NCCHC, 2004a). Such a policy would make it easier for newly released inmates to obtain needed health services and maintain continuity of care (Cuellar, Kelleher, Rolls, & Pajer, 2005).

To offset some of the costs of health care, some correctional systems have instituted copayments for medical and dental services provided. The intent of this practice is to decrease service utilization rates and generate funds. The courts have upheld the initiation of small fees for care, ruling that although government has an obligation to provide care to inmates in correctional settings, there is no obligation to provide free care. In 1996, the National Commission for Correctional Health Care drafted a statement on the appropriate use of copayments for correctional health services. Some of the elements of that statement include the following:

- Copayments should be required only for services requested or initiated by the inmate.
- Copayments should not be assessed for screening, follow-up care for problems identified in screening, emergency services, hospitalization, infirmary care, laboratory or diagnostic services, pharmaceuticals, or mental health services.
- Copayments should be assessed only after services have been provided, not as a prerequisite for services.
- Copayments should be small and should not be cumulative in nature.
- Failure to pay a copayment should not be used as a reason to deny subsequent care.
- Inmates should be provided with a minimum balance in personal accounts to permit purchase of necessary hygiene items and over-the-counter medications, and copayments should not be deducted from this minimum.
- There should be a grievance system in place to address copayment grievances.
- Continuation of a copayment system should be contingent on evidence that it does not impede access to needed care (Vogt, 2002).

Copayments may deter inmates from obtaining needed health care and contribute to the spread of communicable diseases as well as increased costs for care of chronic conditions allowed to deteriorate. Correctional nurses may need to be actively involved in evaluating the effect of copayment systems on the health of inmates and the implications for the health of the general public if legitimate needs for services are not being addressed. They may also need to advocate for elimination of copayments if they are found to impede access to care.

The extent of emergency response capabilities (including suicide prevention programs) is another important aspect of the correctional health system. Emergencies may be inmate-specific or general. Examples of inmate-specific emergencies are medical emergencies (e.g., diabetic coma), psychiatric emergencies (e.g., suicide attempt), or traumatic injury. Systemwide emergencies could include inmate-generated emergencies (e.g., riots) or natural or human-caused disasters affecting the correctional setting. Community health nurses should advocate for and be involved in disaster planning for correctional settings. Disaster planning may include plans for evacuation of inmates as well as staff. For example, in 2005, Hurricane Rita forced the evacuation of more than 10,000 inmates from 10 prison facilities. In addition to plans for safe evacuation and provision for the health and survival needs of inmates and staff, correctional disaster plans must address public safety issues and prevent escape during evacuation (Murray, 2006).

The health care system within a correctional setting should also make adequate provision for efforts to control communicable diseases. This means screening programs, isolation of infectious inmates, and follow-up on contacts both within and outside the correctional system.

For health care services to be adequate to meet clients' needs, health care personnel must be available in adequate numbers and with adequate preparation for practice in correctional settings.

Another consideration related to the health system dimension is inmates' use of health care services prior to their incarceration. For example, the nurse might ask the female inmate when she had her last Pap smear or mammogram. The nurse would also want to explore prior interactions with health care providers related to existing health problems. For example, was the client being seen for hypertension or other health problems? Or has the client not been taking antihypertensive medications because he or she did not have the prescription renewed?

COMMUNITY HEALTH NURSING IN CORRECTIONAL SETTINGS

Correctional or "forensic" nursing is a specialized area of community health nursing with a special target population. **Forensic nurses** are "professional nurses who deliver health care to institutionalized populations in prisons, or to forensic patients in psychiatric facilities" (Weiskopf, 2005, p. 336). Work in correctional settings requires nurses to function within specific security parameters (Stanley, 2004a) and to understand both the legal and public health implications of care in this setting. Correctional settings place constraints on how nurses may care for clients, and nurses must often balance custodial and care functions. Studies of correctional nurses indicated that they are actively involved in advocacy and often take professional risks within the setting to meet inmates' needs or initiate changes in the system (Weiskopf, 2005). Nursing in correctional settings also requires superlative interpersonal skills and skills in collaborating with corrections personnel who often have a philosophical perspective far different from that of the nurse (Stanley, 2004b).

Standards for Correctional Health Care

Standards have been established for both correctional health care systems and for nursing practice within those systems. The American Public Health Association (APHA) (2003) has developed a set of principles that serve as a basis for health care services in correctional settings. Criteria for judging compliance with each of the principles have also been developed. Areas of focus and related considerations are presented in Table 2◆. In addition, NCCHC, a group comprised of 22 national service and professional organizations and service agencies related to correctional health, accredits correctional health systems. Accreditation is based on adherence to specific sets of standards for adult or juvenile correctional facilities (Bell, 2004). Some of the areas addressed by the juvenile standards were presented earlier in this chapter. Similar areas are addressed in the standards for adult correctional facilities.

The first standards for nursing practice in correctional settings were promulgated by the ANA in 1985. These standards were revised in 1995 and are currently undergoing subsequent revision. They address the scope of nursing practice in correctional settings as well as standards of care. Nursing standards for correctional settings are summarized on the next page. The standards of care reflect the expected level of care to be provided to individual clients in the correctional setting as well as system-wide program development reflective of the aggregate focus of community health nursing.

Some of the standards differentiate between basic and advanced nursing practice in correctional settings. Basic nursing primarily involves provision of care to individuals and families. The advanced practice nurse, on the other hand, can execute all of the responsibilities of the basic nurse but is also engaged in formulation of policy and in the development, implementation, and evaluation of programs of care for client groups, again incorporating more of the practice of community health nursing. The responsibilities of basic nursing practice include disease prevention and health promotion, recognition

TABLE 2 Focus Areas of the American Public Health Association *Standards for Health Services in Correctional Institutions*

Focus Area	Considerations	Focus Area	Considerations
Organizing principles of care	• Contribution to community health • Access to care • Ethical and legal issues	Specific clinical issues and services (cont.)	• Tobacco cessation • Sexuality • Dental health • Vision services • Pharmacy services • Distance-based medicine • Food services and nutrition • Palliative care • Hospice care • End-of-life decision making
Organizational principles	• Information systems • Quality improvement • Staffing and organization of health services • Reference libraries • Health care facilities • Health records		
Continuum of clinical services	• Initial medical screening and medical examination • Prisoner-initiated care (sick call) • Follow-up care • Specialty consultation • Urgent and emergency treatment • Hospital and infirmary care • Periodic health assessment • Transfer and discharge	Specific populations	• Women • Children and adolescents • Frail-elderly or disabled persons • Segregation • Transgendered persons
		Restraint	• Physical restraint • Medication as behavioral restraints
Chronic care management	• Identification of inmates with chronic disease • Management and follow-up • Continuity of care • Discharge planning	Wellness promotion and health education	• Injury prevention (intentional and unintentional) • Occupational health • Health education and promotion (mental health, substance abuse, tobacco, safety, nutrition, family life, disease prevention and control, prenatal care, personal hygiene, physical fitness, dental health, discharge planning) • Health maintenance and exercise
Mental health services	• Diagnostic and therapeutic services for acute and chronic psychiatric illnesses • Voluntary services • Separation of health care and custodial functions • Confidentiality • Comprehensive range of services • Suicide prevention • Specialized training for health care and corrections personnel • Institutional mental health promotion		
		Environmental health	• Grounds and structures • Services and utilities (e.g., temperature, lighting, laundry, waste disposal, water supply, vermin control, etc.) • Facilities (recreational, hygiene, etc.) • Safety (fire safety, disaster planning, noise, etc.) • Hygiene and personal requirements (bedding, space, toileting facilities) • Inspections, personnel, and supervision
Specific clinical issues and services	• Communicable disease control and treatment • Drug and alcohol detoxification and treatment		

Data from: American Public Health Association. (2003). Standards for health services in correctional institutions. *Washington, DC: Author.*

and treatment of disease and injury, and counseling. Those of the advanced practice nurse involve supervision of the practice of others, advanced clinical practice (e.g., treatment of minor illness by nurse practitioners), management, and evaluation of the effects of correctional health care programs (ANA, 1995).

Ethical Concerns in Correctional Nursing

There are several ethical considerations that are particularly relevant to nursing in a correctional facility. The right to health care is an ethical as well as legal issue that has already been addressed. Other ethical issues include confidentiality and appropriate use of health care personnel, refusal of care, abuse of prisoners, and advocacy. Many of these issues are addressed in the various sets of standards discussed above, and readers should review the APHA (2003) and NCCHC (Bell, 2004) documents for information on the positions of these organizations with respect to these issues. Confidentiality issues may be a source of conflict in correctional settings when health care providers have access to information that may be of use in criminal proceedings against inmates. Health professionals in correctional institutions may be pressured to divulge client information or to assist with procedures designed to provide evidence for criminal proceedings (e.g., body cavity searches, blood alcohol levels). When these procedures

SPECIAL CONSIDERATIONS

CORRECTIONS NURSING: SCOPE AND STANDARDS

Standard 1. Assessment: The corrections nurse collects comprehensive data pertinent to the patient's health and condition or the situation.

Standard 2. Diagnosis: The corrections nurse analyzes the assessment data to determine the diagnoses or issues.

Standard 3. Outcomes Identification: The corrections nurse identifies expected outcomes for a plan individualized to the patient or the situation.

Standard 4. Planning: The corrections nurse develops a plan that prescribes strategies and alternatives to attain expected outcomes.

Standard 5. Implementation: The corrections nurse implements the identified plan.

> *Standard 5a: Coordination of Care:* The corrections nurse coordinates care delivery.
>
> *Standard 5b: Health Teaching and Health Promotion:* The corrections nurse employs strategies to promote health and a safe environment.
>
> *Standard 5c: Consultation:* The advanced practice registered nurse and the nursing role specialist provide consultation to influence the identified plan, enhance the abilities of others and effect change.
>
> *Standard 5d: Prescriptive Authority and Treatment:* The advanced practice registered nurse uses prescriptive authority, procedures, referrals, treatments, and therapies in accordance with state and federal laws and regulations.

Standard 6. Evaluation: The corrections nurse evaluates progress towards attainment of outcomes.

Standard 7. Quality of Practice: The corrections nurse systematically enhances the quality and effectiveness of nursing practice.

Standard 8. Education: The corrections nurse attains knowledge and competency that reflects current nursing practice.

Standard 9. Professional Practice Evaluation: The corrections nurse evaluates one's own nursing practice is relation to professional practice standards and guidelines, relevant statutes, rules, and regulations.

Standard 10. Collegiality: The corrections nurse interacts with and contributes to the professional development of peers and colleagues.

Standard 11. Collaboration: The corrections nurse collaborates with patient, family and others in the conduct of nursing practice.

Standard 12. Ethics: The corrections nurse integrates ethical provisions in all areas of practice.

Standard 13. Research: The corrections nurse integrates research findings into practice.

Standard 14. Resource Utilization: The corrections nurse considers factors related to safety, effectiveness, cost, benefits, and impact on practice in the planning and delivery for nursing services.

Standard 15. Leadership: The corrections nurse provides leadership in the professional practice setting and the profession.

Reprinted with permission from American Nurses Association. (in press). Corrections nursing: Scope and standards of practice. Silver Spring, MD: Nursesbooks.org.

---

need to be performed by trained personnel (e.g., venipuncture), they should be the task of personnel hired specifically for these types of responsibilities to prevent conflict of interest for health care providers and to avoid jeopardizing a relationship of trust between provider and client. Similarly, health care professionals should not be called on to engage in security measures or to participate in disciplinary decisions or in execution by lethal injection (ANA, 1995). Assuring appropriate use of personnel in the correctional setting may also mean making sure that nonprofessionals (including inmates) are not allowed to perform medical tasks or dispense medications.

Confidentiality, particularly with respect to HIV status, may be more difficult to achieve in a correctional environment. The intensive nature of treatment and the need for multiple doses of medication may serve to label inmates as infected, even when official confirmation of disease is not provided. This potential for lack of confidentiality may act as a deterrent to HIV testing and noncompliance with treatment in infected individuals. Another potential conflict related to confidentiality is the question of whether security personnel should be alerted to inmates' HIV-infection status to ensure their use of universal precautions.

In addition to maintaining confidentiality, nurses may be called on to support an inmate's refusal of care, including forcible administration of psychotherapeutic medications. Inmates have the right to refuse care unless they are determined to be legally incompetent to make that decision. Inmates' right to refuse care, however, must be balanced against state interests in four areas: preserving and protecting life, preventing suicide, protecting the interests of third parties, and maintaining security. Decisions regarding abrogation of the right to refuse treatment should be based on facts in the individual situation, including the inmate's medical condition, prognosis, benefits and burdens of treatment, and the impact of refusal on other inmates. Refusal of care should be carefully documented, including the nature of the care refused, the inmate's stated reason for refusal, the date and time of refusal, provision of education on the possible consequences of refusal, and the inmate's signature or initials (Vogt, 2005).

Aggressive or potentially suicidal inmates may be subjected to physical restraint if they are deemed a danger to themselves or to others. This includes the use of medical isolation when clients suspected of infectious diseases refuse screening procedures or treatment. Medical isolation may also be legitimately employed to protect inmates with symptomatic AIDS from opportunistic

GLOBAL PERSPECTIVES

*I*n 1992, a survey was conducted to determine how health was addressed in European prisons (Gatherer, Moller, & Hayton, 2005). The results of that survey were published in *Prison Health: International Standards and National Practices in Europe*. This and other international corrections efforts led to the development of the World Health Organization's (WHO) Health in Prisons Project (HIPP) to improve health care delivery in prisons through policy change and the development of consensus recommendations on best practices. The underlying principles of HIPP include (a) the right of prisoners to health care at a level commensurate with what is available in the community, (b) the importance of the health of prisoners to society at large, (c) the recognition of the particular vulnerability of prisoners, and (d) the violation of prisoners' human rights with policies for mandatory HIV testing and lack of confidentiality.

HIPP has resulted in several consensus statements that have been accepted by a growing group of European nations. The first HIPP consensus statement focused on communicable disease control, particularly HIV, in prison settings (WHO/UNAIDS, 2001), and subsequent statements addressed mental health (WHO Health in Prisons Project, 2001) and substance abuse issues, including the issue of harm reduction in correctional settings (e.g., providing clean syringes for intravenous drug users) (WHO Regional Office for Europe, 2002). Additional consensus statements have dealt with the needs of minority prisoners, incarcerated youth, and prison health as an aspect of public health practice (Gatherer et al., 2005). Do you think such consensus on best practices in correctional health care could be achieved among correctional systems in the United States? Why or why not?

infection. Although the U.S. Supreme Court has upheld segregation of HIV-infected inmates, many health care professionals suggest that segregation actually increases the potential for the spread of communicable diseases such as tuberculosis (National Center for HIV, STD, and TB Prevention, 2000). For example, segregation may foster the belief that all others in the institution are uninfected and may lead to high-risk activities. Segregation also breaches confidentiality and denies segregated inmates access to programs, such as work release and other programs, available to other inmates. In addition, segregation may contribute to exacerbation of psychoses or depression (Hills et al., 2004).

Because of the imbalance of power inherent in a correctional setting, there is always the potential for abuse of inmates in the name of punishment. For example, pepper spray is occasionally used as a means of forcing compliance among inmates. Punitive use of such chemicals over and above necessary use for subduing violence has been described as constituting torture and falls within the Eighth Amendment proscription of cruel and unusual punishment (Cohen, 1997). Findings also suggest that juvenile inmates may be punished for exhibiting symptoms of mental illness (Coalition for Juvenile Justice, 2000). Preventing this and other forms of abuse of inmates (e.g., denial of health care services) is another ethical aspect of nursing in correctional settings.

Finally, nurse advocacy may be needed in the correctional setting. Advocacy may be required at the level

FOCUSED ASSESSMENT

Assessing Health and Illness in Correctional Settings

Biophysical Considerations

- What is the age, gender, and ethnic composition of the correctional population (inmates and staff)?
- What communicable and chronic health problems are prevalent among inmates? Among staff?
- What is the prevalence of pregnancy among inmates?
- What are the immunization levels in the population?

Psychological Considerations

- What procedures are in place for dealing with suicidal ideation or attempts? Are these procedures followed?
- What is the psychological effect of incarceration? Does the individual inmate exhibit signs of depression? Does the inmate express thoughts of suicide?
- What is the extent of sexual assault among inmates? What are the psychological effects of assault?
- Are there inmates in the setting under sentence of death? If so, what psychological effects does this have? Are there terminally ill inmates in the population?
- What is the prevalence of mental illness among inmates?

Physical Environmental Considerations

- Are there health or safety hazards present in the correctional facility?
- Is there potential for disaster in the area? Is there a disaster plan?

Sociocultural Considerations

- What are the attitudes of health and correctional personnel toward inmates?
- What is the attitude of the surrounding community to the correctional facility and to the inmates?
- What family concerns influence the health of inmates?
- Are there intergroup conflicts within the population? Do these conflicts result in violence?
- What is the extent of mobility in the population?
- Are inmates employed in the correctional setting? Are they employed outside? What health hazards, if any, are posed by the type of work done?
- How do security concerns affect the ability of health care personnel to provide services?

Behavioral Considerations

- Are there inmates with special nutritional needs? How well are they being met? What is the nutritional quality of food served in the correctional setting?

Continued on next page

FOCUSED ASSESSMENT (*continued*)

- What are the health-related behaviors of the correctional population? How do they affect health?
- How are medications dispensed in the correctional setting? Are there procedures in place to prevent inmates from selling medications or accumulating them for use in a suicide attempt?
- What is the extent of sexual activity in the correctional setting? To what extent do inmates engage in unsafe sexual practices? What is the availability of condoms?

Health System Considerations

- What health services are offered in the correctional setting? Are they adequate to meet needs?

- Are there isolation procedures in place for inmates with communicable diseases? Are these procedures followed?
- How are health care services funded? Is funding adequate to meet health needs? Are inmates charged a fee for health care services?
- What is the quality of interaction between internal and external health care services?
- What is the extent of emergency response capability of the correctional facility (e.g., to myocardial infarction, stab wound)?
- What provisions are made for continuity of care after release from the correctional facility?

---

of the individual client to ensure that rights are upheld and that appropriate health care services are received or at the aggregate level to assure adequate health care delivery systems in correctional institutions.

Assessing Health and Illness in Correctional Settings

Features of the correctional setting that influence health are assessed by the community health nurse and used to derive nursing diagnoses. The community assessment guide included in Appendix G on the Companion Website can be used to assess correctional populations. In addition, a comprehensive tool for assessing the health status of correctional populations is provided in the *Community Assessment Reference Guide* designed to accompany this book. Assessment tips for use with correctional populations are provided on the previous page.

The age, gender, and ethnic composition of the correctional population can be derived from system records. Information on existing health conditions, on the other hand, is best derived from a combination of intake assessment data and sick call trends, as well as agency records on the types of treatment provided and the kinds of referrals made for outside care. Incidence and prevalence trends in specific conditions, including pregnancy, should also be noted. Information regarding immunizations can be obtained in intake interviews or early health status assessments. However, in many instances, it may be appropriate to assume that vaccination levels are low in the general population and offer immunization to all inmates. Screening data for specific conditions (e.g., TB and HIV infection) can also provide information on the incidence and prevalence of these diseases in the population.

Assessment of considerations in the psychological dimension should include the prevalence of mental illness determined in intake interviews as well as requests for psychotropic medications during sick call. Triage personnel should also be alert to evidence of mental health problems including mental retardation and psychiatric illness during sick call. Institutional records can

provide information about the incidence of sexual assault and completed or attempted suicides in the population, as well as identifying inmates who are under sentence of death. Assessment in this area should also consider the adequacy of protocols for suicide prevention and for addressing psychiatric emergencies.

Physical environmental conditions in the correctional setting are probably best assessed by observation. Information on accidental injuries brought forward in sick call or treated as emergencies may also highlight environmental safety hazards. The potential for disaster and the extent of institutional disaster preparation should also be assessed by identifying disaster risks in the larger community and discussing them with institutional administration.

Information about many sociocultural factors influencing inmate and staff health can be gleaned from observation or knowledge about the surrounding community, particularly in local correctional settings. For example, if the economic level of the surrounding community is low, the same is probably true of the majority of inmates housed in a local jail. Educational levels are likely to be low in the population overall, but community health nurses working in correctional settings should not assume that all inmates have low levels of education. Intake assessments may or may not address educational and other socioeconomic factors, but health care assessment should include these factors and aggregate data can be derived from such individual assessments. Intragroup conflicts may surface in observations of inmates or of interaction between inmates and correctional personnel. Assessment of sociocultural factors should also consider the extent to which inmates are transferred within settings or among correctional settings and the possible health consequences of these transfers. Information about family issues will probably need to be derived directly from inmates themselves. Experience in the setting will give nurses some idea of how security concerns and procedures promote or interfere with effective health care delivery.

Information about special dietary needs and substance use and abuse should be obtained in intake or health care assessments and aggregate data developed on the incidence and prevalence of such behaviors as smoking and drug use and the need for special diets. Corrections nurses should also assess how medications are dispensed and managed in the correctional setting, particularly for inmate subgroups who require multiple medications. Provisions for directly observed therapy for HIV infection and TB should also be identified. Information related to sexual activity can be interpolated from data on sexually transmitted diseases, but can also be derived from interviews with inmates.

Assessment considerations related to the health system dimension include the adequacy of internal and external systems to meet health care needs identified in the population. Nurses should determine what priority is given to health promotion and illness prevention initiatives and to providing treatment for long-term conditions such as chronic diseases and substance abuse. The extent of funding for correctional health services can be obtained from administrative personnel, and both inmates and health care personnel can provide information on the quality of interaction between internal and external health care services. For example, local health department staff may have insights into the effectiveness of discharge planning for inmates with HIV infection or TB. Morbidity and mortality rates are one indication of the effectiveness of emergency response capabilities. Finally, the nurse should assess the policies and procedures to promote continuity of care on release from the correctional setting, as well as the effectiveness of those processes.

Diagnostic Reasoning and Care of Clients in Correctional Settings

Based on information obtained in assessing the dimensions of health, the nurse in the correctional setting formulates nursing diagnoses. Diagnoses should be validated with the client, significant others, or other health care providers when possible. Community health nurses working in correctional settings determine nursing diagnoses for individual clients as well as diagnoses related to the health needs of the total population of inmates and staff. For example, an individual diagnosis might be "uncontrolled diabetes mellitus due to substance abuse." A diagnosis related to the population group might be "increased potential for violence due to racial tensions and unrest." This second diagnosis would affect facility personnel as well as inmates since all might be involved in any violence that occurs.

Planning and Implementing Health Care in Correctional Settings

Planning to meet identified health problems in correctional settings may be accomplished by the nurse him- or herself or in conjunction with other personnel within and outside the institution. Interventions may take place at the primary, secondary, or tertiary level of prevention.

Primary Prevention

Primary prevention in correctional settings involves both health promotion and illness prevention. Health promotion emphases include adequate nutrition, rest and exercise, health education, prenatal care, and contraceptive services. Preventive efforts center on prevention of communicable diseases, suicide prevention, and violence prevention.

HEALTH PROMOTION Health promotion in correctional settings differs from that in other settings in a number of ways. First, the general purpose of health promotion in correctional settings is to protect the health of others rather than to enhance the health of the particular inmate. Second, group health promotion efforts may be hampered by the compulsory nature of inmates' presence in the institution. For example, inmates may be resistant to health education because they perceive themselves as a "captive audience" with little option regarding participation. Third, the great majority of offenders are men who tend not to be as highly motivated with respect to health promotion as women. Health promotion in correctional settings often needs to focus less on information transmission than on attitude development or change, and behavioral change may not be as easy within the constraints of the correctional setting as in the outside world. In addition, the correctional emphasis on punishment for crimes may result in political interference with health promotion efforts. Finally, given the extensive health problems encountered in this population, there may be little time or few resources available for health promotion efforts, which may receive lower priority than curative activities.

Nutritional intake in correctional settings may be far from adequate. NCCHC recommendations include the initiation of heart-healthy diets as a routine aspect of correctional settings (NCCHC, 2003). The nurse in this setting may need to monitor the diet of inmates and may need to influence administrative decisions regarding the nutritive value of meals served. There may also be a need to suggest changes in food served to facility personnel if meals are provided for them as well. In addition, the nurse may need to make arrangements to meet the special dietary needs of specific inmates based on their health status. Examples include a diabetic diet or a liquid diet for an inmate recuperating from a broken jaw.

Attention should also be given to provisions for adequate rest and exercise by inmates. Nurses may need to advocate for adequate space and facilities for sleeping in inmate housing units. In addition, the nurse should work to assure that time and facilities are provided for inmates to obtain exercise. In some instances, this may mean curtailing certain activities that place inmates at risk because of existing health problems. Nurses can also educate both inmates and staff on the benefits of exercise and suggest forms of exercise congruent with health status and available opportunities.

241

Both inmates and facility staff may be in need of a variety of health education efforts. Areas of importance include the elimination of risk factors for disease. Education programs that may be planned and implemented by nurses may include smoking cessation campaigns or stress management classes. Nurses can also advocate for access to smoking cessation assistance and aids such as nicotine patches. Education regarding problem solving and positive coping strategies may also benefit both staff and inmates.

Prenatal care is a significant health promotion activity for pregnant female inmates. The NCCHC (2003) recommendations include provision of pregnancy screening to all women inmates and further screening of pregnant women for HIV and other STDs. Areas to be addressed in prenatal care include adequate nutrition, the effects of smoking and other substances on the fetus, parenting skills, discomforts of pregnancy, and planning for childcare if the child is delivered while the client is still in custody. HIV prevention education is another area of importance among incarcerated women (and men) who are often at high risk for infection (McClelland, Teplin, Abram, & Jacobs, 2002). Contraceptive education may benefit both pregnant and nonpregnant inmates. There may also be a need for treatment for HIV- or HBV-infected women or those with other STDs. The NCCHC (2003) recommendations also include collaboration between correctional facilities and community health agencies to provide HBV immunization for infants born to mothers with evidence of HBV infection. Similar collaborative efforts should be undertaken to treat the infants of HIV-infected women.

ILLNESS AND INJURY PREVENTION Preventing the spread of communicable diseases in correctional settings is an important primary prevention activity. The concern for public health issues arising in correctional populations has led to the development of a series of "pocket guidelines" for prevention and control of specific diseases in correctional settings. These guidelines are intended to "introduce sheriffs, correctional administrators, correctional health care practitioners, public health leaders, and those who make critical public policy and funding decisions to specific guidelines and recommendations arising out of the interface of public health and corrections" (American Correctional Health Services Association [ACHSA], n.d., p. 1). Guidelines developed as of mid-2006 included TB prevention and control, prevention and control of disease outbreaks, STD prevention, HIV prevention, control of methicillin-resistant *Staphylococcus aureus*, and prevention and control of viral hepatitis. The guidelines are available from the ACHSA Web site at http://www.achsa.org/displaycommon.cfm?an=1&subarticleebbr=23. These guidelines are congruent with the NCCHC (2003) recommendation to the U.S. Congress that correctional health care services make use of nationally accepted evidence-based clinical guidelines.

Possible approaches to illness prevention include the use of universal precautions in the handling of blood and body fluids, isolation of infected persons when appropriate, immunization, and education on condom use during sexual encounters (Bauserman et al., 2003). Isolation is appropriate for diseases spread by airborne transmission such as measles and influenza. Isolation of HIV-infected individuals is not generally recommended. Immunization is particularly recommended for HBV (Division of Viral Hepatitis, 2004a), but other immunizing agents may be needed as well, depending on the incidence of specific diseases in the general community. For example, measles immunizations may be warranted for all inmates and staff during a measles outbreak in the community, and hepatitis A vaccine is recommended for inmates at risk for hepatitis A (e.g., inmates who engage in oral-anal intercourse). Corrections staff, particularly health care personnel, should also receive HBV immunization. Condom use and substance abuse education on harm reduction strategies can also help to prevent the spread of hepatitis B and C in correctional populations (Weinbaum, Lyerla, & Margolis, 2003). Because correctional settings house a large proportion of inmates who are infected with or at risk for hepatitis, provision of HBV vaccine is a good way to minimize disease prevalence within correctional settings and in the larger community (Division of Viral Hepatitis, 2004b). Community health nurses in correctional settings may be actively involved in providing immunizations and advocating their availability to inmates.

Recommended tuberculosis control measures in correctional settings include screening of all inmates for infection, isolation of suspected and confirmed cases, and treatment of persons with active or latent TB infection. Preventing the spread of tuberculosis may also employ engineering controls related to adequate ventilation systems, air filtration, and irradiation of areas where infected persons are housed (Centers for Disease Control and Prevention [CDC], 2004). **TB prophylaxis** is the treatment of persons with reactive tuberculin skin tests but without evidence of active tuberculosis (in other words, those with latent infection), to prevent their development of disease. Prophylactic treatment is also recommended for persons with HIV infection even in the absence of

Think Advocacy

In October 2004, the *San Diego Union Tribune*, the major newspaper in the San Diego area, published an Associated Press story on citizens who were irate that prisoners were being given influenza immunizations when vaccine shortages prevented community members from obtaining protective immunization (Flu shots for inmates, 2004). Who do you think should receive priority access to a limited supply of vaccine? Why? What actions might you take to advocate for access to vaccines for the group you think should receive priority?

evidence of tuberculosis. Corrections personnel with positive skin tests should also receive prophylaxis. In addition, all inmates and personnel should be educated on infection control procedures and universal precautions. Community health nurses are often responsible for providing directly observed TB therapy and in monitoring its effectiveness. They also monitor clients receiving therapy for potential adverse reactions to medication.

Other more mundane avenues for preventing communicable diseases include routine skin screening for infectious lesions and effective wound infection control procedures. Promotion of inmate hygiene, use of alcohol-based hand rubs for handwashing, and effective laundry procedures can also prevent the spread of MRSA infections (Tobin-D'Angelo et al., 2003).

Other avenues for illness and injury prevention include suicide prevention and prevention of violence. The primary mode of suicide prevention is identification of inmates at risk for suicide. Those at risk for suicide should be closely monitored and receive timely referrals for psychiatric services. Suicide assessment involves obtaining information regarding past personal or family history of suicide attempts, the extent of life stress and social support, presence of suicidal ideation, and presence of mental illness (White, 2001). According to the NCCHC, components of an effective suicide prevention plan include identification of inmates at risk, staff training, inmate assessment by qualified mental health professionals, appropriate housing, and referral to needed mental health services. Other elements of effective plans include adequate communication between corrections and health care staff, immediate intervention for a suicide attempt or suicide in progress, and notification and documentation protocols and processes. Finally, an effective plan includes administrative data review and identification of plan weaknesses and improvement processes (Hills et al., 2004).

Suicide prevention may include four levels of monitoring for inmates at risk for suicide. The first level involves continuous observation of an inmate who has made a recent suicide attempt. Level-two observation is for those at high risk and involves placement in a safe room with active observation by staff every 5 to 15 minutes. Level-three observation is used with inmates who are judged to have a moderate risk of suicide or are moving away from level one or two and involves observation every 10 minutes while awake and every 30 minutes while asleep. At level four, inmates have a significant risk history (e.g., history of recent loss) but are not actively suicidal. Inmates at level four are observed every 30 minutes awake or asleep (Hills et al., 2004).

Violence prevention activities may need to be directed to both inmates and corrections staff. The purpose of such activities is to teach alternative behavioral responses to violence. Recommended components of violence prevention programs in correctional settings include incorporation of violence assessment (including prior exposure to violence) in intake screening, referral of inmates with a history of personal violence or violence exposure for counseling, education on alternative responses to potentially violent situations for both inmates and corrections staff, and referral of inmates for continued counseling on release. Primary prevention emphases in correctional health care are summarized in Table 3◆.

Secondary Prevention

Secondary prevention activities in correctional health settings focus on screening and diagnostic and treatment activities.

SCREENING Standards related to screening have been described as some of the more important standards for correctional health care. Screening has a threefold purpose: identifying and addressing the health needs of inmates, promoting early identification of key problems prior to more comprehensive assessments, and identifying and isolating potentially communicable inmates (Stanley, 2004b).

Screening activities in correctional settings typically center on communicable diseases (e.g., hepatitis, HIV infection, other STDs, and TB) and suicide risk. NCCHC (2003), however, also recommends screening of all inmates for hypertension, asthma, obesity, and seizure disorder. Women inmates should also be screened for pregnancy, as noted earlier. Other recommended screening procedures include Papanicolaou smears, mammography, and colorectal cancer screening (Binswanger, White, Perez-Stable, Goldenson, & Tulsky, 2005). However, some authors note that it may be difficult for inmates from minority groups to request such screening procedures that are not conducted routinely

TABLE 3	Primary Prevention Foci and Related Activities in Correctional Settings
Focus	**Related Activities**
Health promotion	• Provision of adequate nutrition • Provision of opportunities for adequate rest and exercise • Health education for self-care, risk factor elimination, stress reduction, etc. • Prenatal care for pregnant inmates • Contraceptive education • Advocacy for available health promotion services in correctional settings
Illness and injury prevention	• Control of communicable diseases • Immunization • Isolation of persons with infectious diseases • Use of universal precautions for blood and body fluids • TB prophylaxis • Education for safe sex • Suicide prevention • Violence prevention • Advocacy for illness and injury prevention service availability

due to the need to make written requests for services in English. Similarly, emergency care needs may receive higher priority than such screening procedures, making them hard to access (Magee, Hult, Turalba, & McMillan, 2005). Community health nurses can be particularly helpful in advocating for routine health screening activities for inmates in keeping with the recommendations of the U.S. Preventive Services Task Force (2005).

As we saw earlier, assessment for suicide risk should be an integral part of every intake interview. Screening for certain communicable diseases may also be warranted based on client health status and the incidence and prevalence of specific conditions in the surrounding community. Screening for tuberculosis has been identified as a need for all employees and new inmates. Inmates who will be in custody long enough for the test to be read (48 to 72 hours) should be given a Mantoux skin test, whereas a chest x-ray is recommended for those in short-stay units. Because of the tendency for HIV-infected individuals to have negative TB skin tests even with active disease, it has been suggested that chest x-ray, anergy testing, and sputum collections may be more appropriate for persons known to be HIV-positive and for those whose HIV status is unknown in areas with high prevalence rates of multi-drug-resistant tuberculosis infection (National Center for HIV, STD, and TB Prevention, 2000).

Screening for HIV infection is also recommended. Voluntary screening programs have not been very effective due to the multiple barriers to screening encountered in correctional settings. These include fear of disclosure and discrimination if HIV status becomes known, isolation, inability to access programs and services available to noninfected inmates, prohibition of conjugal visits, and so on (Braithwaite & Arriola, 2003). For these reasons, routine screening for all inmates on admission to state and federal prison has been recommended. Use of oral screening measures for HIV infection have been found to increase screening acceptability among inmates, particularly those in high-risk groups (Bauserman et al., 2001).

There is also some debate about the advisability of targeted or routine screening for other diseases. For example, one study indicated that targeting HCV screening to inmates with risk factors such as IDU missed 65.5% of infected male inmates and 44.2% of infected women (Macalino, Dhawan, & Rich, 2005), suggesting that routine screening of all inmates might be more appropriate. Nurses in correctional settings are often responsible for conducting routine screenings and interpreting their results for inmates.

Specific screening approaches have also been recommended for juvenile offenders. For example, the Office of Juvenile Justice and Delinquency Prevention (OJJDP) has suggested screening of all incarcerated youth for substance abuse and mental disorders and further assessment of youth with identified problems

(NCCHC, 2005c). The OJJDP has also published a document entitled *Screening and Assessing Mental Health and Substance Abuse Disorders among Youth in the Juvenile Justice System: A Resource Guide for Practitioners*, which includes 42 assessment and screening tools for use with youth. These tools encompass screening for substance abuse; specific psychiatric disorders; psychosocial problems, strengths, and needs; and cognitive ability (OJJDP, 2004). This document is available on the OJJDP Web site at http://www.ncjrs.gov/pdffiles1/ojjdp/204956.pdf.

Screening for mental health problems is another important element of secondary prevention in correctional settings. Mental health screening is needed to identify inmates at risk for harm to themselves or others, determine inmates' functional capabilities, identify the need to transfer inmates to a specific mental health unit, and determine the inmate's potential to benefit from treatment (Hills et al., 2004).

Suggested elements of mental health assessment in correctional settings include an inmate's psychiatric history, current use of psychotropic medications, presence of suicidal ideation, and a history of suicide attempt. Other relevant screening information includes drug and alcohol use, history of violence or victimization, history of special education placement, and history of traumatic brain injury. Assessment also includes evaluation of the inmate's response to incarceration and evidence of developmental disability (Hills et al., 2004).

Data sources for identifying juveniles with mental health problems include self-report, family history, screening measures, observation, collateral information sources (e.g., prior treatment records), and behavior symptom checklists (Boesky, 2003). Similar sources of information may serve to identify mental health problems in adult inmates. Community health nurses working in correctional settings will employ these data sources to identify inmates with mental health problems. They may also assess inmates' readiness and motivation for treatment. Motivational assessment would consider the inmate's perceptions regarding the seriousness of mental health problems (including substance abuse problems), perceived importance of treatment, desire to change alcohol and drug use behaviors, if any, and past attempts to address mental health problems or substance abuse (Hills et al., 2004).

DIAGNOSIS AND TREATMENT Diagnosis and treatment may be required for medical conditions, mental illness, or substance abuse. Correctional nurses may be actively involved in the diagnosis and treatment of existing medical conditions. Many minor illnesses are handled exclusively by nurses working under medical protocols. In other instances, nurses are responsible for implementing medical treatment plans initiated by physicians or nurse practitioners. This may involve giving medications or carrying out treatment procedures. Treatment procedures would be handled in much the same way as in any health care facility. Dispensing medications in a correctional setting, however, requires that the nurse directly observe the client taking the medication, and often only a single dose is dispensed at a time rather than giving the client several doses of medication to be taken at prescribed times. This precaution is necessary because of the potential for inmates to sell medications to other inmates or to stockpile certain medications for use in a suicide attempt. The U.S. courts have upheld the practice of corrections personnel dispensing medications, but significant safeguards must be in place to ensure that corrections personnel dispense medications correctly and accurately document dispensing (NCCHC, 2001a). In some instances (e.g., syphilis outbreaks and epidemics of other communicable diseases) mass treatment of the entire correctional population or subpopulation in a given setting may be warranted (Chen, Callahan, & Kerndt, 2002).

Treatment for tuberculosis and HIV infection in correctional settings is complicated by the long-term nature of the therapies. Inmates with tuberculosis (except those also infected with HIV) should be placed in respiratory isolation in negative-pressure rooms until they are no longer communicable. If negative-pressure rooms are not available in the correctional facility, arrangements should be made to transport the inmate to a local hospital with such facilities. Respiratory isolation should also be instituted for all inmates with respiratory symptoms suspicious of TB. Tuberculosis treatment should involve a multi-drug regimen, particularly when exposure to multi-drug-resistant infection is suspected. Drug susceptibility testing should be carried out on all inmates with active TB, and treatment should rely on directly observed therapy (DOT).

HIV/AIDS therapy is also difficult in correctional settings because of the number of factors that promote noncompliance. As noted earlier, having to receive multiple doses of medication each day may "tag" inmates as infected and leave them open to discrimination and assault. Security practices such as lockdowns and search and seizure may interfere with dispensing of medications or attendance at support group or education programs. A **lockdown** occurs when inmates are locked in their cells at times when they would ordinarily have greater freedom to come and go throughout the facility, usually in response to a security incident or to permit a search for contraband items (drugs, alcohol, weapons) or a **search and seizure** procedure. During search and seizure, all medications are taken away, so clients in some facilities where self-medication is permitted may have their medications removed and be unable to take doses as directed.

Strategies that can increase compliance with HIV/AIDS treatment regimens include simplifying the regimen to include fewer doses or combining medications into a single pill, protecting confidentiality, using medications with fewer side effects, and dealing with those side effects that occur. DOT has also been found to be effective in promoting compliance with highly active antiretroviral therapy (HAART) for inmates with HIV/AIDS (NCCHC, 2005b). Treatment is also more effective if provided by health care professionals who have expertise with HIV/AIDS. In larger systems, inmates with HIV infection may be moved to facilities with this expertise or where this expertise is available in the community.

Treatment may also be needed for a variety of chronic health problems experienced by correctional populations. Again, community health nurses working in correctional settings may provide treatment and monitor treatment effectiveness under approved protocols. They may also be responsible for making referrals for specialty services to outside health care agencies. This may require particular advocacy on the part of community health nurses to assure that outside appointments are kept when they are jeopardized by security concerns or lack of security personnel to escort inmates to community facilities.

Treatment should also be available for substance abuse and mental health problems. There are a number of sound reasons for mental health care in correctional settings. Among these are the need to reduce the disabling effects of mental illness and to maximize the ability of inmates to participate in rehabilitation programs. A second reason is to minimize the suffering of the inmates themselves. Finally, treatment of inmates with mental illness and substance abuse problems promotes the safety of all, both within the correctional setting and in the community when the inmate is released (Hills et al., 2004).

The American Psychiatric Association recommends several aspects of treatment for mental illness and substance abuse in correctional settings. These aspects include:

- Crisis intervention programs with residential beds for stays of 10 days or less
- Acute inpatient care programs for inmates able to care for themselves

EVIDENCE-BASED PRACTICE

*H*ills, Siegfried, and Ickowitz (2004) noted that there is significant research to demonstrate that substance abuse services decrease repeated incarceration. For example, one Federal Bureau of Prisons study indicated that only 3% of prisoners who received treatment were rearrested within 6 months of release, compared to 12% of untreated prisoners. Research also indicates that programs that begin in prison but also include aftercare components are more effective than those that include only in-house treatment. For example, a program in Texas state correctional facilities includes a 9- to 12-month therapeutic community program in prison, followed by 3 months in a residential facility after release and another 9 to 12 months of outpatient therapy. Unfortunately, few correctional systems provide such comprehensive programs for substance abuse. What evidence can you find that supports the effectiveness of such programs? How would you use this evidence to promote such a program in your own state?

- Chronic care programs in housing units for the chronically mentally ill who cannot function in the general population
- Outpatient care programs
- Consultation with other correctional personnel
- Discharge and transfer planning (Hills et al., 2004)

Additional mental health services that should be present in correctional settings, based on the NCCHC standards for correctional health programs, include screening by qualified personnel within 24 hours of admission; information regarding available services; a complete health appraisal, including mental health assessment, within 7 days of admission; and mental health evaluation within 14 days of admission for inmates exhibiting signs of mental disorders. Care should also include development of appropriate treatment plans for inmates with serious mental illness and provision of care by qualified mental health professionals within 48 hours of a request for non-emergent services. Correctional health care systems should also include provisions for dealing with psychiatric emergencies and suicide attempts (Hills et al., 2004).

Treatment modalities can include a broad variety of approaches, including the use of psychotropic medications, individual and group psychotherapy, and family interventions. Another possible approach is therapeutic communities, which are a comprehensive set of interventions in a residential setting separated from the general inmate population, intended to engender lifestyle changes that foster mental health in inmates (Peters & Matthews, 2003). Relapse prevention skills and self-help groups such as Alcoholics Anonymous may also be helpful for inmates with substance abuse problems. It is recommended that substance abuse treatment also include frequent random urine screening for drugs. Mental health care for women inmates should provide an integrated approach to dealing with problems of mental illness, substance abuse, and the frequent history of psychological and physical trauma (Hills et al., 2004).

Methadone maintenance is a special area of consideration in treatment for substance abuse. For many opiate abusers, methadone may be an important step in treatment for addiction. Approximately 10% of persons enrolled in methadone treatment programs will be arrested during their enrollment, yet few correctional settings make provision for continuing methadone treatment except for pregnant inmates. Involuntary cessation of methadone leads to painful withdrawal symptoms and risk of death, as well as relapse to opiate use and subsequent rearrest. Studies have indicated that only 56% of correctional systems ask about opiate addiction during intake. As much as 85% of systems do not continue methadone treatment, and 77% do not use appropriate protocols for methadone detoxification. Further, only 27% of systems routinely contact community methadone programs regarding care of inmates enrolled in those programs. Study recommendations included development of a uniform national policy regarding methadone use with inmates, better coordination between community methadone treatment programs and correctional systems, better education of corrections personnel regarding methadone, and less restrictive regulation of methadone use in correctional settings (Fiscella, 2005).

The Mentally Ill Offender Treatment and Crime Reduction Act of 2004, also known as the Second Chance Act, authorized $50 million per year for mental health programming and services in U.S. correctional facilities and community settings (Bell, 2005). Unfortunately, in spite of the availability of this funding, provision of mental health services in correctional settings is often hampered by variables related to correctional systems, personnel, and inmates (Holton, 2003). System-level variables include limited fiscal allocations for services, privatization of correctional facilities, the institutional climate, and limitations in access to care posed by inmate classification systems. Hopefully, the Second Chance Act will address fiscal barriers to care. Privatization of correctional settings (government contracting with private corporations for operation of correctional facilities) often leads to cost cutting to remain competitive, and cost cutting may eliminate services, such as mental health services, that are considered "nonessential." In addition to entire correctional systems run by private for-profit companies under contract to government agencies, health care services in correctional settings may also be privatized. For example, a county sheriff's department may contract with a private firm for health care personnel and services within the correctional setting rather than hiring health care personnel as county employees. Government service contracts are usually given to the lowest bidder, providing an incentive to decrease the quality or frequency of services in the interests of cost containment. In addition, privatization may lead to less official oversight of correctional facilities and the quality of care provided. On the other hand, privatization has the advantage of services provided by people who have a health care perspective rather than a custodial focus.

The institutional climate is frequently one of punishment rather than treatment, so inmates may not receive needed mental health services. Finally, classification of inmates as security risks may put them at risk for isolation, exacerbation of mental health problems, and lack of access to many services available to other inmates.

Personnel variables that affect mental health treatment services in correctional settings include staff attitudes to mentally ill inmates and training of correctional and health care personnel relative to mental health needs. Cultural diversity and differences between correctional personnel and inmates may make identification of mental health problems more difficult (Holton, 2003).

Inmate-related variables include mental health treatment history, a slower response to medication among inmates than in the general population due to the prevalence of substance abuse, and peer pressure within the setting not to appear weak or vulnerable. In addition, the nuisance side effects associated with psychotropic medications may lead many inmates to be noncompliant with treatment plans (Holton, 2003).

One approach to treatment of mentally ill inmates and those with substance abuse diagnoses is diversion. **Diversion** is the practice of moving mentally ill or substance-abusing offenders from the criminal justice system and placing them in treatment facilities. Diversion may occur prior to booking (before arrest or before criminal charges have been filed) or post-booking (after arrest or conviction). Diversion relies on intersectoral collaboration between legal and mental health care systems to address factors that contribute to **recidivism** (rearrest, reincarceration, or frequent rehospitalization) among mentally ill and substance-abusing inmates. Issues that need to be addressed, in addition to mental health or substance abuse treatment needs, include continuity of public assistance, housing support, and the need for social service referrals and treatment of other medical conditions. In one study of correctional systems, 34% of local jails had some kind of diversion program, but only 18% of them met criteria for true diversion to address recidivism (Broner et al., 2002).

Research has indicated that treatment of substance abuse while an inmate is in prison reduces the likelihood of rearrest and reduces the return to previous drug use patterns. For example, evaluation of one 28-day detention and treatment program in a local jurisdiction demonstrated fewer arrests within 5 years in the treatment group than in a control group (77% versus 60%) (Kunitz et al., 2002). Similarly, youth who receive structured, meaningful, and sensitive treatment for mental illness exhibit 24% less recidivism than those who are not treated (Coalition for Juvenile Justice, 2000), and in-house residential programs of 6 to 12 months have demonstrated a 9% to 18% reduction in criminal recidivism and a 15% to 35% reduction in drug relapse. Unfortunately, only about 60% of mentally ill inmates receive adequate treatment while incarcerated, half receive psychotropic medications, and 44% receive some counseling. Similarly, only a fourth of parole systems include mental health programs (Travis et al., 2001). Community health nurses working in correctional systems can advocate for the availability of adequate mental health and substance abuse programs as well as provide care in such programs.

When physical or mental health services needed by inmates are not available within the correctional health care setting, community health nurses are often responsible for arranging appointments with outside consultants or providers. In addition to arranging for appointments, correctional nurses usually have to arrange transportation and security supervision. This often means that scheduling of appointments can be extremely complicated. Once inmates have been seen by outside providers, correctional nurses also need to follow through on

recommendations for treatment. Because many outside providers do not understand the constraints of correctional systems, nurses may need to be creative in promoting treatment compliance. For example, in some small rural jails, there are no facilities for warm soaks to injuries, and special diets may also be difficult to arrange. Other recommendations that pose security hazards may not be able to be fulfilled (e.g., metal braces that can be converted to weapons) (Johnson, 2006). Community health nurses may need to advocate for treatments that are not typically used in the setting, or may need to explain to outside providers why a particular treatment option is not feasible in a correctional setting.

Nurses will also be involved in emergency response to life-threatening situations. Emergency situations likely to be encountered include seizures, cardiac arrest, diabetic coma or insulin reaction, attempted suicide, and traumatic injury due to inmate violence. The nurse would respond to these situations with actions designed to relieve the threat to life and stabilize the client's condition prior to transportation to a hospital facility either within or outside the correctional system. Correctional nurses may also find themselves involved in emergency care of large numbers of persons injured in human-caused or natural disasters involving the correctional facility. Major foci in secondary prevention in correctional settings are summarized in Table 4◆.

TABLE 4	Secondary Prevention Foci and Related Activities in Correctional Settings
Focus	**Related Activities**
Screening	• Screening for communicable diseases • Tuberculosis • HIV infection • Hepatitis B • Sexually transmitted diseases • Routine screening for chronic conditions • Asthma, hypertension, obesity, seizure disorder • Mammography • Papanicolaou smear • Colorectal cancer • Provision of specialized screening services for inmates at risk (e.g., diabetes) • Screening for suicide risk • Screening for pregnancy • Screening for mental illness and substance abuse • Screening for treatment motivation • Advocacy for availability of routine and specialized screening services
Diagnosis and treatment	• Provision of diagnostic services relevant to inmate needs • Treatment of existing acute and chronic conditions • Treatment of mental illness and substance abuse • Methadone maintenance for opiate users • Emergency care for accidental and intentional injuries • Care for psychiatric emergencies • Emergency care in the event of a disaster • Advocacy for effective and available diagnostic and treatment services in correctional settings

Tertiary Prevention

Tertiary prevention in correctional settings focuses on areas similar to that in any setting, preventing or dealing with complications of disease and preventing problem recurrence when possible. Tertiary prevention directed toward preventing complications of existing health problems depends on the conditions experienced by inmates. For example, tertiary prevention for the inmate with diabetes will be directed toward preventing circulatory changes, diabetic ketoacidosis, and hypoglycemia. For the client with arthritis, tertiary prevention will focus on pain management and prevention of mobility limitations. Community health nurses may also help inmates deal with the long-term consequences of chronic conditions. An example might be providing a walker to an inmate with mobility limitations. Tertiary preventive activities may also be directed toward preventing the recurrence of problems once they have been resolved. For example, the nurse may educate an inmate who has been treated for gonorrhea on the use of condoms to prevent reinfection.

In addition, there are three special considerations in tertiary prevention in correctional settings: long-term care planning, reentry planning, and end-of-life care. Each of these major foci will be addressed briefly.

LONG-TERM CARE PLANNING With the aging of the correctional population throughout the world, there is a need to engage in long-term care planning for elderly inmates and those with chronic conditions. Correctional systems have taken a variety of approaches to long-term care planning for these subpopulations. Older inmates or those with disabilities related to chronic illness may be transferred to appropriate facilities or housing conditions separate from the general inmate population. Usually such facilities have an infirmary where exacerbations of chronic conditions requiring hospitalization can be addressed in-house. In other instances, inmates may be transferred to assisted living facilities that provide assistance with the activities of daily living.

ETHICAL AWARENESS

*F*azal (2005) reported that many states and the federal government have regulations that permit seriously ill or disabled inmates to obtain "medical release" or "medical parole." Many of these regulations exclude those with life sentences or execution orders, sex offenders, or those under 70 years of age. Regulations may also require inmates to have served a certain portion of their sentences and may revoke parole if the inmate's condition improves. Health care coverage for many inmates who receive medical parole is provided under Medicare or Medicaid. Unfortunately, Fazal noted that few jurisdictions employ these laws, even where they exist, to assist seriously ill inmates. Who do you think should be eligible for medical parole? What criteria do you think should be used to determine eligibility? How might you go about advocating for medical parole for an inmate with a serious health condition?

Terminally ill inmates may be transferred to specialized hospice units or to community hospices. Alternatively, hospice services can be provided to inmates housed in the general population, at least until inmates become severely debilitated. Finally, some correctional systems provide continuing care retirement communities for older and disabled inmates similar to comparable institutions in the community, but incorporating the custodial functions of correctional facilities (NCCHC, 2002).

When inmates with chronic illnesses or disability are housed in the general population, correctional systems may provide "home care" services and case management to address their long-term care needs. In such systems, nurses might go to inmate housing units to provide care in the same way that they would provide home care in community settings. Another alternative is to have other inmates function as "personal care attendants" for disabled inmates, assisting them with certain activities of daily living (e.g., bathing). Other systems may create adult day care programs in which inmates with long-term care needs are housed in the general population, but spend a portion of each day in an area of the facility, frequently an infirmary, where these needs can be addressed (NCCHC, 2002).

Other tertiary prevention activities related to long-term care include providing assistive devices, monitoring the status of chronic conditions and treatment compliance, monitoring for adverse effects of treatment, and providing support in dealing with the emotional and physical consequences of long-term physical or mental illness. Community health nurses may be involved in providing these interventions or in advocating their availability in the correctional setting. They may also need to advocate for access to these kinds of services for specific inmates.

REENTRY PLANNING Approximately 98% of the 8 million people admitted annually to correctional settings will ultimately be released back into the community (Conklin, 2004). Annual turnover rates are as high as 800% in jails and 50% in federal and state prisons (Discharge Planning, 2002). In a large metropolitan correctional system like that of Los Angeles County, the inmate population changes completely every 44 days (Inmate Infections Spread, 2005). Many of these inmates reenter the larger society as probationers or parolees. A **probationer** is an adult offender who has been remanded to community-based supervision, often as an alternative to incarceration. Probationers usually are held in correctional facilities for only a short time until their case has been tried in court. A **parolee** is an adult released from a correctional system to community supervision after serving all or part of his or her sentence. Both probationers and parolees are subject to reincarceration if they violate the terms of probation or parole. At the end of 2004, there were 4.9 million U.S. men and women under federal, state, or local probation and 765,400 on parole. Approximately 75% of these former inmates are under active supervision by correctional systems (BJS, 2005g).

The dual process of incarceration and reentry, labeled by some authors as "coercive mobility" (Golembeski & Fullilove, 2005), has been cited as a public health opportunity. In the words of two authors, "Given the inevitability of reentry, every prisoner should be viewed as a future member of free society. Accordingly, the period of time in prison should be viewed as an opportunity to provide health interventions that will yield better health outcomes not only in prison but, equally importantly, after the prisoner's release" (Travis & Sommers, 2004, p. 19). Unfortunately, little planning may be initiated toward meeting inmates' reentry needs. One of the purposes of the federal Second Chance Act is to strengthen community reentry services for released inmates (Pogorzelski, Wolff, Pan, & Blitz, 2005). However, reentry planning should begin, ideally, at admission to a correctional facility, not at the time of or after release (Hills et al., 2004).

Reentry, in the correctional context, is defined as "the process of leaving prison and returning to society" (Travis et al., 2001, p. 1). Two challenges inherent in reentry are protecting the public and promoting effective reintegration into the community. Reentry also poses risks for the spread of communicable diseases within the general population if inmates have not been effectively treated.

Released inmates often have limited job skills and social support networks, so many of them have difficulty reintegrating into the larger community. They may have difficulty finding employment and housing due to the stigma attached to incarceration (Cooke, 2004). At the same time, the social capital or infrastructure of communities that reabsorb large numbers of released inmates are often stretched beyond their capacity. Studies indicate that a small number of communities, and an even smaller number of neighborhoods within those communities, receive the bulk of released inmates. Given the lack of support services, resources, and opportunities for legitimate employment, many released inmates are reintroduced to criminal activities (Golembeski & Fullilove, 2005). An estimated two thirds of inmates released in any given year will be rearrested for a felony or serious misdemeanor within three years of release (Travis & Sommers, 2004). Research, however, indicates that inmates, particularly those with substance abuse problems, who receive health insurance and employment assistance are less likely to return to drug use and be rearrested (Freudenberg, Daniels, Crum, Perkins, & Richie, 2005).

Reentry planning begins with the development of systematic discharge protocols to be used with all inmates to be released from a correctional setting. Such protocols are most effective when they are developed with input from the communities to which inmates will be released (Golembeski & Fullilove, 2005). Community health nurses can be active advocates for reentry planning for all inmates. They can also advocate community involvement in the development of reentry planning protocols and in designing community infrastructures to support reentry.

Planning considerations related to individual inmates are based on an individualized needs assessment and include issues related to health care and social and financial needs. The American Public Health Association (2003) noted a need to provide inmates with a complete copy of their health records, a sufficient supply of medications, referrals (and possibly actual appointments) for physical and mental health services in the community, and assistance with health insurance coverage. This may mean advocacy on the part of community health nurses to get Medicaid, Medicare, or Veteran's Administration benefits reinstated, or assisting inmates to find low-cost health care services. Advocacy may also be required to ensure that inmates have a sufficient supply of necessary medications until they can find employment and purchase medications on their own. This is particularly important for inmates who are receiving long-term therapy for HIV/AIDS or TB. Community health nurses may also need to advocate for continuing therapy for mental illness or substance abuse. There is a particular need for effective communication between the correctional system and community health agencies. Too often, inmates are discharged with ongoing health needs (e.g., HIV/AIDS or TB treatment) without local health authorities being notified. In addition to making referrals and links to community services, community health nurses in correctional settings should also develop systems for monitoring service continuation and its effects on inmate health status.

Reentry planning should also address a variety of social and financial needs of released inmates. For example, many inmates have alienated family members and may not be able to find shelter with their families. In this case, community health nurses may need to assist in arranging housing for former inmates. Referrals may also be needed for employment assistance or job training. Unfortunately, federal spending on employment training in correctional settings was cut by 50% in the 1990s and has never been reinstated (while overall corrections costs escalated by 521%) (Golembeski & Fullilove, 2005). Community health nurses may need to advocate at the societal level for job training programs for inmates and others with low levels of employability. They may also need to advocate for relaxation of restrictions on financial and other assistance benefits for people who have been incarcerated.

For some inmates, reentry planning may entail assistance with family reintegration. Community health nurses may assist families to deal with concerns about bringing a released inmate back into the family constellation, particularly if the inmate was incarcerated for a crime involving family violence. There are also some instances in which inmates should not return to families if their presence may put family members at risk of harm.

END-OF-LIFE CARE End-of-life care for inmates with terminal illnesses may be similar to that on the outside. For example, community health nurses may need to discuss advance directives with inmates and help those who wish to execute advance directives. Community health nurses may also need to advocate adherence to advance directives when they have been executed by an inmate. According to the NCCHC (2005a) data, discussions of advance directives have been undertaken with less than 1% of inmates. In some cases, seriously ill inmates have chosen not to execute advance directives, possibly out of a fear of being abandoned as they are dying. In addition to discussing advance directives with inmates, correctional health care personnel need to develop policies regarding the timing of advance directives, communicating information about advance directives when inmates are transferred to outside hospitals or hospice settings, and addressing effective pain control for seriously ill inmates (NCCHC, 2005a). Correctional health systems also need to develop policies for notifying family members and significant others of imminent death (APHA, 2003).

Just as in the general population, referral for hospice care may be appropriate for terminally ill inmates. Some correctional facilities have in-house hospice units, and others may transfer inmates to community hospices when there is no security risk to the public (NCCHC, 2002). Whether in a hospice setting, in an infirmary, or in the general correctional population, terminally ill inmates are likely to need assistance in setting their affairs in order. For some inmates, there may also be a need to reconcile with family members. Community health nurses can be instrumental in facilitating these end-of-life activities. For example, they may advocate with family members for reconciliation or assist inmates to obtain legal assistance in settling any assets they may have on their heirs. Symptom control and palliative care are also important aspects of end-of-life care in correctional settings.

There are also two unique aspects to end-of-life care that need to be addressed in correctional settings. The first is the concept of "compassionate release" or "medical parole." **Medical parole** is the release of a seriously ill or disabled inmate back into the community (Fazal, 2005) to receive needed health care services from community agencies and, often, to permit time with family members. Medical parole is most often used for terminally ill inmates. As noted in Table 5◆, community health nursing advocacy may be required to initiate or support a medical parole decision. In addition to advocating for medical parole when appropriate, community

health nurses will assist with arranging for follow-up care after release.

The second unique aspect of end-of-life care in correctional settings relates to inmates who have been sentenced to death. In 2002, more than 3,500 inmates were facing the death penalty (U.S. Census Bureau, 2005). These inmates have the same needs for psychological end-of-life care as those with terminal illnesses, but their care is often complicated by feelings of hopelessness and attendant security measures (e.g., the use of handcuffs and shackles and constant supervision) (Boisaubin, Duarte, Blair, & Stone, 2004). Aspects of tertiary prevention in correctional settings are summarized in Table 5◆.

TABLE 5	Tertiary Prevention Foci and Related Activities in Correctional Settings
Focus	**Related Activities**
Long-term care planning	• Transfer to appropriate facility as needed • Provision of "home care" in general population • Assistance by a personal care attendant • Use of assistive devices as needed • Adult day care services • Continued monitoring of the status of chronic conditions • Monitoring treatment compliance • Monitoring for adverse effects of treatment • Provision of support in dealing with long-term consequences of chronic illness • Advocacy for effective long-term care service availability
Reentry	• Development of systematic discharge protocols • Development of individual discharge plan • Provision for continuity of health care • Arrangement for a supply of necessary medications on discharge • Arrangement for health insurance coverage • Provision for housing and financial assistance needs • Assistance with job training and employment as needed • Assistance with family reintegration as needed • Coordination of community health care and correctional activities • Advocacy for effective prerelease planning for all inmates • Advocacy for development of community infrastructure to support reentry • Advocacy for civil rights of released inmates
End-of-life care	• Development of advance directives as desired by inmates • Symptom control and palliative care • Advocacy for medical parole and arrangement for follow-up care • Advocacy for use of advance directives by personnel • Provision of emotional and spiritual support to inmates and significant others • Referral to hospice care • Assistance with setting life in order • Assistance with family reconciliation as needed

Evaluating Health Care in Correctional Settings

The principles that guide the evaluation of health care in correctional settings are the same as those applied in other settings. The nurse evaluates the outcomes of care for individual clients in light of identified goals. Correctional nurses may also be involved in evaluating health outcomes for groups of inmates or for the entire facility population, including staff. In addition, the nurse examines processes of care and makes recommendations for improvements in terms of quality, efficiency, and cost-effectiveness.

Correctional facilities present a useful setting in which community health nurses can engage in health-promotive and illness-preventive activities with clients who may have little knowledge of these activities. Clients in correctional settings may be less motivated than those in other settings, but can realize substantial health benefits through the efforts of community health nurses during incarceration and in promoting follow-up on release. Community health nursing efforts in correctional settings also help to prevent the flow of health problems back into the larger population, thereby benefiting society as a whole.

Case Study

Nursing in the Correctional Setting

You are the only nurse on the night shift in a county jail housing 150 male inmates. A new inmate is admitted to the jail for driving under the influence of alcohol. During your initial history and physical, the inmate tells you that he is on kidney dialysis and missed his last dialysis appointment, which was yesterday. It is Sunday night and your facility does not have dialysis capabilities. The dialysis unit at the local hospital does not function on Sundays except in the case of emergencies. The inmate appears to be in no immediate distress and has normal vital signs and no evidence of edema. He is appropriately alert and oriented despite the odor of obvious alcohol consumption. The watch commander tells you he has no one to spare to transport the inmate to the hospital, and if he goes it will have to be by private ambulance. Your back-up physician is out of town for the weekend and the on-call physician is tied up with an emergency.

1. What are the biophysical, psychological, physical environmental, sociocultural, behavioral, and health system factors operating in this situation?
2. What are your nursing diagnoses? How would you prioritize those diagnoses?
3. What action would you take in this situation? Why?

Test Your Understanding

1. What are the implications, for inmates and for the general public, of providing health care in correctional settings?

2. Describe some of the ethical considerations facing nurses in correctional settings. What values are in conflict in each of these areas?

3. How do basic and advanced nursing practice in correctional settings differ?

4. What are some of the biophysical, psychological, physical environmental, sociocultural, behavioral, and health system factors that influence health in correctional settings? How might these factors differ for inmates and correctional staff?

5. What are the major aspects of primary prevention in correctional settings? What activities might nurses perform in relation to each?

6. What are the main aspects of secondary prevention in correctional settings? How might community health nurses be involved in each?

7. Discuss considerations and community health nursing involvement in tertiary prevention in correctional settings.

EXPLORE MediaLink

http://www.prehall.com/clark
Resources for this chapter can be found on the Companion Website.

Audio Glossary
Appendix G: Community Health Assessment and Intervention Guide
Exam Review Questions
Case Study: Penitentiary Nursing

MediaLink Application: Puppetry in Prison (video)
MediaLink Application: Interview with Author of *Acres of Skin* (video)
Media Links

Challenge Your Knowledge
Update *Healthy People 2010*
Advocacy Interviews

References

Abrahams, N., & Jewkes, R. (2005). Effects of South African men's having witnessed abuse of their mothers during childhood on their levels of violence in adulthood. *American Journal of Public Health, 95*, 1811–1816.

American Academy of Pediatrics. (2001). Health care for children and adolescents in the juvenile correctional care system. *Pediatrics, 107*, 799–803.

American Correctional Health Services Association. (n.d.). *Pocket guide series*. Retrieved March 30, 2006, from http://www.achsa.org/displaycommon.cfm?an=1&subarticlenbr=23

American Nurses Association. (1985). *Standards of nursing practice in correctional facilities*. Kansas City, MO: Author.

American Nurses Association. (1995). *Scope and standards of nursing practice in correctional settings*. Washington, DC: Author.

American Public Health Association. (2003). *Standards for health services in correctional institutions*. Washington, DC: Author.

Bauserman, R. L., Richardson, D., Ward, M., Shea, M., Bowlin, C., Tomoyasu, N., et al. (2003). HIV prevention with jail and prison inmates: Maryland's prevention case management program. *AIDS Education and Prevention, 15*, 465–480.

Bauserman, R. L., Ward, M. A., Eldred, L., & Swetz, A. (2001). Increased voluntary HIV testing by offering oral tests in incarcerated populations. *American Journal of Public Health, 91*, 1226–1229.

Bell, C. C. (2004). *The sanity of survival: Reflections on community mental health and wellness*. Chicago: Third World Press.

Bell, C. C. (2005). Mentally ill offender law brings help . . . and hope. *Correct Care, 19*(1), 3.

Binswanger, I. A., White, M. C., Perez-Stable, E. J., Goldenson, J., & Tulsky, J. P. (2005). Cancer screening among jail inmates: Frequency, knowledge, and willingness. *American Journal of Public Health, 95*, 1781–1787.

Boesky, L. M. (2003). Identifying juvenile offenders with mental health disorders. In T. J. Fagan & R. K. Ax (Eds.), *Correctional mental health handbook* (pp. 167–198). Thousand Oaks, CA: Sage.

Boisaubin, E. V., Duarte, A. G., Blair, P., & Stone, T. H. (2004). "Well enough to execute": The health professional's responsibility to the death row inmate. *Correct Care, 18*(4), 8.

Braithwaite, R. L., & Arriola, K. R. J. (2003). Male prisoners and HIV prevention: A call for action ignored. *American Journal of Public Health, 93*, 759–763.

Braithwaite, R. L., Treadwell, H. M., & Arriola, K. R. J. (2005). Health disparities and incarcerated women: A population ignored. *American Journal of Public Health, 95*, 1679–1681.

Brodie, J. (2000). Caring—The essence of correctional nursing. *Correct Care, 14*(4), 1, 15, 18.

Broner, N., Borum, R., & Gawley, K. (2002). Criminal justice diversion of individuals with co-occurring mental illness and substance use disorders: An overview. In G. Landsberg, M. Rock, L. K. W. Berg, & A. Smiley (Eds.), *Serving mentally ill offenders: Challenges and opportunities for mental health professionals* (pp. 83–106). New York: Springer.

Brunswick, M. (2005). "Meth mouth" plagues many state prisoners. Reprinted from *Star Tribune*, Minneapolis-St. Paul in *Correct Care, 19*(1), 7.

Bureau of Justice Statistics. (2003a). *Prevalence of imprisonment in the U.S. population, 1974–2001*. Retrieved March 30, 2006, from http://www.ojp.usdoj.gov/bjs/abstract/piusp01.htm

Bureau of Justice Statistics. (2003b). *Reentry trends in the United States*. Retrieved March 30, 2006, from http://www.ojp.usdoj.gov/bjs/reentry/reentry.htm

Bureau of Justice Statistics. (2005a). *Crime characteristics*. Retrieved March 30, 2006, from http://www.ojp.usdoj.gov/bjs/cvict_c.htm

Bureau of Justice Statistics. (2005b). *Criminal victimization*. Retrieved March 30, 2006, from http://www.ojp.usdoj.gov/bjs/cvictgen.htm

Bureau of Justice Statistics. (2005c). *Jail statistics*. Retrieved March 30, 2006, from http://www.ojp.usdoj.gov/bjs/jails.htm

Bureau of Justice Statistics. (2005d). *Prison and jail inmates at midyear 2004*. Retrieved March 30, 2006, from http://www.ojp.usdoj.gov/bjs/pub/pdf/pjim04.pdf

Bureau of Justice Statistics. (2005e). *Prison statistics*. Retrieved March 30, 2006, from http://www.ojp.usdoj.gov/bjs/prisons.htm

Bureau of Justice Statistics. (2005f). *Prisoners in 2004*. Retrieved March 30, 2006, from http://www.ojp.usdoj.gov/bjs/pub/pdf/p04.pdf

Bureau of Justice Statistics. (2005g). *Probation and parole statistics*. Retrieved March 30, 2006, from http://www.ojp.usdoj.gov/bjs/pandp.htm

Centers for Disease Control and Prevention. (2004). Tuberculosis transmission in multiple correctional facilities—Kansas, 2002–2003. *Morbidity and Mortality Weekly Report, 53*, 734–738.

Chen, J. L., Callahan, D. B., & Kerndt, P. R. (2002). Syphilis control among incarcerated men who have sex with men: Public health response to an outbreak. *American Journal of Public Health, 92*, 1473–1475.

Coalition for Juvenile Justice. (2000). *Handle with care: Serving the mental health needs of young offenders*. Retrieved June 2, 2001, from http://www.juvjustice.org

Cohen, M. D. (1997). The human health effects of pepperspray—A review of the literature and commentary. *Journal of Correctional Health Care, 4*, 73–88.

Conklin, T. (2004). Medicaid a must for new releasees. *Correct Care, 18*(3), 3.

Conklin, T., Lincoln, T., Wilson, R., & Gramarossa, G. (2003). Innovative model puts public health services into practice. *Correct Care, 17*(3), 1, 14–15.

Cooke, C. L. (2004). Joblessness and homelessness as precursors of health problems in formerly incarcerated African American men. *Journal of Nursing Scholarship, 36*, 155–160.

Coolman, A., & Eisenman, D. (2003). Sexual assault: A critical health care issue. *Correct Care, 17*(4), 3.

Cuellar, A. E., Kelleher, K. J., Rolls, J. A., & Pajer, K. (2005). Medicaid insurance policy for youths involved in the criminal justice system. *American Journal of Public Health, 95*, 1707–1711.

Cutler, D. L., Bigelow, D., Collins, V., Jackson, C., & Field, G. (2002). Why are severely mentally ill persons in jail and prison? In P. Backlar & D. L. Cutler (Eds.), *Ethics in community mental health care: Commonplace concerns* (pp. 136–154). New York: Kluwer Academic/Plenum.

Discharge planning: Reintegrating inmates living with HIV/AIDS into the community. (2002). *HIV Inside, 4*(1), 1–11.

Division of Viral Hepatitis. (2004a). Hepatitis B vaccination of inmates in correctional facilities—Texas, 2000–2002. *Morbidity and Mortality Weekly Report, 53*, 681–683.

Division of Viral Hepatitis, National Center for Infectious Diseases. (2004b). Incidence of acute hepatitis B—United States, 1990–2002. *Morbidity and Mortality Weekly Report, 53*, 1252–1254.

Division of Viral Hepatitis. (2004c). Transmission of hepatitis B virus in correctional facilities—Georgia, January 1999–June 2002. *Morbidity and Mortality Weekly Report, 53*, 678–681.

Durose, M. R., Harlow, C. W., Langan, P. A., Motivans, M., Rantala, R. R., & Smith, R. L. (2005). *Family violence statistics: Including statistics on strangers and acquaintances*. Washington, DC: Bureau of Justice Statistics.

Fagan, T. J. (2003). Mental health in corrections: A model for service delivery. In T. J. Fagan & R. K. Ax (Eds.), *Correctional mental health handbook* (pp. 1–19). Thousand Oaks, CA: Sage.

Fazal, S. (2005). Medical parole: With safeguards, a practical solution. *Correct Care, 19*(3), 19.

Fiscella, K. (2005). Methadone treatment absent in many jails. *Correct Care, 19*(1), 1, 14.

Fiscella, K., Pless, N., Meldrum, S., & Fiscella, P. (2004). Alcohol and opiate withdrawal in US jails. *American Journal of Public Health, 94*, 1522–1524.

Flu shots for inmates upset people seeking vaccine. (2004, October 20). *San Diego Union Tribune*, A9.

Francis J. Curry National Tuberculosis Center and National Commission on Correctional Health Care. (2003). *Corrections tuberculosis training and education resource guide, 2004–2005*. Chicago: Authors.

Freudenberg, N., Daniels, J., Crum, M., Perkins, T., & Richie, B. E. (2005). Coming home from jail: The social and health consequences of community reentry for women, male adolescents, and their families and communities. *American Journal of Public Health, 95*, 1725–1736.

Fry, R. L. (2003). Transsexualism: A correctional, medical or behavioral health issue? *Correct Care, 17*(1), 1, 20.

Fulco, S. D. (2001). Babies behind bars: The rights and liabilities of babies and mothers. *Correct Care, 15*(1), 6.

Gatherer, A., Moller, L., & Hayton, P. (2005). The World Health Organization European Health in Prisons Project after 10 years: Persistent barriers and achievements. *American Journal of Public Health, 95*, 1696–1700.

Gershon, R. R. M., (2002). Infectious disease risk in correctional health care workers. *Correct Care, 16*(3), 3.

Golembeski, C., & Fullilove, R. (2005). Criminal (in)justice in the city and its associated health consequences. *American Journal of Public Health, 95*, 1701–1706.

Hammett, T. M., Harmon, M. P., & Rhodes, W. (2002). The burden of infectious diseases among inmates of and releasees from US correctional facilities, 1997. *American Journal of Public Health, 92*, 1789–1794.

Hayes, L. M. (2004). Juvenile suicide study finds gaps in prevention. *Correct Care, 18*(4), 13.

Head, G., Kelly, P. J., Bair, R. M., Baillargeon, J., & German, G. (2000). Risk behaviors and the prevalence of chlamydia in a juvenile detention facility. *Clinical Pediatrics, 9*, 521–527.

Heines, V. (2005). Speaking out to improve the health of inmates. *American Journal of Public Health, 95*, 1685–1688.

Hills, H., Siegfried, C., & Ickowitz, A. (2004). *Effective prison mental health services: Guidelines to expand and improve treatment.* Retrieved March 30, 2006, from http://www.nicic.org/misc/URLshell.aspx?SRC=Catalogue&REFF=http://nicic.org/library/018604&ID=018604&Type=PDF&URL=http://nicic.org/pubs/2004/018604.pdf

Holton, S. M. B. (2003). Managing and treating mentally disordered offenders in jails and prisons. In T. J. Fagan & R. K. Ax (Eds.), *Correctional mental health handbook* (pp. 101–122). Thousand Oaks, CA: Sage.

Inmate infections spread. (2005). *NurseWeek, 18*(1), 7.

Johnson, D. (2006). Don't let outside consultations be a liability minefield. *Correct Care, 20*(1), 9.

Kahn, A. J., Simard, E. P., Bower, W. A., Wurtzel, H. L., Kristova, M., Wagner, K. D., et al. (2005). Ongoing transmission of hepatitis B virus infection among inmates at a state correctional facility. *American Journal of Public Health, 95*, 1793–1799.

Kim, S., & Crittenden, K. S. (2005). Risk factors for tuberculosis among inmates: A retrospective analysis. *Public Health Nursing, 22*, 108–118.

Kunitz, S. J., Woodall, G., Zhao, H., Wheeler, D. R., Lillis, R., & Rogers, E. (2002). Rearrest rates after incarceration for DWI: A comparative study in a southwestern US county. *American Journal of Public Health, 92*, 1826–1831.

Kushel, M. B., Hahn, J. A., Evans, J. L., Bangsberg, D. R., & Moss, A. R. (2005). Revolving doors: Imprisonment among the homeless and marginally housed population. *American Journal of Public Health, 95*, 1747–1752.

Macalino, G. E., Dhawan, D., & Rich, J. D. (2005). A missed opportunity: Hepatitis C screening of prisoners. *American Journal of Public Health, 95*, 1739–1740.

Macalino, G. E., Vlahov, D., Sanford-Colby, S. Patel, S., Sabin, K., Salas, C., et al. (2004). Prevalence and incidence of HIV, hepatitis B virus, and hepatitis C virus infections among males in Rhode Island prisons. *American Journal of Public Health, 94*, 1218–1223.

MacNeil, J. R., Lobato, M. N., & Moore, M. (2005). An unanswered health disparity: Tuberculosis among correctional inmates, 1993 through 2003. *American Journal of Public Health, 95*, 1800–1805.

Magee, C. G., Hult, J. R., Turalba, R., & McMillan, S. (2005). Preventive care for women in prison: A qualitative community health assessment of the Papanicolau test and follow-up treatment at a California state women's prison. *American Journal of Public Health, 95*, 1712–1717.

Maruschak, L. M., & Beck, A. J. (2001). *Medical problems of inmates.* Retrieved June 2, 2001, from http://www.ojp.usdoj.gov/bjs

McClelland, G. M., Teplin, L., Abram, K. M., & Jacobs, N. (2002). HIV and AIDS risk behaviors among female jail detainees: Implications for public health policy. *American Journal of Public Health, 92*, 818–825.

Mertens, D. J. (2001). Pregnancy outcomes of inmates in a large county jail setting. *Public Health Nursing, 18*, 45–53.

Meyer, J. A. (2003). Improving men's health: Developing a long-term strategy. *American Journal of Public Health, 93*, 709–711.

Morgan, R. (2003). Basic mental health services: Services and issues. In T. J. Fagan & R. K. Ax (Eds.), *Correctional mental health handbook* (pp. 59–71). Thousand Oaks, CA: Sage.

Murray, O. (2006). Hurricane Rita leaves lessons in its wake. *Correct Care, 20*(1), 3.

National Center for HIV, STD, and TB Prevention. (2000). Drug-susceptible tuberculosis outbreak in a state correctional facility—South Carolina, 1999–2000. *Morbidity and Mortality Weekly Report, 49*, 1041–1044.

National Center for HIV, STD, and TB Prevention. (2005). *What is the difference between jail and prison?* Retrieved March 30, 2006, from http://www.cdc.gov/nchstp/od/cccwg/difference.htm

National Commission on Correctional Health Care. (1999). A summary guide to revisions in the 1999 Standards for Health Services in Juvenile Detention and Confinement Facilities. *Correct Care, 13*(2), 18–19.

National Commission on Correctional Health Care. (2001a). COs passing meds passes court—but wise wardens will mandate controls. *Correct Care, 15*(2), 6.

National Commission on Correctional Health Care. (2001b). Study released on health needs of detained youth. *Correct Care, 15*(1), 19.

National Commission on Correctional Health Care. (2002). Long-term care planning needed, say PA researchers. *Correct Care, 16*(2), 15.

National Commission on Correctional Health Care. (2003). Policy recommendations for better health care. *Correct Care, 17*(1), 17–18.

National Commission on Correctional Health Care. (2004a). CMS asks states to maintain Medicaid enrollment for inmates. *Correct Care, 18*(2), 15.

National Commission on Correctional Health Care. (2004b). Hasta la vista, cigs! *Correct Care, 18*(3), 7.

National Commission on Correctional Health Care. (2005a). Advance directives study shows room for improvement. *Correct Care, 19*(4), 15.

National Commission on Correctional Health Care. (2005b). DOT for HAART shows promise. *Correct Care, 19*(1), 15.

National Commission on Correctional Health Care. (2005c). Guidance on tools to screen, assess youth mental health. *Correct Care, 19*(1), 13.

Newkirk, C. F. (2003). The unique needs of incarcerated women. *Correct Care, 17*(1), 3.

Norman, A., & Parrish, A. (2000). Prison health care. *Nursing Management, 7*(8), 26–29.

Office of Juvenile Justice and Delinquency Prevention. (2004). *Screening and assessing mental health and substance use disorders among youth in the juvenile justice system: A resource guide for practitioners.* Retrieved April 12, 2006, from http://www.ncjrs.gov/pdffiles1/ojjdp/204956.pdf

Paris, J. E. (2005). New thinking on "appropriate" approaches to HIV care. *Correct Care, 19*(3), 3.

Patterson, G. T. (2002). Overview: The law enforcement response to social problems: Mental health as a case in point. In G. Landsberg, M. Rock, L. K. W. Berg, & A. Smiley (Eds.), *Serving mentally ill offenders: Challenges and opportunities for mental health professionals* (pp. 47–50). New York: Springer.

Peters, R. H., & Matthews, C. O. (2003). Substance abuse treatment programs in prisons and jails. In T. J. Fagan & R. K. Ax (Eds.), *Correctional mental health handbook* (pp. 73–99). Thousand Oaks, CA: Sage.

Pogorzelski, W., Wolff, N., Pan, K.-Y., & Blitz, C. L. (2005). Behavioral health problems, ex-offender reentry policies, and the "Second Chance Act." *American Journal of Public Health, 95*, 1718–1724.

Porter, J. (2005). Clearing the air on tobacco use in corrections. *Correct Care, 19*(2), 1, 22.

Reisig, M. D., Holtfreter, K., & Morash, M. (2002). Social capital among women offenders. *Journal of Contemporary Criminal Justice, 18*, 167–186.

Restum, Z. G. (2005). Public health implications of substandard correctional health care. *American Journal of Public Health, 95*, 1689–1691.

Richardson, L. (2003). Other special offender populations. In T. J. Fagan & R. K. Ax (Eds.), *Correctional mental health handbook* (pp. 199–216). Thousand Oaks, CA: Sage.

Shimkus, J. (2004a). Corrections copes with health care for the aged. *Correct Care, 18*(3), 1, 16.

Shimkus, J. (2004b). Juveniles in jails: Different models, similar outcomes. *Correct Care, 18*(1), 9.

Snyder, H. N. (2004). *Juvenile arrests 2002.* Retrieved March 30, 2006, from http://www.ncjrs.gov/html/ojjdp/204608/contents.html

Stanley, J. A. (2004a). Teamwork vital to meeting the medical autonomy standard. *Correct Care, 18*(4), 16.

Stanley, J. A. (2004b). The most important standard: Receiving screening. *Correct Care, 18*(3), 20–21.

Stringer, H. (2001). Prison break. *NurseWeek, 14*(6), 13–14.

Teplin, L. A., Abram, K. M., McClelland, G. M., Washburn, J. J., & Pikus, A. K. (2005). Detecting mental disorder in juvenile detainees: Who receives services? *American Journal of Public Health, 95,* 1773–1780.

Teplin, L. A., Mericle, A. A., McClelland, G. M., & Abram, K. M. (2003). HIV and AIDS risk behaviors in juvenile detainees: Implications for public health policy. *American Journal of Public Health, 93,* 906–912.

Thigpen, M. L., Hunter, S. M., & Watson, B. P. (2002). *Services for families of prison inmates: Special issues in corrections.* Longmont, CO: National Institute of Corrections Information Center.

Tobin-D'Angelo, M., Arnold, K., Lance-Parker, S., La Marre, M., Bancroft, E., Jones, A., et al. (2003). Methcillin-resistant *Staphylococcus aureus* in correctional facilities—Georgia, California, and Texas, 2001–2003. *Morbidity and Mortality Weekly Report, 52,* 992–995.

Travis, J., Solomon, A. L., & Waul, M. (2001). *From prison to home: The dimensions and consequences of prisoner reentry.* Retrieved September 25, 2003, from http://www.urban.org/URL.cfm?ID=410098

Travis, J., & Sommers, A. (2004). New perspectives foster better health outcomes. *Correct Care, 18*(1), 1, 19.

Treadwell, H. M., & Ro, M. (2002). Poverty, race, and the invisible men. *American Journal of Public Health, 92,* 705–706.

U.S. Census Bureau. (2005). *Statistical abstract of the United States: 2004–2005.* Retrieved May 12, 2005, from http://www.census.gov/prod/2004pubs/04statab

U.S. Preventive Services Task Force. (2005). *The guide to clinical preventive services, 2005.* Retrieved August 13, 2005, from http://www.ahrq.gov/clinic/pocketguide.htm

Vogt, R. P. (2002). Inmate co-pay finds support in the courts. *Correct Care, 16*(3), 8.

Vogt, R. P. (2005). When an inmate refuses medical care. *Correct Care, 19*(3), 8.

Wagaman, G. L. (2003). Managing and treating female offenders. In T. J. Fagan & R. K. Ax (Eds.), *Correctional mental health handbook* (pp. 123–143). Thousand Oaks, CA: Sage.

Wakeen, R., & Roper, J. (2002). Good eatin': Sensible guidelines for medical diets. *Correct Care, 16*(2), 17.

Weinbaum, C., Lyerla, R., & Margolis, H. (2003). Prevention and control of infections with hepatitis viruses in correctional settings. *Morbidity and Mortality Weekly Report, 52* (RR-1), 1–36.

Weiskopf, C. S. (2005). Nurses' experiences of caring for inmate patients. *Journal of Advanced Nursing, 49,* 336–343.

White, T. W. (2001). Assessing suicide risk: Taking it step by step is your best bet. *Correct Care, 15*(3), 1, 21.

Wolfe, M. I., Xu, F., Patel, P., O'Cain, M., Schlinger, J. A., St. Louis, M. E., et al. (2001). An outbreak of syphilis in Alabama prisons: Correctional health policy and communicable disease control. *American Journal of Public Health, 91,* 1220–1225.

World Health Organization Health in Prisons Project. (2001). *Consensus statement on mental health promotion in prisons.* Retrieved July 10, 2006, from http://www.hipp-europe.org/events/hague/0040.htm

World Health Organization Regional Office for Europe. (2002). *Prison, drugs and society: A consensus statement on principles, policies, and practices.* Retrieved July 10, 2006, from http://www.hipp-europe.org/downloads/England-prisonsanddrugs.pdf

World Health Organization/UNAIDS. (2001). *HIV in prisons.* Retrieved July 10, 2006, from http://www.euro.who.int/document/E77016.pdf

Index

Page references followed by "f" indicate illustrated figures or photographs; followed by "t" indicates a table.